THE PHILOSOPHY OF MEDICINE

THE PHILOSOPHY
OF MEDICINE

THE EARLY EIGHTEENTH CENTURY

LESTER S. KING, M.D.

HARVARD UNIVERSITY PRESS

CAMBRIDGE, MASSACHUSETTS

AND LONDON, ENGLAND

1978

Library of Congress Cataloging in Publication Data

King, Lester Snow, 1908-
  The philosophy of medicine.

  Includes bibliographical references and index.
  1. Medicine — 15th-18th centuries. 2. Medicine —
Philosophy — History. I. Title.
R148.K515   610'.1   77-24645
ISBN 0-674-66585-6

PREFACE

Twenty-five years ago I wanted to write a history of medicine of the eighteenth century, but I soon relinquished the idea as quite visionary. The subject matter refused to remain limited. I could not determine what medicine was. Quite obviously there were the practical activities — restoring the sick person to health or, if he enjoyed good health, keeping him well. With equal obviousness, such activity drew its support from medical theory. The practice of medicine had its rationale — the concepts that served to validate particular actions. Medicine in the eighteenth century, as in every other era, had its practice and its theory. Today the practice rests on what we fondly call the basic sciences; in the eighteenth century the foundation was called natural philosophy.

A history of medicine, then, must tell what the doctor did and why he did it. My own interests inclined me more toward the latter facet. But natural philosophy — the philosophy of nature — was merely a part of philosophy in its wider sense, a subject that included metaphysics and logic and ethics, as well as what later was called science. In the seventeenth century many leading physicians dealt explicitly with metaphysics, and many others did so by implication. As the seventeenth century progressed into the eighteenth the metaphysical aspects tended to recede into the background. Yet they never disappeared but instead kept intruding themselves in annoying fashion into the development of science. This was especially true in that movement usually called the scientific revolution, when the philosophical presuppositions changed markedly, to affect all areas of intellectual endeavor, including medical theory.

However, if we want to understand the medicine of a given era, we cannot stop with the practice and the theory, which offer a far too limited view. The sick patient, the physician who tries to cure him, and the philosopher who provided the theoretical rationale, are only a part of a larger community. Society includes much more than patient, doctor, and philosopher (or scientist). People in the aggregate offer a vast array of special problems that relate to such disciplines as sociology, economics, and politics. These, with the various subsidiary aspects like national conflicts and wars, have intense relevance to medicine. We need only regard the increase in population, the growth of industry, the spread of poverty, the occurrence of epidemics, the need for public health measures. All these have to do with what we today call social medicine, all are intimately relevant to medical practice, and so too are various economic considerations. As a simple example, the establishment and growth of hospitals illustrate the interaction of many social and economic factors that have converged on the medical scene to bring about marked transformation.

The history of medicine does indeed consider the one-to-one relationship of doctor and patient but cannot rest there. The historian must take into account the one-to-many relationship of the doctor with society, an interaction that affects the practice of the healing art as well as the theory on which this practice rests. Medical history must take into account a host of disciplines: philosophy, science, sociology, economics, and politics, for medical theory and medical practice make contact with virtually all branches of knowledge, all phases of human activity.

This realization compelled me to give up any idea of writing a comprehensive medical history of the eighteenth century. Since the subject as a whole was far too broad, I chose to limit my studies to one small aspect, namely, the theories that underlay the practice. But then I encountered another difficult hurdle in the question, when was the eighteenth century? We cannot understand theories if we confine them in a temporal straightjacket. Theories have deep roots, lost in antiquity, and nowhere is this more true than in medicine.

I take as my premise that the medical theory of the eighteenth century rests in philosophy, and I suggest that the major battle lines were already clearly arrayed in the fifth century B.C., when Platonic doctrine confronted the Democritean. Plato emphasized the primacy of the immaterial—of the soul, mind, ideas, qualities, and relationships. Democritus, on the other hand, emphasized the primary reality of the material, of minute particles in endless combination, while mind and ideas were a spin-off from the combinations of a more primary stuff. These two contrasting views dominated Western thought for 2,500 years, undergoing modifications, to be sure, yet influencing all subsequent philosophy. They might alternate in their dominance, but whichever was subordinate was merely subdued, never eliminated.

When I decided to limit myself to analyzing medical theory of the eighteenth century, I found a complex interweaving of philosophic doctrine, tracing back eventually to Plato and Democritus but more directly to the

thinkers of the seventeenth century, whose influence determined the course
of eighteenth century thought.

Whoever tries to trace influences must plead guilty to arbitrary selection. As I regarded the complexities of seventeenth century thought and
tried to distinguish certain strands that had the most effect on eighteenth
century medical theory, I paid special attention to the problem, how real is
the immaterial? — a problem that came to a focus in the concept of the substantial form. This I discuss in great detail later, and I will not define it
here. Suffice it to say that the concept derived from Aristotelian doctrine.
In medicine, the scientific revolution brought about the decline of the substantial form and the correlative rise of corpuscular philosophy. Yet the
notion of the substantial form did not vanish. It remained disguised within
the concept of "mind" and the later growth of psychology as a discipline, as
well as the doctrine of vitalism.

The history of thought reveals a series of overlapping trends: concepts
may show a slow rise and development as they struggle against the prevailing modes of thought; then a triumph, of variable duration, and then a
decay as competing modes grow in force and effect. What was once dominant becomes subordinate and loses its manifest power. Yet decay is rarely
total, for the same concept may show a new growth under different circumstances and emerge again under a different guise. In any given period
many trends are conflicting simultaneously and show different degrees of
rise and decline.

To expound the trends in eighteenth century medical theory I go back to
the middle of the seventeenth century, when the reality of the immaterial
was a vigorous concept. As we proceed forward in time, we realize that the
intellectual trends of the late seventeenth century cannot be separated
from those of the early eighteenth. A significant division came not around
1700 but about a half century later. Between 1740 and 1750 the modes of
thought of the early eighteenth century declined and new trends surged
into prominence. In my title I indicate "Early Eighteenth Century." This
period, made deliberately vague, extends from about 1660 to about 1740
or 1750, with pseudopods extending forward or backward in a fluid manner as occasion arises.

Originally I felt that medical theory fell within the general field of the
history of ideas, but soon I realized that this was too broad. My interests are
more specifically in the philosophy of medicine, especially in its metaphysics and logic. Philosophy deals with generalizations of increasingly greater
scope, progressing toward ultimate or first principles. Philosophy deals
with the great questions to which there are no definite answers. For example, what is the real and what do we mean by reality? What can we understand by nature? What are the relationships of man, nature, the universe,
God? What is true and what is false? And how do we know? These are prob-

lems of inexhaustible depth and perhaps of insoluble character. From our present-day vantage point we may say that there are no answers to such ultimate questions. But as historians we must say that there have been abundant answers buttressed by much argument, although neither the answers nor the argument have carried conviction beyond a limited group, in a limited time span. These questions did find answers. The answers given in the seventeenth and eighteenth centuries are an intrinsic part of medical history. And to this part I devote this book.

In addition to questions that we call metaphysical, there are cognate problems of method and of logical validity, of truth and error, of topics such as causality, and explanation, or reductionism, analogy, proof, and other subjects that we designate as the logic of medicine. These I discuss in the last three chapters, although I realize that I merely explore the surface.

This book makes no attempt at comprehensive coverage. I am reminded of the apology that Barbara Tuchman made in the foreword to *The Proud Tower*. She was aware, she said, that after finishing her book she could have written it all over again, under the same title, but with an entirely different subject matter. And she added, that she could have done this a third time, still without repeating. Such a statement would not apply literally to a book on the philosophy of medicine, but I fully realize that I could have written a quite different volume, paying much more attention, say, to Descartes, or Locke, or Leibniz, or even Spinoza, and to a large number of physicians whom I ignored. I could also have touched on other philosophic problems. However, my selection of physicians and scientists and philosophic topics, while arbitrary, accords with my specific interests. I have deliberately avoided the subject of medical ethics, even though this branch of philosophy is receiving increasing attention at the present time.

It is with great pleasure that I express my thanks to Alan Donagan, of the University of Chicago, who read a draft of Chapter 8 and offered many helpful suggestions for revision. However, the responsibility for the opinions expressed is entirely my own. I also want to thank George Rousseau, of the University of California, who kindly shared with me his vast knowledge of eighteenth century literature and made many suggestions regarding readings that bear on the imagination.

My secretary, Mrs. Merry Uchida, has, by her care and skill, made this book possible, and to her I owe an immeasurable debt.

Finally, I must gratefully acknowledge the financial aid provided by a grant from the Department of Health, Education and Welfare, LMO 1804.

CONTENTS

THE PHILOSOPHY OF MEDICINE

ONE

THE OLD ORDER CHANGETH

Whoever wants to study the medicine of the eighteenth century will find the plays of Molière (1622-1673) an excellent point of entrance. Jean Baptiste Poquelin, called Molière, one of the greatest of all satirists, was particularly severe on doctors. In several of his plays he attacked the personal behavior of physicians as well as their intellectual bankruptcy and thus impugned both their character and their doctrines. Pompous ignorance, avarice, reactionary adherence to tradition and stubborn resistance to change, narrow guild restrictions, quarrels and jealousies of the medical faculty, absurd etiquette, all were sharply etched, as were the empty verbalisms of book learning, quite out of touch with the newer science. Since all good satire rests on a foundation of truth, Molière was merely exaggerating a real situation. Certainly, in the third quarter of the seventeenth century the medical faculty of the University of Paris was vulnerable to critical needling.

In *Le médecin malgré lui*, Sganarelle, a woodcutter masquerading as a physician, is called to treat a young girl who supposedly has lost the ability to talk. The girl's father has great faith in doctors, and Sganarelle offers a long harangue that purports to explain how the patient lost her speech. The rascally fraud declares,

> These vapors of which I was speaking, passing from the left side, where the liver is situated, to the right side where the heart is, finds that the lung, which we call *armyan* in Latin, communicating with the brain, which we call *nasmus* in Greek, by means of the vena cava, which we call *cubile* in Hebrew, meets in its path the above-mentioned vapors, which fill the ventricles of the omoplate.[1]

Géronte, father of the patient, is much impressed but timidly questions the positions of the liver and heart. "It seems to me that you place them opposite to where they are, that the heart is on the left side and the liver on the right." To which Sganarelle airily replies, "Oh yes, it used to be that way, but we have changed all that and now we practice medicine according to a quite new method" — a clear reference to the new seventeenth century discoveries in medical science and the claims of the "moderns" or neoterics.

In *Monsieur de Pourceaugnac* we again find long medical harangues.[2] The physicians, this time real members of the faculty, express themselves in circumlocutions and repetitions, always using three or four words to say

what a single well chosen word might convey. Since the audience knows
that the physicians are actually treating a perfectly healthy man, the trivi-
alities of the therapy and the completely inappropriate medical approach
are especially piquant. The two doctors toss long-winded compliments at
each other while making known their own different points of view. After
listening to the interminable opinions the bewildered "patient," Monsieur
de Pourceaugnac, asks, "What are you trying to say with your galimatias
and stupidities?" — a query in which the reader joins. The word "galimatias" has gone out of fashion, but if we look it up in the dictionary we see
that it conveys volumes and indicates Molière's opinion of the learned physicians.

Molière's undoubted masterpiece is *Le malade imaginaire,* first produced in 1673. The characters of Doctor Diafoirus and his booby son,
Thomas, a fledgling doctor, are triumphs of satire, but the greatest glory
rests on the third intermezzo where, in the combination of ballet, recita-
tion, and song, we see burlesqued a medical examination and the confer-
ring of a medical degree.[3] The dialogue, in neologistic Latin and French,
cannot be properly translated but is readily intelligible in the original
form. Here occur the immortal verses that have done more to pillory the
absurdities of seventeenth century medicine than any other single text. The
scene is an examination wherein the faculty subjects the candidate to rigorous questioning. One examiner asks,

> Demandabo causam et rationem quare
> Opium facit dormire.

To which the bachelor candidate replies,

> Mihi a docto doctore
> Demandatur causam et rationem quare
> Opium facit dormire.
>
> A quoi respondeo,
> Quia est in eo
> Virtus dormativa,
> Cujus est natura
> Sensus assoupire.

And with this trenchant answer the candidate received the admiring plau-
dits of the audience:

> Dignus, dignus est intrare
> In nostro docto corpore.
> Bene, bene, respondere.

When the question concerned the reason why rhubarb and senna purge
and drive out two types of bile, the candidate again declares,

Quia est in illis
Virtus purgativa
Cujus est natura
Istas duas biles evacuare.

The *virtus,* especially the *virtus dormativa,* has been a byword to indicate the absurdity, the futility of seventeenth century medical doctrines, before the "scientific revolution" steered medicine into its modern course.

Molière directed his medical satire against two rather different aspects of medicine. One concerned the physician as a person, his reactionary attitude, selfishness, vanity, pride, ignorance, and pomposity; the other condemned medical doctrines of the times, the science that underlay the practice. To some extent, of course, these two coincide.

We must not, however, allow Molière's satire, brilliant as it is, to distort our view. Let us examine a closely contemporary but quite different description of the medical scene, this time written by a physician. I offer the writings of Johann Peyer (1653-1712), best known today for the lymphoid accumulations that bear his name, the Peyer's patches in the intestine. His book, *Merycologia,* was published in 1685, twelve years after *Le malade imaginaire.* Certain sections of his work offer a praiseworthy ideal for the physician.[4]

Peyer was an excellent physician and a modest man who emphasized the glory of God and exhibited considerable religious fervor. He also emphasized the study of nature rather than of books, and he depicted the physician as an admirable character. Philosophy, he declared — and by philosophy he meant what we today call the natural sciences — is the subject "by which a man acquires a firm and wise aptitude for judging all things that pertain to reason. Wisdom, moreover, is the knowledge of truth through first causes. But no one will ever find truth and first causes who does not seek God. From which it is clear that they are all mistaken who consider philosophy something to be understood from books . . . for wisdom is far more noble and divine than can be shut up within the confines of books." Emphasis on the book of nature rather than on medical texts is definitely within the Paracelsian tradition.

The true philosopher is not the one who remembers all the opinions of others and who can recite what the Egyptians and Greeks, what Plato and Pythagoras, Socrates and the Stagyrite, Lucretius, Cicero, and Pliny taught, and among the moderns, what Descartes and innumerable others had in mind. No, the philosopher is not the one who is skilled in all these things; rather is he a person not restrained by human authority or the opinions of others, who comes to his own conclusions with a mind free of prejudice (*pace* Thomas Diafoirus). Peyer would eliminate the controversies of the schools and the futile disputations, for the nature of truth is immutable.

The good teacher is the one who roots out from the mind erroneous preconceived opinions and, when fallacious perceptions are eliminated, gives over the mind to be instructed by God. The good physicians cultivate reason so that nothing escapes the attention that man can bring about through the "natural light." Peyer praised mathematics, especially algebra, as the way that leads to the stars, the ladder by which we ascend into heaven. Without mathematics no one can be learned or wise or a philosopher.

Physicians, continued Peyer, are made, not born. The art of healing is discovered by human industry and experience rather than by reason. The acquisition of this art involves a great deal of labor. Medicine is the faculty of properly curing human ailments, and the physician should know everything that pertains to health and whatever maintains it and to diseases and their remedies. Knowledge is acquired through anatomy, whereby the structure of membranes, of both the surface parts and the deep recesses, is made clear. We regard the heart, the kidneys, and the viscera, and we distinguish veins, arteries, and nerves that carry the animal spirits, blood, chyle, and lymph. Anatomy studies the muscles—the instruments of motion—and the bodily connections of bones and joints, all so carefully arranged for fine movements. Nor is it enough to be skilled in the structure and position of the parts, but the way these separate parts function must also be considered. Then the physician must also study the nature and movement of the spirits; and lastly, the temperaments, varying according to the differences and changes of sex, age, and individuality.

Pathology teaches a thousand kinds of diseases and their causes and symptoms. It is more important to attend patients in hospitals than to learn from books alone. And of great importance is the diligent examination of diseased cadavers. Then there is therapeutics, which deals with medications and surgery, and also with the search for medicinal plants. Animals, too, must be distinguished for their value in natural science and for their medical uses. Nothing that nature produces is foreign to the physician and nothing that the industry of man prepares. Peyer praised chemistry as producing important medications and pleaded for experiments, the testing of medicines, and the search for new ones through reason, which can seek the causes for their effectiveness. Philosophy examines the causes of things and "fulfills" medicine. Nor can the physician who lacks a knowledge of philosophy be considered a complete physician.

Surely no one, not even Molière, could find fault with an evaluation such as this. It is a program for sound medicine, which emphasizes our going directly to nature and using observation and reason aided by rational inference. Peyer was an enlightened and forward-looking devotee of the new science of medicine.

He emphasized nature rather than books, observation rather than tradition, but he nevertheless stressed the importance of reason in achieving knowledge, especially of causes. Futhermore, when Peyer emphasized the dependence of medicine on God and pleaded for the recognition of divine power, he was reflecting a major concern of his era, namely, a basic religious attitude and a dread of atheism. Peyer was, to be sure, combatting atheism; but more than that, he was revealing his dependence on the immaterial, on the reality of what is not corporeal. The newer mechanical philosophy was turning its back on those immaterial aspects of reality that played so important a part in the Aristotelian and neo-Galenic concepts. Peyer did not turn his back on what was old. Rather, we see in him a blending of old and new, an admission of previous excesses and at the same time a program directed toward the future, a program that retains the best of the old.

The medical scenes that Molière portrayed, even though exaggerated, probably represented the nadir of medical practice and medical theory. The very success of Molière's writings and their continued popularity suggest that popular regard for physicians was at a low ebb. In retrospect we realize that in any given era physicians as persons are much like other people. There have always been the "good guys" and the "bad guys," the genuine altruists and the selfish opportunists, and one of the great merits of Molière lies in the universality of his characters. Making allowances for changes in temporal environment, his satire is as applicable today as in the seventeenth century. The reactionary who resists change is not a seventeenth century invention, nor is he restricted to medicine. For our purposes we need only indicate that in Molière's time organized medicine — manifested especially by the medical faculty of Paris — was open to widespread criticism.

The image did gradually improve. By the middle of the eighteenth century even Voltaire, as Gusdorf points out, had a few good words to say about doctors.[5] Voltaire declared that Molière was quite right to make fun of physicians — of one hundred physicians, ninety-eight were charletans. He indicated that the profession had been mercenary and subject to many abuses. But then he asked the rhetorical question, whether anything was more estimable than a physician who, having studied nature in his youth, knows what makes the human body work, the evils that torment it, and the remedies that can offer relief. This, coming from Voltaire, was high praise indeed. However, even this praise was tempered with sneers. Voltaire stressed the healing power of nature and put into the mouth of the physician the words that the doctors "infallibly cure all those [evils] that get well by themselves," and that nature, the *premier médecin,* accomplishes everything. Nevertheless, even this admission marks a vast step forward when compared with the imbecilities of a Thomas Diafoirus. Undoubtedly the physician had made real progress in public esteem, a progress especially significant when acknowledged by so critical a writer as Voltaire.

Medical history includes not only the theoretical doctrines of medicine and the actual modes of medical practice but also the relationships of medicine to the contemporary science and technology and, further, the relationships of doctors to society, taken in a very broad sense. This comprehensive field I regard as an essential unity, which we must fragment for ease of analysis, while admitting that such a fragmentation necessarily introduces distortion. In this book I concentrate on the intellectual background of medicine and the changes therein that occurred from about 1660 to about 1740.

In general, changes in medicine arise along two interconnected paths. A new discovery can markedly alter existing technology. For example, the invention of the microsope or the vacuum pump, the discovery of methods for vascular injections, the practice of auscultation, were technical advances that permitted the accumulation of many new facts and then the creation of new theories. We can more easily appreciate the impact of technological advance when we look at present day medicine and the progress initiated through, say, tissue culture or x rays or the electron microscope. Investigators glimpse new lands to conquer. Only long painful struggle can realize the possibilities that a new technique can offer, yet through such struggles come both practical and theoretical advances.

There is, however, a quite different route to progress. Someone may attain a new point of view, and a new way of looking at things may be quite as revolutionary as a specific invention. To use a homely example: the copybook maxim states that the early bird catches the worm. Clearly, therefore, it is desirable to *be* the early bird, to get up early and attend to the tasks at hand. But sooner or later some bright child will point out that the early worm is eaten by the bird. Clearly, with the very same maxim, getting up early is fraught with danger and certainly is to be avoided. Nothing has changed but the point of view. Yet this means that everything has changed.

Harvey's great discovery of the circulation of the blood illustrates this second type of progress. Harvey had an idea, a point of view which was profoundly revolutionary. It was not enough merely to have the idea; there must be proof. Through his physiological experiments, Harvey found proof sufficient to convince most of the world outside Paris and eventually even the medical faculty in the University of Paris. But the evidence that he offered did not derive from any new gadgets nor did it depend on any new technique or apparatus hitherto unknown. Harvey's experiments could have been performed by anyone, if only he had thought of the idea. In contrast, the discovery of the rings of Saturn or of "animalculae" depended on the development of the telescope and microscope, respectively, that is, on the appropriate technical apparatus.

Techniques and attitudes interact. A new technique must incite new ideas and a new point of view must lead to new technical advances. At any given moment there are several determinants for change. One we may call attitude, another apparatus or technique. Attitude, however, involves far more than the narrow discipline of any given investigator: it diffuses broadly to include social, religious, economic, and political aspects and the value judgments underlying them, together with some particular philosophic orientation. And all these, in turn, are influenced by technical advances. With this as a framework let us examine the so-called scientific revolution, a central feature in the history of seventeenth century science.

There are many ways of studying the phenomena embraced by this concept of a revolution. We can, perhaps, regard it as the decline of the Aristotelian philosophy. Certainly there was a shift in metaphysics, from the once dominant teachings of Aristotle to the atomism that derived from Democritus, Epicurus, and Lucretius. In my own thinking I regard Aristotle as part of the tradition derived from Plato, namely that reality—basic and irreducible existence—includes an immaterial component or character, wherein mind and intelligence and qualitative distinctions have a primary status. This view, while it formed an essential part of Christianity and the social and political establishment arising therefrom, was not very successful in explaining the data of experimental physics and astronomy.

Many great minds of the early seventeenth century realized that in physics the atomistic philosophy in one or another version was far superior to the Aristotelian views that participated in the Platonic tradition. Experimental and scientific observations could be better explained by the Epicurean doctrines that basic reality consists of material atoms in motion, combining and recombining endlessly. Criticism of Aristotle became the fashion.

The major impetus in the decline of Aristotle came from astronomy and physics, especially kinetics. Aristotelian doctrine proved vulnerable indeed to the competition engendered by more precise observation, an experimental approach, and imaginative theories. All texts on the history of science recount the triumphs of sixteenth and seventeenth century investigators and philosophers, culminating, perhaps, in Galileo (1564-1642), Descartes (1596-1650), and Gassendi (1592-1655). By the middle of the seventeenth century much of Aristotelian teaching in the physical sciences was discredited among scientists, and his metaphysics was also being replaced. Hand in hand with all this was a more empirical attitude, for which Francis Bacon (1561-1626) was the most articulate spokesman.

The various advances in knowledge and the change in attitude at first affected a few intellectuals, but the new views became gradually more pervasive. Mary Hesse described the progress, although with some rhetorical exaggeration: "In 1600 natural philosophers were discussing the same problems that had exercised the scientific minds of Greece, using the same arguments and the same categories of thought . . . By 1700, most of these problems had either been solved, often as trivial special cases of newly formulated physical laws, or had been shelved as lacking in interest." So rapid was progress that by the end of the seventeenth century "not only had every type of explanation known to the Greeks, with the exception of atomism, been entirely discredited, but the new orthodoxy, an alliance of Cartesianism and atomism, was already in decline." By the end of the century, Hesse claimed, "A particular type of subject-matter and a particular method of investigation were taking charge of science, and critics, though vocal, were ineffective."[6]

Hesse is quite obviously dealing with a specific branch of science, and so persuasively that if we do not make explicit qualification, we would quite naturally speak of the "scientific revolution of the seventeenth century." And generations of historians of science have done so in line with the tradition that Hesse has so well expressed. In this connection we have the recent influential work of Kuhn, who tried to expand the concept of revolution in science and provide a generalized analysis.[7]

Unfortunately, some severe drawbacks attend this attitude. I have previously pointed out that this concept of scientific revolution, as Kuhn expounds it, does not apply to medicine.[8] One obvious response might be a cavalier assertion that medicine is not a science, or at best is only a protoscience, a view that simply ignores much of seventeenth century intellectual history. I do not want to touch here the vexing problem, what do we mean by science? I would declare, however, that while the massive changes in physics might justify the notion of "revolution," this should not be unjustifiably extended. When we are talking specifically about physics, we should speak of revolution in physics rather than in science generally. The distinction is not trivial, for the rash extension of terms has done much to prevent a sound understanding of seventeenth century medicine.

The term revolution, useful in a broad and vague fashion, finds a place in many disciplines. We hear of many different kinds of revolution — political, scientific, industrial, social — in any field of study that shows substantial change in a relatively short time. In politics revolution connotes sudden and violent change. Such events as the American or French or Russian revolutions permit us to point not only to violence but also to a fairly specific date that we can construe as a beginning. Yet in any extended usage we cannot equate revolution with either violence or suddenness. The "industrial revolution" was obviously not sudden. And although riots did occur in many places, so that we might conceivably make out a case for violence, this would be only peripheral and not part of the essence. In the so-called scientific revolution not even the most vigorous proponent of that nomenclature can point to violence.

If we must retain the concept of revolution and if we eliminate suddenness and violence as necessary components, what, then, would be the essential features? I suggest this explication, applicable to all fields where the term finds any acceptance: revolution is a change so profound that what formerly was dominant is toppled to become markedly subordinate; while some opposing factor (the terminology would vary with subject matter, whether political struggle, philosophical doctrine, scientific theory, or social custom), hitherto markedly subordinate, becomes dominant. The essential features, then, consist of an intense opposition and the reversal of an original subordination. The changeover might occur rapidly or slowly, quietly or with violence. These factors are unimportant. Significant is what we can call the transfer of dominance to some markedly opposed alternate.

We should also ask what distinguishes revolution from evolution. And to this there is no clear answer. Obviously, the one is more rapid than the other, but this does not make an adequate demarcation. If, for example, we regard the institution called feudalism — a system based on land tenure — we see that it gave way to an economy based on money and trade. The change, involving strongly opposed social and conceptual schemata, was indeed profound, but since it took place over several centuries and at different rates in different locales, we think of it as evolution. On the other hand, when British agriculture gave way to an industrial economy, the change occurred much more rapidly, and the major determinants were much more clearly defined, so that the term revolution found ready acceptance.

Kuhn's influential book leads us to query: why all the concern with what is or is not included in the term revolution? The answer, I believe, lies in a faulty attempt to explain change. There is, perhaps, the feeling that if we can circumscribe certain clusters of events and characterize them as revolutions, we would then have a concrete data-base for analysis. But this involves methodological error, namely, a circumscription that is so entirely arbitrary that it has only ad hoc value. If, for example, we must distinguish paradigm stage from pre-paradigm stage, mature science from immature science, and small revolutions from large ones, we have lost all generality. We hinder, rather than help, any understanding of the profound changes we find, for example, in medicine.

My earlier comments on this subject, published in 1970, were written before the second edition of Kuhn's book appeared or the publication of the relevant *Criticism and the Growth of Knowledge*.[9] In the latter symposium one critic pointed to 22 different meanings in which Kuhn used the crucial term paradigm.[10] Kuhn tried to dispel the confusion but in my opinion without success.[11] In the second edition of his book, as he restated his position in the attempt to blunt various criticisms, he devoted himself principally to the philosophy of science so far as it rests on modern physics. He did refer somewhat to the history of physics, but he ignored biology almost completely and medicine totally.[12] We must not equate physics, especially modern physics, with science in its historical context.

The concept of paradigms does indeed call attention to the phenomena of change but does not adequately illuminate the dynamics of change. And though Kuhn's term may have validity in physics, it does not have any validity in medicine. I believe we would acheive a better understanding if we ignore the concept of revolution altogether.

We can study the changes in medicine through a different approach, one that admits complexity and confusion and that nevertheless seeks at least a few relevant factors, whose interaction is admittedly incompletely understood. To appreciate the changes in medicine we should study the ecology of ideas — the complex relationships where a shift in one component can produce subtle alterations elsewhere. Any attempt at a neat formulation is doomed to failure.

In the history of medicine, we try to find out how the changes came about or, differently phrased, what are the "dynamics" involved. My conception of the way a historian can approach the problem I can illustrate by two extended metaphors.

We are watching a growing boy. Over a period of time we note that his wrists seem to be extending out of his sleeves, that his coat is too narrow for his chest, the cuffs of his trousers are too high above his shoes. Clearly, his suit no longer fits. Then one day we see him attired in a new suit that does fit. Our problem is not a Carlylean concern with clothes. We do not trouble ourselves with, say, the name of the manufacturer, or whose decision it was to get the new suit. Rather are we concerned with the physiological mechanisms responsible for the relatively rapid growth of the boy. The real problem concerns the physiology of growth or perhaps we might say, of metabolism. The number of relevent factors, internal and external, can ramify without limit, and any investigation will at best unravel only a small part.

As a second metaphor I would point to a phenomenon in floriculture. At one time in my garden I planted adjacent beds of creeping phlox and creeping sedum. After a few years the sedum had overrun both beds and the phlox had almost, but not quite, disappeared. If a botanist wanted to know why this happened, he would need to study a variety of topics, ranging from plant genetics and plant physiology to soil chemistry. He could implicate various factors in the environment and various activities and components in the plants themselves — and the way in which they all interact. It is a complex phenomenon of comparative plant metabolism.

The growing boy, after he gets a new suit, presents to the world a much more pleasing aspect than he did before. There is a better fit all around. But paying attention to the suit distracts us from the really important question, which concerns the dynamics of growth and metabolism. And similarly, the triumph of the sedum over the phlox illustrates the competition found in nature.

If we return to medical history at the turn of the eighteenth century, these metaphors can serve as models for various changes, particularly when one set of concepts replaces another, such as the decline of the Aristotelian philosophy and the rise of the corpuscular philosophy. This we can regard as a competition between two systems of thought within a particular environment, wherein one triumphed over the other. The challenge for us lies in identifying some of the factors involved, the dynamics at work, and their relationships to medical theory and medical practice. The phenomena offer a problem in what I would call the metabolism of ideas.

In the past there has been an overly narrow view of what constitutes medicine. Obviously the subject includes theory — science in the narrow sense — and practice, sometimes called the *methodus medendi*. But there are also involved vast other areas wherein physicians interact with social, intellectual, economic, religious, and political environments, all of which bear on both theory and practice. If we want to understand how one set of medical concepts gets replaced by another, we cannot neglect this varied environment that shapes the climate of thought and determines the attitude of physicians. In this present volume I try to analyze a small part of this environment, especially certain topics that fall within the general area of philosophy. In this connection I must enthusiastically endorse the statement of Pagel: "No historian of science or medicine is safe from the need — sudden or sustained — for full information on philosophic concepts — their meaning today and their history. Such fundamental *topoi* include Cause and Effect, Analysis and Synthesis, Aristotelianism, Form and Matter, Existentialism, Phenomenology, Experimentation and Empiricism, Atomic Theories, Positivism, Semantics, Progress, Sociology, Social Anthropology, and a legion of similar '-isms' and '-ologies.' "[13] I would add that we must also maintain a historical perspective throughout, so that concepts are evaluated within their own intellectual environment and not dissected in the hothouse surroundings of present-day problems.

Such a program as Pagel suggests is, of course, far beyond the scope of any one person. But a historian can at least look at topics that hold especial interest for him and try to understand them in the framework of seventeenth and eighteenth century thought.

Philosophy, as Pagel envisions it, comprises far more than physics. For example, the influential thinkers of the era were all exposed to the social and intellectual pressures of organized religion. Philosophic systems could not ignore the divine power and glory but had to find a place for God in a total scheme of things. Bacon had figuratively shrugged his shoulders; anything connected with God he wanted to separate off and hand back to the theologians, contenting himself with the material objects of this world. Other philosophers, like Descartes and Gassendi, in the Continental tradition of rationalism, dealt far more subtly with the problem of God, the immaterial, and other-worldliness and tried somehow to combine the mechanistic aspects of atomism with certain minimal attributes of divinity.

Philosophers tried to harmonize traditional religious concepts with the new science, but what seemed harmonious to some ears sounded quite discordant to others. The new philosophy was suspected of being atheistic. It is difficult to appreciate today the revulsion that such an epithet produced in the seventeenth century. We can find a twentieth century parallel, perhaps, in the epithet Communist during our own McCarthy era.

In the seventeenth century the point at issue involved the basic tenet of Platonism as embodied in Christian doctrine: is the world created by an intelligent being, an immaterial conscious mind? Or is the world an eternally existing heap of material particles in motion? The distinction was not merely an excercise in logic chopping. It concerned the fundamental attitude toward the universe, toward Christian doctrine, toward the establishment with its social and economic and intellectual sanctions, with its overtones in medicine.

Another aspect that profoundly affected medicine was the attitude toward evidence. What, for example, were physicians willing to accept as evidence? Why did a given datum appear important and significant at one era and a century later seem quite inconsequential? The difference, for example, between a vitalistic or a mechanistic viewpoint would lie precisely in this area — that a protagonist was willing to accept certain data as reliable, while his antagonist saw no cogency therein. A discrepancy might bother one investigator but another might not even see discrepancy, let alone worry about it. What one physician might regard as important another might ignore. What to accept, what to disregard? There was no adequate agreement on these important points. Perhaps even more basic was the question, what constitutes a problem? How to recognize a significant problem? Events do not carry placards saying, "I am a problem. Solve me."

These questions, although they perhaps allow no ready solution, are nevertheless important. In the seventeenth and eighteenth centuries various writers offered many elaborate hypotheses. It is a great error to think that these hypotheses were purely imaginative, for they were always based on evidence. Since these theorists were not fools but very intelligent men, we must believe that the evidence seemed to them sufficient, the problems significant, and the answers adequate. The critic, however, can ask how good is the evidence? how acceptable or reliable? how real the problem? how well grounded the hypothesis? how valid the solutions? The original theorists believed that their hypotheses were well grounded and adequate; the critic believed they were not. Different ideas of adequacy mean that the climate of opinion has changed. How did this change come about?

The changes in the seventeenth and eighteenth centuries reflect different ways of looking at evidence, that is, different attitudes. The medical historians who deal primarily with discoveries and inventions may find the eighteenth century rather disappointing. But those who study primarily ideas and attitudes find the turn of the eighteenth century fascinating indeed.

Descriptions of the eighteenth century often use rather formalized phrases that may degenerate into cliches like reason or nature, or the age of system or the cult of order. When, for example, we call the eighteenth century an age of reason, that word serves only as a facade that conceals a vibrant and changing reality. Any epithet will indicate only a few properties, leaving behind an important and elusive residue. Any given term may be incomplete, for it may imply an opposite and then cannot be understood in isolation. There is a natural dialectic, an opposition, a moving forward in time. A so-called classical era will imply a romanticism somewhere in the neighborhood. Rationalism is quite meaningless without empiricism, natural without artificial, and the like.

Whatever a given term may mean—and often we must remain in considerable doubt—we must also seek out the opposite. Most of Western thought shuttles back and forth between pairs of opposites: yes and no, good and bad, up and down, in and out, are among the first words a child learns. When he becomes older he appreciates such pairs as pleasure-pain, conservative-radical, benign-malignant, virtue-vice. Somehow we better understand the meaning of a word by referring to its opposite. Some dictionaries give antonyms as part of their definitions.

Of course, all this pairing off of concepts is only a trick of language and does not necessarily reflect the nature of the universe. This I have no desire to dispute. But trick or not, a great deal of our thinking is clothed in sharp contrasts. For over 2,500 years certain pairs recur again and again. God and the devil, war and peace, love and hate have furnished themes for drama and song through all recorded history. The actors, the costumes, and the stage settings all have changed, but the basic oppositions remain. Similarly with other contrasts — Apollonian and Dionysian, idealist and realist, rational and empirical, mechanist and vitalist are pairs that have produced factions from early times right up to the present. The tendency to carry on our thinking by means of opposites was especially marked in Greek philosophy.

Some of these pairs, especially relevant to medicine, can furnish a frame of reference within which medical history may be analyzed. In any pair of opposites the separate terms cannot be understood one without the other, and yet together are highly meaningful. The pairs that have an especial appeal for me are nature and the supernatural, materialism and the immaterial, rationalism and empiricism. These concepts provide a way of looking at the data, a pair of spectacles, so to speak, through which I examine, in the following chapters, some of the conceptual background of early eighteenth century medicine.

TWO

THE CONCEPT OF NATURE

The phrase "healing power of nature," a heritage from Greek medicine, can serve as a whole text of medical history as well as philosophy.[1] The word heal raises few problems, but what does the word nature mean? We probably think first of the world around us with its orderly sequences, the world that the scientists study and the philosophers try to explain. In the older formulations, nature would be the realm of coming into being and passing away, of generation and corruption.

In the latter part of the seventeenth century and the first part of the eighteenth, the concept of nature loomed especially important. "The word nature," wrote Boyle in 1682, "is every where to be met with in the writings of physiologers: but though they frequently employed the word, they seem not to have considered what notion ought to be framed of the thing." He went on to indicate "of how vast importance it is in philosophy, and the practice of physick too, to have a right notion of nature."[2]

But what is the right notion? Aristotle had indicated several senses of the word but these have become more numerous and intricate since his time.[3] Quite obviously, the meaning of the word will change, depending on the context. This we readily see when we consider the many different words derived from the single root *physis*. Thus, physics and physicists, physick, physician, and physiology, all derive from *physis*, or "nature," and all show different meanings.

There would be no value for us to note the several dozen shades of meaning that nature exhibits today, nor to trace the historical development of the different senses. It is important, however, to gain some insight into the way the word was used in the second half of the seventeenth century. Robert Boyle conveniently gathered together a number of meanings, without any intent of making the list exhaustive. For the senses of nature that he deemed important, he compiled a list of eight concepts or clusters of meanings. His different senses are: God, the author of nature; the essence of a thing—the important attributes; the temperament or constitution of a living creature; the internal determining cause—the internal principles of locomotion; the established order of things; the aggregate of powers belonging to a body; the universe, the phenomena of the world; a semi-diety, in certain pagan religions.[4]

Gassendi also discussed the meanings of nature and distinguished several senses. Apart from the phenomenal world around us—the world in its entirety as we perceive it—there may also be involved some force or activity at work in this totality, something perhaps divine within the whole. There is also a contrast between nature and art. Or there may be involved certain patterns relative to certain goals, that we may regard as according to nature, in contrast with chance. Nature may also indicate the entirety that contains within itself the principle and cause of action.[5]

We cannot simply latch on to one of these various meanings, analyze it exhaustively, and neglect all others. Yet neither can we analyze all the meanings. We must instead try to see some genetic relationship among the different senses and try to appreciate some of the basic oppositions, either latent or expressed. I would emphasize one particular opposition, between those definitions that somehow refer to God (or *naturam divinam,* or deity, or even semi-deity); and other definitions that have to do with the realm of sense perception, the phenomenal world, the realm of change, of coming into being and passing away. This would be the world studied in physics.

But what about man? Is he part of the world of physics or does he have relationship to some higher realm associated with the deity or with the supernatural. Is man wholly within nature or is he in part above nature? We have the opposition between mind and body, between soul and body, between matter and spirit. Are spirit, mind, soul parts of nature? Or do they belong to the supernatural, quite different from the world of physics? These are problems commonly designated as metaphysical, and physics in the latter seventeenth century cannot be understood without bringing in metaphysics. And nature with its host of different senses must relate to metaphysics as well as physics.

At this point we might recall that philosophy traditionally embraced a wide content. It included moral philosophy and logic, which we can for the present ignore. It included metaphysics and the rational aspects of theology (as distinguished from revelation). It also included the philosophy of nature that later became transformed into "natural science." The separation between these different branches was relative only, more a matter of convenience than of inner necessity.

The distinction between the natural and the supernatural we can regard as closely akin to the distinction between natural and speculative philosophy. The study of mind and soul and their properties and relationships hovered uneasily in the total domain of philosophy, uncertain whether to rest in metaphysics or in natural philosophy. The concepts of the living and the nonliving; mind and soul and the nature of man; God, immanence and transcendence; causality and change; matter and motion; elemental particles and ultimate constituents; these had long been the domain of metaphysics. These all impinge in one or another way on the various concepts that fall into the realm of physics and hence into the realm of nature. The key point in the study of nature is, perhaps, the conviction that we cannot separate physics and metaphysics.

Correlative to nature is the supernatural. Or, to phrase this in a somewhat more sophisticated fashion, we can refer to phenomena and to the forces behind them and responsible for them. For the sake of simplicity let us designate the world of phenomena as nature. The forces behind the phenomena may be part of nature or else part of the supernatural realm or possibly belonging to both. And the position of man in this rough dichotomy remains to be decided.

We can illustrate the problems by reference to medical history, as found in the beginning of the *Iliad*. Agamemnon, the Greek leader, had taken captive a beautiful Theban maiden whose father, Chryses, was a priest of Apollo. When the father tried to secure the release of his daughter, he was crudely rebuffed. Thereupon he prayed to Apollo to wreak vengeance on the Greeks. Apollo answered the prayer and to punish the Greeks let loose his arrows against them, afflicting them with a grievous pestilence that affected both men and animals. The Greeks in despair consulted their own priests. One soothsayer indicated that the pestilence resulted from Apollo's anger at Agamemnon and that the god must be appeased. After bitter quarrels among themselves, the Greeks finally returned the captive girl to her father and made appropriate sacrifices to Apollo. Chryses then prayed to Apollo, who, satisfied, removed the pestilence.

We can call this an example of animistic thinking, wherein various phenomena are controlled by personalities, by individuals called gods, similar to man but more powerful, who can, by their volition, control the course of events. Nature, the world of phenomena, is under direct supernatural control. Apollo, by deliberate acts of will, caused the pestilence that afflicted the Greeks, and he also brought it to an end. Yet even though possessing such vast powers, he acted from motives like those of men.

A sharply contrasting view we find in the familiar Hippocratic text, "The Sacred Disease," describing epilepsy. This condition is not "any more divine or sacred than any other disease but, on the contrary, has specific natural characteristics and a definite cause," that is, it is not due to any volition of the gods.[6] Hippocrates did not expressly reject the concept of gods, but he did deny that they produced the symtoms in patients and further denied that special healers could cure the ailment through sacrifice, incantations, or magical rites. Persons who alleged a divine origin were merely covering up their own ignorance.

This attitude, carried to its logical extreme, we find expressed in the *Rubáiyát* of Omar Khayyám,

> And that inverted bowl they call the Sky,
> Whereunder crawling coop'd we live and die,
>   Lift not your hands to *It* for help — for It
> As impotently moves as you or I.[7]

These lines deny any personality to the forces that work in nature, deny any voluntarism in these forces, and indicate a course of events beyond the influence of prayer. This, indeed, is the same message that we find at the beginning of "The Sacred Disease."

In my single example of the Homeric pantheon I am not trying to over-simplify a complex situation. Among the multiple divinities the personalities varied and the powers are from from clear. Furthermore, the concept of necessity and fate, *ananke* and *moira,* vague at best, cast a shadow over the ultimate degree of voluntarism that divinities may have exerted. I use the incident in Homer merely as one phase of the distinction between the natural and the supernatural, a distinction important in the seventeenth and eighteenth centuries as well as among the early Greeks.

The religious thought of the Greeks was not confined to simple dichotomy that we can force into the categories of natural and supernatural. Indeed, the contrast between these two terms is far from being a simple opposition. The relations of magic, animism, mysticism, and advanced religious thought, and the stages of naive, mature, and sophisticated science are all intertwined.

Yet if we compare the Homeric account of disease with the text of Hippocrates, we can note a broad line of distinction between nature and supernature, a distinction that centers on the term autonomy. This has to do with the degree to which phenomena are dependent on any outside control. The phenomena around us show considerable order and predictability. To what extent is this order self-contained, autonomous, dependent on forces entirely within the phenomena? And to what extent is it all directed by agencies outside the flow of events? Are the gods constantly engaged in regulating the events in nature or do the events run themselves, with the gods interfering only at particular times or not at all? To what degree are observed phenomena dependent on personal will greater than that of man?

When we try to untangle the relationship between the natural and the supernatural, we find variation in three different lines: the degree of autonomy in nature; the degree to which divinity may be in the world or remote from it; and the degree to which divinity resembles man, particularly in regard to the attribution of will and foresight, as well as susceptibility to influence.

However, it is wrong to make a sharp disjunction between divine personality affecting events and impersonal forces acting within the phenomena. The two aspects may blend. This we see in certain phases of ancient medicine, particularly in the cult of Aesculapius, the god of healing.[8] In the temples of Aesculapius, the patient submitted to various rites of purification, following which there might occur different kinds of interaction between the god and the patient. In the simplest stage there was a direct personal and individual relation between the god and the patient, with the priest ordinarily as the intermediary. The patient supplicated, the god answered, removing the illness by fiat analogous to the way Apollo removed the pestilence from the Greeks.

But Aesculapius also acted in a more indirect fashion. Instead of exercising a divine fiat the god might recommend to the patient certain drugs that would cure the illness. The actual cure would have been achieved by the virtues within the medicine, while the god merely indcated which medicine to use to bring about the favorable outcome. The priest transmitted the information. The god was counselor rather than manipulator, entering into each treatment as adviser rather than as direct agent.

For present purposes we can regard nature as the realm of uniform events that are autonomous, uniform, self-contained within certain limits. The regulatory action is independent of any divine will. The supernatural, on the other hand, exerts a controlling power over the observed phenomena, a power that expresses personality or, perhaps we should say, personhood.

Some of the relations between natural and supernatural can be illustrated by an extended figure of speech. Let us imagine that Agamemnon suddenly reappeared in the late twentieth century and confronted an automobile for the first time. He might at first consider the entire machine to be alive, in all its parts. In our terminology there would be complete immanence of deity. Furthermore, Agamemnon would speedily note that the indwelling god was propitious only so long as he received sacrifices and gifts, known as gasoline and oil and the like. Furthermore, a cult of priests, who dwelt in special temples, would preside over the ceremonies of sacrifice.

As Agamemnon became more sophisticated his thinking might develop along these lines: he would give up the idea that the whole auto was alive but would feel that a god still controlled the engine, to which the chassis responded in a natural fashion. The engine would be divine, the chassis part of nature. Still later Agamemnon would change his views of deity from a being partly immanent to a being totally transcendent. Because of this change, the entire auto would be regarded as a natural phenomenon. The divine agent no longer dwells in the car but is regarded as creator or, in the barbarian language, manufacturer, who resided "out there," far beyond direct sense perception. "Out there" would seem to be Detroit, the barbarian word for Olympus. Regardless of the god's locus, his will would continue to be interpreted by the priests who, after receiving the appropriate sacrifices, would cure or prevent the various ailments.

Agamemnon would study philosophy and become acquainted with other religions and other modes of approaching important problems. He would realize that the deity in Detroit did not really create the automobile but merely transformed already existing materials into particular forms. This deity, far from being supreme, was then merely a synonym of the demiurge of Plato. This particular demiurge worked with metals and plastics and wires, according to certain immutable laws—for example, that friction produces heat, that electricity will pass through some materials but not others, that gasoline will not flow uphill by itself, and the like. The god in Detroit is clearly subject to *ananke,* necessity.

As Agamemnon studied still more philosophy he would begin to speculate on certain other problems. How did the metals and plastics come into existence? What was their ultimate composition? Who established the law that gasoline would not flow uphill? Furthermore, what is the relation between the automobile and the man who is driving it? Questions of purpose and value would arise. And then the thought would occur to Agamemnon, how much difference is there *really* between the man who is driving the automobile and the automobile? This problem he would tuck away in his mind for future meditation.

But perhaps we have carried this little fable far enough, even though there is ample scope for further analogies. I want merely to indicate some basic philosophic problems that have always found some sort of solution, but the solutions have changed over the centuries.

To provide a basis for eighteenth century concepts, let us now examine some major formulations of the seventeenth century in regard to nature. In the history of thought there are two major doctrines that differ fundamentally: the teachings of Democritus and his disciples, on the one hand, of Plato and his followers, on the other. Democritus, Epicurus, and Lucretius represent the atomistic philosophy that eventually had such a profound influence on modern science. For the atomists, material particles in ceaseless motion, combining and recombining endlessly, formed the ultimate stuff of the universe. All change consisted of the coming-to-be of new combinations and the passing away of old combinations. Meanwhile the atoms persisted—uncreated, indestructible, the really real. These are the attributes that theologians attributed to God. The atomists, as Hooykaas points out, pulverized the divine being into atoms which "bear unmistakably divine attributes; they are eternal, unchangeable, self sufficient."[9]

In contrast the Platonic philosophy holds that material objects—the material world—have only a secondary or subordinate reality. The highest reality is immaterial, of the nature of mind (a term open to various interpretation). But in any case, ultimate reality lies in the realm of eternal ideas or forms. We may think of them as hypostasized qualities—redness, hardness, beauty, animality, goodness, justice. For Plato the qualities were real, while for the atomist the qualities represented a spin-off—to use a modern term—from particles in motion rather than something real in their own right.

This basic contrast in philosophic thought, already significant in the fifth century b.c., has persisted with variations and has profoundly affected all branches of philosophy up to the present. In the seventeenth century the conflict was especially acute, and the special battleground was the area we call natural philosophy.

Cudworth and Neoplatonism

In the seventeenth century the representative of Platonism most important for our discussion was Cudworth, one of the group commonly known as the Cambridge Platonists.[10] The British divine Ralph Cudworth (1617-1688) lived during troubled times, yet his personal life seemed relatively serene. The conflicts between Crown and Parliament, the establishment of the Protectorate, the Restoration, and the events leading up to the Bloodless Revolution in the year of his death, affected him little. His was an essentially academic life, as a doctor of divinity, master of Christ's College at Cambridge, and Anglican clergyman. His most important work, *The True Intellectual System of the Universe,* published in 1678, is a work of stupendous learning, dealing with theological and philosophical controversy that even in his own day seemed often remote from the urgent problems of the times.[11] The title page indicated that this volume was the first part, but he never wrote a sequel.

When his book appeared the intellectual and political climate in Great Britain was stormy. Politically, the conflict between Puritan and cavalier, between Commonwealth and monarchy, had been resolved in favor of the monarchy, for after the death of Cromwell only the restoration of the monarchy could achieve peace and security. In the field of religion the established church faced dissenters of many different types. Religious controversy and pamphlet wars often revolved around narrow doctrinal points, no less bitter, however, for their narrowness.

To conservative churchmen the whole basis of religion seemed under attack. Thomas Hobbes had published his *Leviathan* in 1651, thereby antagonizing conservatives and provoking them to strong defensive reactions. The new science was beginning to play a major role in intellectual life, and this new philosophy was coming perilously close to materialism and atheism. It seemed to leave little scope for spiritual values. The Royal Society grew in influence, and as it did so, the materialistic philosophy seemed even more threatening. The Society members were aware of this and apologists like Spratt and Glanvill could allay some fears. Yet other forms of counterattack were needed. The Cambridge Platonists, and especially Cudworth, aloof from the practical workings of science, tried to maintain and elaborate the traditional values and at the same time react against the atheistic trends.

Cudworth expressed his intent in the subtitle of his book: "Wherein, All The Reason and Philosophy of Atheism Is Confuted; And Its Impossibility Demonstrated." Since there are many shades and varieties of atheism, he distinguished and refuted each type in turn, with long and wearisome arguments, often raising what seem like straw men serving only to be knocked down. All this he did with enormous learning and detailed quotations from classical authors. Nevertheless, the major points of his exposition are intensely relevant to the concepts of nature.

Unlike many controversialists Cudworth insisted on defining his terms and made perfectly clear what he meant when he referred to deity. "The true and genuine idea of God in general, is this, a perfect conscious understanding Being (or Mind) existing of it self from eternity, and the cause of all other things."[12] God is transcendant, above the world and separate from it, the conscious all-powerful creator, with foresight and providence, the source of all life and of all else in the universe. Whatever philosophical doctrine denied the existence of a God such as this, Cudworth characterized as a form of atheism.

Cudworth minutely expounded the different forms of atheism, which ranged from the crudest atomism, where everything happened by chance, to various types of pantheism. For our purposes the essence of atheism lies in the assertion, "There is no conscious intellectual nature, presiding over the whole universe." To appreciate this view we must keep in mind certain basic distinctions in Cudworth's thought. First we must distinguish between corporeal and incorporeal, material and immaterial, matter and mind. The atoms, for example, are corporeal; mind and consciousness are not, yet a "corporealist" is not necessarily an atheist. He becomes one if he maintains that "animality, sense, and consciousness" are *derivative* from matter, that they are "a secondary, derivative, and accidental thing, generable and corruptible, arising out of a particular concretion of matter organized and dissolved together with them."[13] Matter and mind are distinct. Mind cannot be derived from matter.

Cudworth also distinguished sharply between life and mind. A mere vegetative form of life, a vital energy without any self-awareness, without perception or understanding, lacks the attributes characteristic of mind. He distinguished between "dead" matter, which lacks any sort of vital force, and "stupid" matter, which has a low grade of vital energy. And this in turn he distinguished from "mind," which has understanding and reason. The atheist might consider mind as a derivative of matter, a development of "stupid" matter. But this is wrong. Life and understanding "can never possibly rise out of any mixture or modification of dead and stupid matter whatsoever."[14] They come directly from God. For the atheist, mind is a derivative. For Cudworth it is primary. God is the ultimate mind and the cause of all else.

Then Cudworth faced the problem of explaining nature. The atheists, particularly the atomists, might find a satisfactory explanation in the blind play of atoms — "senseless atoms, fortuitously moved." By "making successively several encounters and consequently various implexions and entanglements," the atoms chanced at length "into the form and system of things, which now is, of earth, water, air and fire; sun, moon and stars; plants, animals and man." With this viewpoint "life and understanding . . . could only be accidental and secondary results from certain fortuitous concretions and contextures of atoms."[15] To these doctrines Cudworth was diametrically opposed. God is true substance, eternal and primary, above change and corruption, the source of all other beings. God involves consciousness, personality, intelligence, in other words, mind. But then arises the problem, how to get from God to the world. The answer, as befitted a Christian theologian, was creation. But at this point Cudworth showed his kinship to Neoplatonism. Creation took place not directly but indirectly through an intermediary, and this intermediary was "plastic nature," not as an independent force but as a subordinate agent carrying out the will of God.

According to Cudworth there are clear-cut alternatives. The universe is either "nothing else but a mere heap of dust, fortuitously agitated" — and this is atheism — or else it is subject to "divine causality," divine planning and execution. Then, since divine causality is the obvious answer, we have a further pair of options. One is that "God himself doth all *immediately,* and as it were with his own hands, form the body of every gnat and fly, insect and mite."[16] The alternative is an intermediary agent that would carry out the will of God, a sort of executive secretary. Cudworth would not go directly from God to the created nature but insisted on intercalating an additional being to carry out the divine plan. This concept of an intermediary who actually brought the world and its contents into being derives from the Platonic demiurge, as discussed in the *Timaeus,* but modified by the teachings of Plotinus.

The biblical account of creation presents quite an opposite view. God brought all things out of nothingness by his word alone. The biblical God "was not opposed by any matter that had to be forced into order, and He did not have to reckon with eternal forms."[17]

In contrast, Cudworth did not go directly from God to created nature. There was a gap — at least a logical gap — between divine intent and actual material activity. All the works of nature did indeed come about through "a divine law and command, yet this is not to be understood in a vulgar sence, as if they were all effected by the mere force of a verbal law or outward command, because inanimate things are not commandable nor governable by such a law." Words—even the word of God—cannot act on things. An intermediary is necessary: there must be some *efficient* cause to act on the inanimate object. Either God himself is the efficient agent for every activity in the universe, even for the smallest and most insignificant event, or He delegates that responsibility. "Not so much as a stone . . . could at any time fall downward, merely by the force of a verbal law, without any other efficient cause; but either God himself must immediately impel it, or else there must be some other subordinate cause in Nature for that motion." The divine command sets into activity "some energetick, effectual and operative cause for the production of every effect."[18] And this efficient cause is plastic nature.

Thus, intermediate between God and the world is plastic nature, the "subservient or executive instrument," while mind is "the principal and directive cause." Nature is not all powerful or "irresistible," for it must deal with matter, and matter can be "inept and contumaceous." As a result nature, although guided by a divine plan, may be "sometimes frustrated and disappointed by the indisposition of matter." Hence we have those "errors and bungles in nature" that an omnipotent agent would have avoided.[19] Here we have a doctrine of extreme importance. The apparent imperfections of nature are not due to the direct will of God, not to some inscrutable intent beyond our comprehension, but to the inadequate power of plastic nature as it faced the "indisposition" of matter. Nature works against resistance, which is sometimes excessive.

Nature, servant not master, is a living agent. It "acts upon matter as an inward principle . . . not . . . from without mechanically, but from within vitally." Nature, although alive, is only a lowly form of life without any understanding of what it does. It acts purposefully "yet it self doth neither intend those ends, nor understand the reason of that which it doth." Cudworth mentioned instinctive behavior, as of bees, spiders, and birds, to illustrate this point, that there may be actions toward ends although the animals do not comprehend the reasons for those actions. Plastic nature, then, is a vital force, an energy without awareness. It "cannot act electively nor with discretion."[20]

At this point we can appreciate the "healing power of Nature," as Cudworth understood it. Plastic nature regulates activity in an orderly fashion. Body has no internal energy of its own. Plastic nature supplies this energy as the living directing force for the vegetative functions. It heals and repairs as well as regulates normal physiological processes. It "restores flesh that is lost, consolidates dissolved continuities, incorporates the newly received nourishment and joyns it continuously with the preexistent parts of flesh and bone; which regenerates and repairs veins consumed and cut off."[21]

This healing power of nature reflects the immaterial regulating force of plastic nature. As we shall see in the next chapter there is a certain degree of kinship with the "form" on which neo-Galenism rests and also with the archeus of van Helmont and of Stahl, discussed in Chapter 6. Plastic nature seems to be *in* things as a dynamic regulating power, distinct from intelligence and mind and reason, acting for goals and ends of which it is unaware ("stupid" rather than intelligent). It affects the totality of phenomena as well as the individual living being.

Cudworth relied heavily on intermediaries as a means of connecting dissimilar entities. He assumed that these intermediaries, if numerous enough, can provide a smooth transition. We can, for example, derive matter from mind by virtue of intermediaries, wherein the immaterial aspect decreases while the material component progressively "thickens" and increases. I suggest an illustration drawn from histologic technique. If we want to examine specimens under the microscope, we ordinarily embed them in paraffin. This process involves first of all subjecting the tissue to an aqueous fixative. How, then, to get the tissues into paraffin, which is not miscible with water? To achieve this goal the tissues are passed through a graded series of alcohols, up to absolute alcohol. This process removes the water. Then we pass from absolute alcohol to chloroform, which can mix with alcohol but not water. From chloroform we are able to go to paraffin, which mixes with chloroform but not alcohol. The intermediate steps enable us to pass from water to paraffin and thus achieve a transition between incompatibles.

Intercalation allows gradual transition whereas sudden breaks can outrage the sense of order. Transitions permitted seventeenth and eighteenth century physicians to "explain" numerous physiological and psychological phenomena and to pass, for example, from mind to body. In this transition the concept of spirit serves as an intermediary. Then, when "spirit" becomes readily interchangeable with "spirits" having varying degrees of fineness and subtlety, all difficulties seem to disappear.

The process of transitions was a basic tenet of biological theory in that era. Plato had provided the germ of this doctrine of transition, but the principal development came from Plotinus (204-269), the major figure in Neoplatonism.[22] Cudworth embraced Neoplatonic teachings, but the mechanists also used what I call "Neoplatonic maneuvers."

Although we are specifically concerned with nature, yet the doctrines of Plotinus form a well-integrated system, and we cannot understand any part without an overview of the whole. Plotinus was a monist who derived all existence from the transcendent ineffable One, beyond human description or prediction, yet the ground of all being and reality. The first problem is to get from the One to the Many. From the plenitude of its being, the One overflows by a process that is called emanation; that is, without itself changing in any way, it gives rise to all else. This was compared to the activity of radiation where, according to ancient doctrine, the sun gives off light without itself becoming altered.

This first emanation gives rise to *nous,* mind or intellectual principle, corresponding in a rough sort of way, to the Platonic realm of ideas and the realm of the universals. It can be approached and described through reason. Since ideas are multiple, the One has already become differentiated to some degree. In this first emanation, there is no longer pure unity but rather a one-many. However, being cannot rest; just as light rays must continue to travel, being must continue its process of emanation. Mind, therefore, or intellectual principle, undergoes a further emanation to produce soul, psyche, or vital principle. In this realm multiple souls exist. Differentiation has progressed. The one-many has become one and many, receiving unity from above, becoming multiple and passing further multiplicity to the next stage below.[23]

The One, the intellectual-realm, and the realm of soul are all immaterial. How does the concrete material world arise? According to the principle of emanation the world necessarily comes into being. "In the absence of body, soul could not have gone forth, since there is no other place to which its nature would allow it to descend. Since go forth it must, it will generate a place for itself; at once body, also, exists."[24] Thus, the material world, in all its multiplicity, *necessarily results from the continued process of emanation.* The One has become many and the immaterial has become corporeal, and it all happened through an unbroken chain that links the world to the realm of souls directly above, then to the realm of mind somewhat further removed, and then to the ineffable One.

What proceeds from the world of souls "downward" into matter is nature. When Plotinus spoke of nature he thus had in view not only material objects but also a spiritual, immaterial force that draws from the "upper" realms and transmits to the "lower." There is thus a hierarchy, a ladder or chain of being.[25] For Plotinus nature was an immaterial being that acted relatively blindly and, without conscious awareness, transmitted the ideas of the intellectual realm into matter, that is, imposed on matter the laws and regularities of the world as we know it. This notion that an immaterial force can, out of the fulness of its being, "produce" a material substance or body which it then proceeds to direct, is a Neoplatonic concept that will reappear in the eighteenth century, in the explanation of birth defects and of the mother "marking" her unborn child, as discussed in Chapter 7.

The philosophy of Plotinus, highly influential in the Renaissance and the seventeenth century, had surprising ramifications. Without going into all the complexities, we can appreciate how clear was Cudworth's debt to Plotinus, in regard to the concept of nature.

Neoplatonism is a branch of the Platonic tradition, whose views on nature are characteristically expressed by Cudworth. The contrary view we find in atomism, and for the seventeenth century version of this doctrine, and the concept of nature derived therefrom, I will refer to Gassendi and to Boyle.

Pierre Gassendi (1592-1655) combined classical atomism with a more or less orthodox Christian theology. While his eclecticism was not, perhaps, fully successful, he created a system that found a place for both atoms and God, harmonized pagan doctrine with religious orthodoxy, brought religion and science together, and served as a model for later theorists. Gassendi's general framework of explanation antedated that of Robert Boyle, whose formulations had a more direct influence on modern science and medicine, but the French cleric and philosopher played an important part in establishing what came to be the dominant point of view for the early eighteenth century.

Although Gassendi pursued a theological career, he showed a talent for mathematics and served as a professor of mathematics at the Collège Royale of Paris. Furthermore, he had a life-long appreciation of the physical sciences and closely followed the discoveries of Galileo and Kepler. He became a doctor of theology in 1616 and took holy orders in 1617. Early in his career he turned against the Aristotelian philosophy, but not until late in life did he write extensively on the Epicurean philosophy. His most important work, the *Syntagma Philosophiae Epicuri,* was published in 1649, and his collected works were first published, posthumously, in 1658.

Gassendi wrote in Latin and until very recently his writings have not been available in English. At one time a French abridgement[26] was widely used, but unfortunately this conveys a distorted and misleading view. Good accounts of Gassendi's teachings can be found in some excellent secondary sources.[27]

In the *Syntagma,* Part II Book IV, Gassendi expounded his views on atomism, drawn from the writings of classical authors, especially Lucretius, and from later supporters.[28] He makes a distinction between matter (*materia*) and body (*corpus*).[29] Body is matter with certain properties — magnitude or quantity, which consists of extension — length, width, and depth. Body or corporality comprises nature — what Gassendi calls *res naturales.* Different bodies are distinguished one from another by their forms, but form cannot exist by itself. It must necessarily inhere in matter or body.[30] These relationships of form and matter will be discussed in detail in the next chapter. For the moment let us consider body as a particular kind of matter, one that has extension and three-dimensionality.

The atoms constitute matter, uncreated and indestructible, out of which all things are created and into which they are ultimately dissolved. The atoms have certain properties. They are not mathematical points but they have magnitude or size. They are *bodies*. As such they have configuration or shape and they differ in shape and size. Some are larger and some small-er, but all are invisible. They can be identified only by reason. The in-equality in size and shape helps explain the different properties that we ob-serve in things. In modern terms we can say that a variety of atomic shapes provides a sufficient number of variables to allow specific correlations with specific phenomena. If all atoms were the same size, we would not be able to account readily for the variety of things.[31]

Atoms vary in their configurations, an imperceptible property that can be understood only by reason. Gassendi offered an interesting analogy. The finest granules of dust might appear round and smooth to the naked eye but if examined under a microscope (*engyscopium*) they are seen to have an angular configuration and vastly many different shapes and sizes. The variety of sizes and shapes of atoms is large but not infinite. While there is a limit to the number of sizes and shapes of atoms, for any particu-lar size and shape there is an unlimited number of examples.[32]

Another property of the atoms is *pondus* or *gravitas*. The translation of these terms is not easy, for Gassendi provided synonyms that in our usage do not have the same meaning. Thus, "weight" or "gravity" is nothing other than the "natural internal power or force, by which an atom by itself can agitate and move itself." This is an inherent, intrinsic, and eternal propensity or impulse to motion. The concepts of gravity, of weight, and of intrinsic eternal motion are deemed equivalent. Hence, in simplistic terms the properties of atoms consist of size, shape, and motion, and the particles possessing these attributes comprise matter, or the substrate for forms.

Although Gassendi expounded with great sympathy the doctrines of Epicurus and the classical atomists, he could not accept the metaphysical implications. Atomism, in its ancient guise, had atheistic and materialistic overtones quite at odds with Christian doctrine. Gassendi wanted to intro-duce various modifications that would harmonize atomism with orthodox theology. He rejected the idea of atoms as eternal, uncreated, and infinite. They were, however, the prime matter which God created at the beginning and which formed the basis of all things.[33]

The atoms, then, do not exist from all eternity. Gassendi discussed a second doctrine to be rebutted—the tenet that atoms have an intrinsic motion or motor force existing from eternity. These small primary bodies are indeed mobile but this motion is not an intrinsic property. Instead it is a force that God implanted when he created the atoms. Matter does not possess motion of its own right.

God, of his own free will, created matter. It consisted of small bodies or atoms, in whatever number was necessary, in indefinite variety, of many shapes and sizes, and having a force suitable for moving, combining, intertwining and separating out, to accomplish all the ends and purposes He intended. Furthermore, at the creation God made the first seeds of living things from special atoms and from these seeds, the *semina,* there occurred propagation. The seeds were made appropriate for the regions where they were to propagate and grow. These seeds can disintegrate into their component atoms, but these same atoms can easily come together again to form seeds.[34] Gassendi indicated an unending series of generation and corruption, the atoms always furnishing the matter from which bodies were composed, as well as the motion by which they were arranged. God created the atoms and endowed them with motions appropriate for the ends they were to serve.

However, the mind and soul of man fall into a quite different category and are not to be equated with the concourse of atoms. Man is quite distinct from all other living creatures.

Despite his interest in natural science and the empirical attitude that this implied, Gassendi approached philosophy in a thoroughly rationalistic manner and reached conclusions dictated by reason. For him the atomistic hypothesis logically explained the material world, that is, the world of nature. We cannot directly perceive the atoms, but through reasoning we can grasp their principal characteristics—they are indivisible and indestructible, solid (resistant), and they have weight.

But material nature is not the totality of the universe. Whence came the atoms, and the force and direction that they exhibit? For the classical atomists who followed the doctrines of Epicurus, the atoms in motion existed from eternity and the combination of atoms occurred by chance. For Gassendi the atoms and their motions and properties were created by God. Thus, to understand the world as we see it—nature, the world of atoms— we must gain some understanding of God.

As an accomplished theologian, Gassendi engaged in subtle reasoning to demonstrate the existence and characteristics of God. He "proves" the existence of God, as one, eternal, infinite, characterized by intelligence, absolute power, goodness, and freedom. God created the world of nature, the realm of atoms with its admirable harmony and wonderful properties. Creation manifests intelligence, goodness, and foresight.

Gassendi helped popularize the atomistic philosophy that was to become so successful as an explanation. In addition he brought the atomistic philosophy into complete harmony with Christian theology. He created a *system,* a unified intellectual construct that, like a curled-up hedgehog, could repel any hostile probings. Instead of prickly spines his intellectual hedgehog used formidable reasoning deduced from the premises. His methodological approach we call rationalism, and he falls within the tradition that includes Descartes, Spinoza, and Leibniz among the great seventeenth century figures. For them the universe is rational and its essence can be reached through intellectual probings.

Boyle

Robert Boyle (1627-1691) was one of the most influential of the seventeenth century atomists. Living a full generation after Gassendi, he grew up in a markedly different tradition. In contrast to the French Catholic theologian, who was a good mathematician but without practical expertise in science, Boyle was an English Protestant layman and an eminent practicing scientist. Despite the differences, Boyle owed a great deal to the doctrines of Gassendi, a debt which Kargon has especially emphasized.[35] Yet in contrast to the rationalist Gassendi, Boyle belonged to the philosophic tradition that we call empiricism, along with such giants as Bacon and Locke. Whether the contrast between the two philosophical approaches is really as sharp as is often claimed will form a topic for later discussion.

Boyle adhered to the corpuscular philosophy, but as a deeply religious man he had to harmonize religious doctrines and natural philosophy. He devoted an entire treatise specifically to the subject of nature.[36] This was originally published in 1686 but presumably was written at intervals at some earlier time. The preface is dated 1682.

The term nature, as he pointed out, has had many different meanings, with much resulting confusion. As a clear thinker he indicated the limitations that he ascribed to the term and offered, if not a strict definition, at least a fairly consistent circumscription. Nature for him was the "aggregate of bodies, that made up the world, framed as it is." These bodies act "according to the laws of motion prescribed by the Author of things." Boyle explicitly rejected the concept of an intermediate entity or force, intervening between God and the concrete world. He declared, "I see no need to acknowledge any architectonic being, besides God, antecedent to the first formation of the world."[37] And he repeatedly returned to this denial.

These views, baldly stated, have various corollaries and implications and raise many problems. Boyle's definition refers to "bodies"—material entities. He did not draw any distinction between grossly visible bodies like trees and houses, and the invisible and only postulated bodies like atoms. They were all material. But what about immaterial entities? Are there any? If so, what is their status? In his discussion of nature, Boyle made a specific disclaimer: he sharply limited his universe of discourse and explicitly excluded "the rational soul or mind of man," for this is "an immaterial spirit."[38] Immaterial beings exist but he excludes them from his discussion. It is Boyle the physicist who was speaking.

The realm of the immaterial, which he excluded from nature, does include God and the rational souls of man and, as he sometimes suggested, souls not joined to human bodies. Such a realm has different properties from the aggregate of material particles, which obey the laws of motion. But from this immaterial realm he expressly rejected any being resembling a Platonic demiurge, any created being subordinate to God and carrying out the will of God.

In rejecting such a concept, Boyle indicated his nominalism. This is the philosophic position that carefully distinguishes between names and things, between an abstract word drawn from a mass of particulars and any reification of that word (that is, granting to it some real existence in its own right). Abstract terms, for Boyle, had no independent reality but were merely names or notions. So with nature. It was not an *ens,* not an existing being in its own right, not in any sense an independent force, but only a name.

The commonly used expression "Nature does this or that" represents a manner of speaking and not any real entity that performs an activity. A favorite example of this error — using a name as if it were a real agent — is "Nature abhors a vacuum." This expression does not in any way explain the concrete event that "really" depends on the pressure relationships between particles of air. Boyle refused to "ascribe to a notional thing that, which, indeed, is performed by real particles." A comparable expression would be "The law punishes murder." Law is only a notional rule and does not concretely perform anything.[39]

His concern with material particles led Boyle to place immaterial beings in a separate category, and this in turn yielded a dualism as troublesome in its way as that of Descartes. The rational soul of man was not material, not subject to mechanical laws. But man was a complex creature and Boyle had eliminated from the discussion only man's rational soul, not the "sensitive soul." This had to do with physiological processes of bodily organs, including sense organs, nerves, and brain. All these are material and obey the causal laws governing material particles in motion. The body of man was a machine — an "engine" — and that part of the soul related directly to the machine, the sensitive soul, would be under mechanical rule.[40] But is the rational soul subject to *any* law? Later in the century Locke helped establish the science of psychology, but this is not relevant here. The rational soul had never been adequately analyzed. Reason, free will, religious aspiration and moral sense, all were confused. Boyle did not attempt any analysis but accepted the rational soul as an indefinite entity, immaterial, distinct from the sensitive soul which, as part of the body, was material. Nature was concerned with material particles in motion.

This motion of material particles was "skillfully guided" by the Creator, but the laws that God imposed on matter were not invariable. Here we confront the troublesome problem of miracles. Boyle was somewhat apologetic to the "strict naturalists" for saying that "events may sometimes be varied by some peculiar interposition of God." Yet he emphasized his firm belief that God does perform miracles — God "does seldom manifestly procure a recession from the settled course of the universe, and especially from the most catholic laws of motion." Such actions are supernatural, or miracles.[41]

Boyle was dealing, although rather gingerly, with that major philosophic problem, the relationship of the immaterial to the material. In a somewhat obscure but, in my opinion, extremely significant passage, he declared that "the sovereign Lord and Governor of the world, doth . . . give, by the intervention of rational minds, as well united, as not united, to human bodies, divers such determinations to the motion of parts . . . as by laws merely mechanical those parts of matter would not have had." Thereby there occur many "things conducive to the welfare or detriment of man."[42] God, clearly, may alter the laws of motion for the welfare of mankind. But somewhat less clear is the phrase "rational minds, as well united, as not united, to human bodies." I interpret this to mean not only the rational soul of man but also such creatures as angels, and possibly devils, or other immaterial beings that can have special control over material events.

In another passage Boyle rather confusedly returned to this topic, that the ordinary laws of motion can be changed. Man has under his command "the direction of many local motions in the parts of his own body." And, "since man himself is vouchsafed a power to alter, in several cases, the usual course of things, it should not seem incredible, that the latent interposition of man, or perhaps angels, or other causes unthought by us, should sometimes be employed to the like purposes by God." However, Boyle cautioned against using divine intervention as a ready explanation for phenomena. God does indeed sometimes "interpose in the ordinary phenomena and events . . . but . . . this is done so seldom . . . that we are not hastily to have recourse to an extraordinary providence."[43]

Another cautious statement mentioned that "all motions, where no intelligent spirit intervenes, are made according to catholic, and almost, if not more than almost, mechanical laws." Or again, in the "hydraulico-pneumatical engines we call human bodies, when neither particular problems, nor the rational soul, nor over-ruling impediments interpose, things are generally performed according to mechanical laws."[44]

Passages such as these indicate, I believe, Boyle's ambiguous and uncertain attitude. As a scientist he believed that mechanical laws govern the behavior of material particles, yet these laws *seem* to have loopholes. They may not be *entirely* mechanical, and intelligent minds may be able to alter them on occasion. God, of course, may do so; and perhaps to some extent so can the mind of man — that is, his rational soul; and perhaps angels or other spirits may also do so.

Boyle has a great deal to say about the traditional concept of the healing power of nature, or as he phrased it, *natura est morborum medicatrix*. He rejected the notion of "a certain provident or watchful being" that acts "by its own endeavors, as well as by any occasional assistance, that may be afforded it by the physician, to rectify what is amiss, and restore the distempered body to its pristine state of health."[45] Instead, Boyle insisted, the human body is an automaton. He drew analogies between the tendency of the human body to maintain itself and similar tendencies in inanimate objects which, when distorted, return to their former state (as, a compass or a spring). Similarly in the body there are forces that act to preserve the original structure. These forces, or causes, are mechanical.

The body, as a machine, has not only solid parts but fluids. It is a "hydraulopneumatical engine," and a living man is "so constituted that in certain circumstances the liquors are disposed to be put into a fermentation or commotion, whereby either some depuration of themselves, or some discharge of harmful matter by excretion, or both, are produced so as . . . to conduce to the recovery or welfare of the body."[46]

Of course, in all this Boyle is simply repeating the old Hippocratic concept, that the healing power of nature, acting by coction and excretion, eliminates the peccant matter. To this familiar concept Boyle added the hypothesis that the coction is a chemical process acting chiefly by fermentation, that the body is a "hydraulopneumatical engine," that its laws are similar to those of the inorganic world. He added further that no immaterial being, no individual directing force exists to achieve the end result. He thus denied any "archeus."

But the laws of mechanics, hydraulics, and pneumatics do not apply to the rational mind of man; furthermore, in the realm where they do apply the laws are almost but not quite invariable. Intelligence, divine or human, may produce alterations. Then, slipping back into metaphor, Boyle declared that the physician, far from being the servant of nature, is an assistant who must use his judgment and promote those activities he considers helpful to recovery and oppose those he considers harmful.[47]

Much of Boyle's reasoning rests upon analogy, upon the resemblances between man-made machines and the human or animal body. Man, the human artificer, can, however, make only imperfect products, markedly

inferior to the products of God. What justification do we have for calling
the living body a machine, when the automata to which it is compared are
so limited? Boyle touched upon this difficulty and solved it by simply
begging the question. If anyone objected to the examples drawn from
automata as not adequate, Boyle admitted the charge. But the bodies of
living animals are "engines of God's own framing, and consequently effects
of an omniscient and almighty artificer. So that, it is not rational to
expect, that in the incomparably inferior productions of human skill, there
should be found engines fit to be compared with these, which in their
protoplasts had God for their author."

The assumptions are magnificently circular. The human body *is* a machine like those that are man-made, but incomparably better. How do we
know? Because God is so much better a mechanic than is man. As for logical cogency, this argument will appeal only to someone already convinced
on other grounds, while those not already convinced would hardly be
swayed.

The writings of Boyle show the unsettled state of science and philosophy.
"Nature" meant both the living and the nonliving. The latter was the
world of physics, of law and mathematical formulations, of laboratory
investigation and rational explanation. And apart from man, the world of
the living could be squeezed into the same framework. But man was in a
unique category, having to do not only with the world of physics but also
with religion and metaphysics. The relationships between nature, man,
and God—or man, nature, and the supernatural—were far from clear.
Boyle gave equivocal and uncertain answers, derived from the atomism of
Gassendi under the influence of Protestant theology.

Hoffmann

A rather different approach to nature and the supernatural is offered by
Friedrich Hoffmann, who will appear frequently in this book in various
contexts. His views diverge somewhat from those of Boyle and reflect continental rationalism. In addition they analyze in striking fashion the crucial
features in the relationship between the natural and the supernatural,
namely, the problems of witchcraft.

Hoffmann, the son of a physician, was born in 1660 in Halle. From early
childhood he had had a deep interest in the new science and he decided to
study medicine, receiving his M.D. degree in 1680. A few years later he
traveled extensively and visited England, where he became friendly with
Boyle. Then, on returning to Germany, he practiced medicine for a number of years in Minden and in Halberstadt. In 1693 the Elector Frederick
III (later Frederick I of Prussia), who had established the new University at
Halle, called Hoffmann to be the first professor of medicine. Georg Stahl

later became the second professor. These two formed one of the strongest faculties in Europe and, with Boerhaave, dominated medical thought for the first forty years of the eighteenth century.

Hoffmann's most influential text was his massive *Medicinae Rationalis Systematica,* which contained his most mature thought.[48] But an earlier and much smaller text, a virtual primer of medicine, he published in 1695, shortly after he accepted the professorship at Halle. This small text, in aphoristic form, is now available in English.[49] In his terse statements, Hoffmann indicated his views on nature, mind, and soul. He adhered to the corpuscularian philosophy but followed that of Descartes rather than of Gassendi.

Medicine, he said, depends on nature, and nature is mechanical. The first principles of mechanics are matter and motion. The essence of matter is extension, and Hoffmann accepted the Cartesian division of matter into three grades, of which, for our purposes, the finest or extremely subtle matter is especially important. Correlative to matter is motion, "the first and most universal principle of things and the efficient cause of all forms. As matter gives the essence, to things, so motion provides them with specificity." Size and shape, motion and rest are the "basic states of simple bodies." Matter is passive and requires an agent as the source of motion. This source is God, who impressed motion on the extremely subtle matter in nature. All motion takes place by pressure.[50]

Living bodies are machines or automatons whose parts are either solid or fluid. Life "consists in the continuous and appropriate movement of the fluid parts through the solids. The fluid parts, moreover, are the primary cause of motion."[51] Of all the fluids the most important are the "animal spirits," the blood, and the lymph.

The life of man involves "the uninterrupted communion of mind [*mens*] and body." Hoffmann distinguished between soul (*anima*) and the mind (*mens*). All philosophers agree, he declared, "that in our machine the first principle of motion is the soul [*anima*] which you may, if you want, designate as nature, or spirit endowed with mechanical powers, or a most subtle ethereal matter acting in an ordered and specific fashion." This vital principle, "apart from its mechanical capacities and power of performing ordered movements, is endowed with a more noble power, namely of thinking and reasoning, which the vital principle of brutes does not have; and by virtue of this power it is called mind [*mens*], an immortal substance stemming from the decree of God himself." God is the first cause of those powers that exist in the soul. The animal spirits are not the vital principle itself, but the soul uses the spirits "as instruments for achieving its functions." The soul moves the spirits and directs them. The spirits, or subtle ethereal matter, are intermediate between soul and body.[52]

Hoffmann described the structure and functioning of the body in detail.

He paid particular attention to the "animal spirit" in the brain and nerves. This spirit "is an *ens activum,* producing, in matter, movement which is limited and orderly." Since matter by itself is passive, it cannot produce any motion "without an active spirit and prime mover." This prime mover, contained in nerves, "is nothing but very fine matter, endowed with a limited mechanical power suitable for bringing about ideational and ordered motions in the body. Hence it can properly be called spirit."[53]

We can see, perhaps, how the Cartesian metaphysics, with its three grades of matter, actually harmonizes with the Neoplatonic tradition as elaborated by Cudworth. For Hoffmann, who claimed to be a mechanist, the key to life is the extremely subtle matter. If matter is fine enough it can harmonize with the commands of God and the rational soul and also serve as motive force for matter that is somewhat coarser. It thus acts as an intermediary that shuttles between the rational soul, the sensitive soul, and more crude matter.

We see this in Hoffmann's account of the brain and nervous system. The nerve fluid — the very finest material particles — "is the finest of all and most suited for producing very rapid movement." These "animal spirits, provided with the utmost fineness and elasticity, have a power impressed by God, not only of moving themselves mechanically but doing so by choice, purposefully and toward a definite goal. This power is called the sensitive soul."[54] The sensitive soul is mechanical. But the mechanical activities of the nerves are transmitted to the "common sensory" — not the pineal gland, as Descartes had claimed, but the "centrum ovale" (in modern terminology, the striate body). Here, "In the common sensory, as in the highest tribunal, all sensory impressions of external things gather together and are perceived by the mind. And then, from this highest place for guiding the will and decisions of the mind, the animal spirits are directed and pass out to all the parts which should be animated by sensation and motion."[55]

In this early work Hoffmann has not specifically tried to solve the knotty philosophical problems that cling to his concepts of nature. However, his views emerge by indirection and indicate an ordered hierarchy. God, the rational soul, and the vital principle or *anima,* form a gradation. The *anima* controls the extremely subtle matter or animal spirits, which in turn control other bodily motions involving particles that are coarser in various degrees. The analogy to the Neoplatonic hierarchy is close, even though the nomenclature is different. Hoffmann claimed to be a mechanist, explaining the world through matter and motion. But to explain life and the immaterial mind he adopted the Neoplatonic maneuver wherein extremely subtle matter served as intermediate between the realm of the immaterial and the coarser grades of extended matter. The very subtle matter could be deemed to have a minimal real extension. And since, for the

Cartesian philosophy, there are no atoms and no lower limit of divisibility, minimal extension can be construed as merging with the immaterial.

In this work Hoffmann merely skirted the subject of the immaterial. But in a slightly later study this problem came to the fore. He chose to discuss witchcraft, and in so doing he could not avoid coming to grips with the problems of the immaterial and the supernatural.

The concept of witchcraft has a venerable lineage. Well established in biblical times, it had a checkered course ever after. Belief in witchcraft flourished with special intensity in Europe between the late fifteenth and early eighteenth centuries. Many outstanding historians have studied the phenomena and the associated persecutions, and the literature is enormous. Good historical overviews will be found in many excellent recent secondary sources.[56] The rise of persecutions during the Renaissance is generally associated with the activities of the Dominican friars Kraemer and Sprenger and their book, *Malleus Maleficarum.*[57] Witch hunting grew progressively for about 150 years to reach its maximum intensity and then gradually diminished as religious passions abated and skeptics gained more and more ground. By the early eighteenth century persecutions had virtually disappeared and apologists and critics alike could speak with greater calmness. Rational discussion could replace fanaticism.

Friedrich Hoffmann has given us a detailed analysis of these problems, an analysis that illuminates medical thinking at the beginning of the eighteenth century. The work in question is a dissertation originally published in 1703, with the title *De potentia diaboli in corpore,* bearing on the title page, *praeside Friederico Hoffmann . . . submittit Godofredus Bueching, Halle, Gruner.* Customarily, at that time, a dissertation represented the work of the professor, and the student defended the thesis at a public disputation where the professor served as presiding officer or *praeses.* From the bibliographic standpoint dissertations are ordinarily included among the collected works of the *praeses.* In the present instance the monograph is included in the *Opera Omnia* of Hoffmann.[58]

Concerning the real existence of the devil there was no doubt. The initial problem involved not his existence but his characteristics. By general agreement, said Hoffmann, the devil is considered to be a created spirit, finite, very evil, provided with certain powers over man. In this context Hoffmann used the word spirit in a sense somewhat different from that discussed earlier. Here he meant a creature—a created being—that lacks extension, spatial circumscription, divisibility or impenetrability. The devil lacks all corporality, yet has the faculty of understanding, knowing, and willing—the properties of mind.[59]

God established the laws of nature that science studied, but God can alter these laws at will. When he does so he brings about an event that transcends nature and constitutes a miracle, which, by definition, is a supernatural occurrence brought about by an act of will. The devil, subordinate to God, cannot perform miracles. He cannot violate the laws of nature that God has established and which only God can abrogate.[60] This principle serves as a touchstone for understanding the powers of the devil in this world and also the role that the devil may play in the alleged phenomena of witchcraft.

Since the devil cannot perform miracles he cannot, for example, transport bodies through the air.[61] This reasoning struck at the very heart of popular demonology, for one of the characteristics claimed for witches was their power—with the help of the devil—to fly through the air to attend the witches' Sabbath. Since such an alleged action would run counter to natural law, the claim must be rejected. Although alleged witches, in their confessions, claimed that they did fly through the air to participate in the orgies, such claims must be attributed to disordered imagination, perhaps due to drug action.

Hoffmann similarly rejected comparable allegations that ran counter to natural law. The devil cannot transmute base matter into gold or change the inner essence of a body. He cannot create life nor transform an inanimate object into a living body. These would be miracles and beyond the power of the devil. Hoffmann referred to the biblical account of Moses, who, when he appeared before Pharaoh, transformed a rod into a live serpent. But Moses, as the servant of God, was performing a true miracle. The Bible tells us that the magicians of Pharaoh, to discredit Moses, apparently performed the same act. But the magicians were tricksters who produced only the image (Hoffmann's term is *simulacrem*) and not a real serpent.[62] The change, then, was nothing but a trick, not a real transformation, although Hoffmann did not tell us how the trick was accomplished.

By logical reasoning Hoffmann has shown us what the devil cannot do— he cannot perform miracles or act counter to the laws of nature. Any allegations to the contrary must be rejected.

All this merely indicates the negative aspect of demonology. While the devil cannot perform miracles, he nevertheless has power in the world and can affect both immaterial objects and man. To explain the way the immaterial devil can act on the material world, Hoffmann gave the analogy of the human mind willing a voluntary action—mind, which is immaterial, acts on the body not directly but through the mediation of the animal spirits, the finest possible material substance. This permits a smooth transition from immaterial to material. Through the nerve fluid the mind, which is of "spiritual stock," excites and directs the motor activity.[63] Mind acts on body through the intervention of another agent.[64]

In comparable fashion the devil, totally immaterial, can act on the material world through an extremely subtle intermediary. In this connection we can distinguish the macrocosm or great world from the microcosm or man. In the macrocosm the devil acts by affecting the ether, an extremely subtle substance. He produces effects on the atmosphere and hence the weather. As part of his evil activities he can produce winds and storms, rain, hail, and cold.[65] In acting on man, the microcosm, the devil exerts his power by affecting the animal spirits, which are so finely material that they can be acted on by immaterial substance. There is an excellent symmetry involving macrocosm and microcosm. The devil, immaterial, affects each of them through the medium of the extremely subtle matter—the ether in the one case, the animal spirits in the other.

The devil exists as pure spirit, above nature yet limited by its laws which he cannot contravene. Yet while the devil cannot break the laws of nature, he can bend or direct them to serve his own evil purposes. He harms mankind by a chain of interactions wherein his evil will, purely immaterial, acts on extremely subtle matter, which in turn acts on progressively coarser matter. The actual movement of the subtle matter falls within the laws of nature, but the will of the devil, which initiates the action, is supernatural.

Acts of will initiate chains of causation. Ordinary human volition offers a familiar example. The will of the devil, although far more powerful than that of man, would seem to be analogous in its essence. After that first step of initiation, the activities set into motion are restricted by the laws of nature, which God has established. The powerful will of the devil can initiate chains of causation far beyond the scope of man. A human, for example, cannot affect the atmosphere to bring about a storm, nor can one man interfere with the animal spirits of another. The devil, however, can readily do these things. We might say that God created natural laws and can suspend them at will—thus performing miracles; the devil cannot suspend natural laws but has vast power to direct them to harmful goals; man has free will to initiate certain chains of events but can apply this will only to a limited range of activities.

At the beginning of this chapter I noted the animistic religions of the Homeric Greeks and the control that the will of the gods exerts over disease. In contrast, nature came to mean a series of forces that act autonomously, not affected by volition. In orthodox religion, however, nature is limited, and under certain conditions its forces can be either set aside or influenced through immaterial will.

The place of man in nature remains rather indefinite. The soul of man participates in the realm of the divine; the will is a property of the soul; but the will of man can act only within rather strict limits, whose relationship to nature is not clear.

In the seventeenth and eighteenth centuries the discussions of nature

involved problems that had already exercised the greatest minds of antiquity. Who will say that these problems have been solved by the twentieth
century? To what degree is nature synonymous with the universe? Is man
completely part of nature, or do some aspects of man transcend nature?
The question of nature and its relations to the supernatural is part of a
larger problem, what aspects of the universe are material, and what
aspects immaterial? And what are the relations of the immaterial to the
material? Some facets of this topic we have considered in the present
chapter. A rather different facet of the same problem involves the "substantial form," an important part of our medical heritage. This we will
study in the next chapter.

THREE

SUBSTANTIAL FORM

Most children, I hope, have played a game often called "animal, vegetable, or mineral," or sometimes "twenty questions." In this game one player thinks of some object and the other players, by asking questions capable of a yes or no answer, try to identify that object. The first question ordinarily would be, "Is it animal?" If not, "Is it vegetable?" And if not, "Is it mineral?" For example, if the chosen object were "the coins in my pocket," this would be mineral; "my brother's shirt" would be vegetable (cotton); "my mother's fur coat" would be animal.

After determining the general class, the interlocutors have to narrow down the field by finding successively more precise categories—for example, Is it something to eat? something to wear? something ornamental? something useful? Or the questions might narrow down the locus. Is it in this city? in this house? in this room? The course of the questioning would reflect the logical acumen of the interlocutors.

This game also appeals to adults who can bring a much higher degree of sophistication. The categories of "animal," "vegetable," or "mineral" are far too restrictive. They exclude all but simple entities—"things"—and eliminate anything abstract or conceptual or imaginative.

For example, a player might want to choose a fictional character like Mr. Pickwick. Here we become entangled with ontology and complex philosophic problems. With such a choice, how can a player answer the question "Is it animal?" The answer would be "no," and the same answer would apply to "Is it vegetable?" and "Is it mineral?" The interlocutor would then be mightily puzzled until he enlarged his categories. He would need to ask, "Is it corporeal (or material)?" or perhaps, "Is it fictional?" or perhaps, "Is it real?"

Fictional characters are relatively easy to deal with. But suppose a player chose "the shadow on the wall," or "the reflection in a mirror" or "the square root of -1" or "a unicorn" or "Banquo's ghost" or "the dream I dreamed last night" or "the thoughts that Newton had when the falling apple allegedly hit him on the head." How could these be categorized? What sorts of questions must be asked to determine the most general classes and then the progressively subordinate classes? When we have such categories as real or unreal, conceptual or material, we are dealing with ontology. But we do so not in any deliberately self-conscious way, not as professed philosophers, but as ordinary people playing a parlor game for

fun. Yet our ordinary speech patterns necessarily have philosophic overtones, which sometimes we must make explicit.

There is certainly a significant difference between Mr. Pickwick as a fictional character and my brother; between a reflection in a mirror and a sea
serpent; between a unicorn and a thought that occurred to Newton or
Pascal. Those who play this game do not spend their time in metaphysical
discussion but speedily come to some sort of agreement about the categories of real and conceptual and material; and then they use these categories
in a meaningful fashion.

However, those who are argumentative and who want to make more
precise the ontological status of, say, a dream or a sea serpent, will speedily
find themselves enmeshed in discussions that will remind us of twelfth century philosophers and the realist-nominalist controversy of that era. How
real is an immaterial or conceptual entity? I am not so foolhardy as to attempt any answer, but I do wish to point out the relevance of this problem
to the medical conflicts of the seventeenth century, especially as it concerns
the topic of substantial form, the core of neo-Galenic medicine.

As I mentioned in Chapter 1, the best entry into eighteenth century
medical thought lies in the plays of Molière. *Le malade imaginaire,* with its
virtus dormativa, gives us a splendid problem in ontology, a problem that
might tax the ingenuity of those who want to use this concept in the game
of twenty questions. If the *virtus dormativa* were selected for a game of
twenty questions, what could the interlocutors ask? and what kind of
answer could they accept? Is it real or, in the words of the nominalists, is it
merely *flatus vocis?* Obviously, the answer would depend on whom we ask.
I use this example of a fascinating game to illustrate the importance of the
immaterial, a topic of fundamental significance in seventeenth century
thought.

In 1747, when La Mettrie published his *L'homme machine,* he mentioned the "old and unintelligible doctrine of substantial forms."[1] It is not
always safe to take La Mettrie at face value, but if we do so in this instance
we must stand amazed at the changes during a single century. In 1647 substantial form was the central core of the prevailing medical doctrine. It
was, to be sure, under strong attack from corpuscularians and chemists
and soon would fall from its dominant position, helped by Molière's satire
on powers and virtues. A century later, to believe La Mettrie, the term was
unintelligible. To call substantial form unintelligible tells us a great deal
about La Mettrie but nothing at all about the concept itself.

The substantial form, derived from Aristotle and Galen plus the influence of 1,500 years of accretion and modification, had extreme importance among the orthodox physicians of the seventeenth century. These
doctors, along with those of the sixteenth century, I prefer to call neo-

Galenist and I make no attempt to identify the specific ways in which the teachings of such men as Sennert diverged from the original texts of Galen himself. The substantial form is perhaps the central core of neo-Galenic philosophy.

We can approach the subject through the topic of nature, which I discussed at length in the last chapter. The study of nature is the study of change and transformation, a meaning we perceive in the term physiology. Today this word has only a medical sense, but for the neo-Galenists physiology was a standard subject that dealt with the general nature of things, provided a background for a future analysis, and in a sense corresponded to the basic sciences that underlie modern medical education. The present-day sense of physiology—the functioning of the living body—was a later and more restricted meaning. In the various institutes and medical texts, physiology—the science of nature—was the introductory subject, essential for the understanding of medicine.

Physiology had seven divisions that in the aggregate went by the name *res naturales,* or things according to nature.[2] These divisions or aspects are: the elements, the temperaments, the humors, the spirits and natural heat, the parts, the faculties and functions, and finally the generation of man. These subjects included the structure and function of the human body and also the basic sciences of that day. In addition they included the metaphysical background on which all this rests. When the student had a firm grasp on these fundamentals, that is, when he understood nature in general, he could then go on to study disease and its cure, namely, the subjects of pathology, hygiene, semeiology, and therapeutics.

While the substantial form has intimate connection with all the "naturals," it has special relevance to the "parts," the elements, and the faculties or functions. These correspond to present-day anatomy and physiology, with their background in physics and chemistry.

Then as now, physicians were concerned with the problem, what is the body made of, what are the parts of the body and of what are they composed? Obviously this relates closely to the more general problem, what are the building stones out of which everything is composed? And this leads immediately to the further question, what makes them work?

If we want to learn how things are put together and what they are made of, the simplest procedure is to take them apart. In anatomy we call this dissection; in logic, we call it analysis. Dissection is an empirical process. We start with what we see. This we divide into smaller and smaller portions, reflecting all the while on their properties and relations, until we get to portions that we cannot further divide. Then we say that we have reached the limit of visibility. By the late seventeenth century the primitive microscopes were able to enlarge the realm of our direct vision, but the neo-Galenic teachings had been well established long before the primitive microscope had any influence. Indeed, microscopic findings were one of the factors that helped bring down the neo-Galenic edifice.

Limits to visibility do not bring an end to the process of dissection, for this we can continue by inference, through intellectual analysis rather than through any physical manipulation—that is, we can engage in reasoning. The twin processes of direct observation and of reasoning were the tools with which the philosopher explored the world.

The human body, like all other perceptible objects, is a composite that can be subdivided into parts. Certain major subdivisions are obvious—the head, thorax, abdomen, and extremities. These in turn are further divisible—the upper extremity can be divided into an upper arm, forearm, and hand, together with the joints. Continuing the process the physicians could identify component parts, such as skin, veins, arteries, flesh, tendons, bone, and the like, comprising what later became known as tissues. So far as concerns gross dissection, these marked the end stage, for each of the tissues—they went by the name of "similar parts"—seemed homogeneous with itself. One fragment of bone, for example, seemed identical with any other fragment, one portion of ligament identical with another portion, just as one particle of gold was quite identical with another particle, and further subdivision could not produce anything different. Thus, we start with a composite that gets divided into smaller components and eventually into something simple—or apparently simple.

Although the similar parts, or tissues, make up the body, there is nothing ultimate about them. They come into being and pass away, and they reflect process and change. We eat food, the food becomes changed into the tissues and organs of the body (the similar and dissimilar parts) and in time the body itself dies and its parts disintegrate. There is interaction between the living and the nonliving. Thus, the tree becomes lumber which is made into a house through the agency of man and in time the house may burn and become ashes. The lump of iron becomes a horseshoe through the agency of man, then again through some particular agency gets transformed into a sword. This process of transformation demands explanation and philosophers from the earliest times have labored to find one.

The explanations current among the neo-Galenists had their origin in Aristotle, with his concepts of form and matter and elements. Aristotle offered an explanation for manifest changes. Reality consists of concrete objects which undergo change. In this process something remains constant: this is *matter*. What changes is the aggregate of properties and qualities, the pattern. This makes up the form—the distinguishing properties that make a thing what it is. We can know an object only under one or another form—a house, a table, a statue. Each has the special qualities or properties that render it what it is and distinguish it from all other objects. The matter is that which receives the form, that on which form is imposed. A statue made of wood has wood as the matter and a specific statue as the form. A table can also have wood as its matter but embodied in a different form. The same matter can appear in many different forms.

In analogous fashion a given form can be imposed on different materials. A statue may be made of wood or stone or bronze. The form is the same, the matter is different. Whatever serves as the matter for the statue has its own form as well. Bronze, before it is cast, is molten metal, which previously was solid ore; the block of marble was solid rock before it was quarried; the wood was a tree. Each of these, as an object, consists of form imposed on matter, and each of them can serve as matter for some form to be subsequently imposed. If a tree is cut down and converted into timber, the properties and qualities have changed — there is a new form — but there is something that continues, the matter. The timber is made into, say, a boat. The boat is eventually broken up and the wood is carved into a statue, which is eventually discarded into the fire to become ashes. In transformation one form has given way to a different form, with different characteristics. Each object in turn — the tree, the timber, the boat, the statue — becomes the matter on which some new form is imposed.

Matter, then, is that which gets determined by form; form is the determination imposed on matter. Form and matter are completely correlative. They do not exist separately but (with the exceptions to be noted later) are always united in the concrete objects. Aristotle's term for matter is *hyle,* which means wood, and by an easy extension of meaning the material or stuff of which something is made.

With this preliminary sketch of form and matter we can go back to the dissection of the body and the similar parts disclosed thereby. Each of these similar parts or tissues, such as skin, flesh, tendon, bone, has its own characteristic properties and qualities, which, in the aggregate, relate to the form of that part. However, these similar parts identified in dissection are themselves parts of a larger whole — the bones, flesh, and other components are parts of the larger whole we call the arm. The arm in turn is part of the whole body with its own characteristics. The arm has its form, the body has its form. The similar parts or tissues serve as matter for the organs (the dissimilar parts); the separate organs serve as matter for the body. John Fernel said explicitly that similar parts are like matter for the dissimilar parts.[3] Any composite has its own form and its constituents make up its matter. Each constituent, in turn, may be a composite whose constituents also have their form and matter.

Form

Before we can pursue this chain of reasoning further, we must study more closely the notion of form. This we must not construe in too narrow or static a sense. Any material object can be analyzed into form and matter but if we stop with this simple opposition, we remain on a superficial level. In the seventeenth century the usage was far more complex, packed with meanings that, in the aggregate, brought together a large part of the Aristotelian philosophy of nature.

Daniel Sennert made this clear.[4] He indicated that "form" represented something for which the Greeks used many different terms — *morphe, eidos, logos, entelecheia,* and *to ti tin esti.* In a similar context, Gassendi indicated a comparable multiplicity.[5] Each of these various terms is, of course, complex in its own right; and if we aggregate them and pack the entire aggregate into a single word, *form,* we can readily understand what confusion may result when that single word is used now in one sense, now in another.

To appreciate the meaning of form in seventeenth and eighteenth century thought we must determine how the authors in that period actually used the word, examine the different contexts in which it occurs, and so far as we can, see what they intended through its use. Sometimes the authors provided actual definitions, but not often enough, so that we must also gather the sense by indirection and inference. In the present account I draw principally on the writings of Sennert, Fernel, Lazar Riverius, and Gassendi.

First of all, the form provides specificity to an object, makes the object what it is rather than something else. An oak tree differs from a radish because the form of the oak is in the one, the form of the radish in the other. Whatever characterizes natural objects derives from their forms. As Sennert declared, "All natural objects are what they are because of their form, and from the form is derived all bodily structure."[6] This concept of specificity we see emphasized in Fernel, who frequently used the term *species,* sometimes to be rendered as appearance or kind but sometimes also as *form.*

The form is immaterial, a statement true by definition: form and matter are distinct and irreducible aspects of all things, and neither can be derived from the other nor from anything else. Hence, whatever is not material is by definition immaterial. Besides the forms, other examples of the immaterial would include mind and soul. The immateriality of the form becomes especially significant when we make a further distinction between material and corporeal, a problem I will discuss later.

The form is qualitative. In neo-Galenic philosophy qualities had primary status and were responsible for the appearance and specificity of any object. An object long and thin, flat, smooth, and green is different from something rough, brown, hard, and irregular. Through qualities or properties such as these we distinguish kinds of objects and discriminate a blade of grass from the bark of a tree. The qualities inhere, so to speak, in the form. The form carries or provides the qualities, bestows them on the object to make it what it is. This attribution is, of course, metaphorical, but in the metaphorical sense we must regard the form in its minimal sense as that in which inheres a bundle or collection of qualities.

But form, far from being a passive bundle of qualities, is active, dynamic, and functional. It is intimately bound with development, change, generation, transformation, and passage from potential to actual. Time and process are of the essence, and to these are joined the concepts of goal and purpose. Form is responsible not only for what a thing is but what it becomes.

Form thus involves organization in both a spatial and a temporal sense. It is not enough to regard single objects as static or isolated. If we speak of the form of an oak tree, we refer to the tree we perceive here and now, but we also deal with a progression from an acorn to a seedling to a mature tree, which in turn produces more acorns. Furthermore, the tree has many parts — roots, trunk, branches and leaves, flowers and fruit, as well as wood and sap and other components. Each part has its own form but these are not independent. There is an interrelation, a hierarchy. Some forms are subordinate to others, and the hierarchy, like a pyramid, leads to a master or controlling form. The form of the oak, considered as a whole, obviously dominates and controls the forms of the leaves or the roots or the bark and their respective functions. The master form controls the activity and the development of the parts. Each part has its function but the functions are under progressively higher control. This concept of a hierarchy of forms is a crucial aspect of neo-Galenic thought.

Hierarchy is perhaps most obvious in a biological framework. Fernel spoke of many orders of form arranged according to their functions. The forms of elemental objects are imperfect and lowest in the scale; the forms of plants are more perfect and nobler; of animals, still higher and nobler. The highest of all and most perfect is the form of man. This, he said, results from the divine mind, as the gift of the immortal gods.[7]

The higher and more complex the function, the more perfect the form. The form of an elemental particle of nonliving material is lowest on the scale; in a plant with vital functions of nutrition, growth, and reproduction, the form is higher and nobler; in animals, with complex physiological functions, still higher; and the form of man is highest of all. The degree of perfection or nobility relates to the complexity of function which the form regulates.

This same hierarchal arrangement and subordination of forms we see in the purely inorganic world. Riverius, in discussing what we may regard as chemical combinations, mentioned the elements and their combinations. He pointed to this problem: in any "mixed body" the component elements have their forms, while the "mixture" (chemical compound) has *its* own form. The forms, however, are not equal, nor is it true that "no one may lord it over the rest." Instead, "in mixt bodies there is a herauldry, one form being nobler than another: it is the form of the mixt body it self, to the commands of which the forms of the elements . . . pay the tribute of obedience."[8]

It is easy to see the extreme difficulties to which this doctrine could lead, difficulties by no means inapparent to the philosophers of the seventeenth century. But at this point I want only to characterize the form; its difficulties and fate I will discuss later.

Other characteristics help define the concept. The form is indivisible. Its essence remains just as entire in a small mass as in a large; the form of water is equally perfect in the single drop as in the largest quantity; the appropriate form is just as entire in the individual acorn as in the whole oak tree; in the poppy seed as in the whole plant.

As a further property the form extends to all the material components and to every identifiable part. Whatever is alive has the power of the whole form in every living part. In a living creature all portions are alive, and the chief form, the *anima,* is present in all of them. As we progress in the scale of complexity, wherever there is not only nutrition and growth but perception, the *anima,* with all its faculties, is present in all parts.[9]

Third, although the form is indivisible, it undergoes multiplication. This may take place in different ways, in plants, in animals, and in inanimate objects.[10] When we have material division as the partition of water into many drops, or a mass of gold into grains, the form becomes dispersed into each part and it exists entire in each part: the form is divided not in its essence but only in its extension.[11] That is, the material aspect is divided but the essential or formal component continues to fill every material particle just as it filled the undivided mass.

Form and matter cannot exist separately. Each needs the other. The function of form is to "inform matter and determine a particular kind, giving the specificity and distinction from other kinds; and finally to furnish and bring about all activities."[12]

Substance

One additional property requires discussion: the form is *substantial,* a qualification that has contributed greatly to misinterpretation of seventeenth century medical thought. The word substance is currently used to mean something corporeal, something palpable, possessing mass. But this meaning we must totally reject if we want to understand substance in its earlier scholastic sense.

The root of the problem lies with the concept of substance and its relation to the terms matter and body (or corporality). The word substance, like a chameleon, takes on a different appearance according to the context in which it finds itself. At the present time, when used in the naive or ordinary sense — that is, without special reflection or historical sophistication — substance conveys a sense of body or mass, something that you can readily get hold of and that will not vanish while you look at it. "A man of substance," "a substantial amount," "a chemical substance" are a few of the different senses popular today.

In times past it was quite otherwise. The term had quite specific philosophical meanings deeply imbedded in Greek philosophy, especially in the doctrines of Aristotle that formed the basis of Galenic thinking and have remained influential with varying intensity up to the present. Aristotle, however, was not consistent and used the term substance (Greek *ousia*) in two different senses.

The first meaning refers to the truly real or the ultimate existence. For Plato true and ultimate reality lay in the realm of the forms or Ideas. These, eternal and unchanging, could be grasped by the mind but not by the senses. Objects in the material world, the world of change, generation, and corruption, had a secondary or derivative reality. Aristotle denied this and, modifying the doctrine of his teacher, considered the individual object to be truly real. Socrates is real, this horse, this statue, this table, this ship are all real. They all represent substance, and Aristotle defined this in logical phraseology, as that which could serve as subject but never as predicate. You can say a great many things about Socrates or about this table or this statue, but you can never say "Socrates" or "this table" *about* any other thing. The individuals, that is, the substances, are subjects and never predicates. This is what Aristotle meant by substance, taken in the sense of the ultimately existent.

This meaning — substance is the real — we may call the ontological sense, that is, concerned with existence. The second meaning has to do with the description of reality. When Aristotle analyzed the individual object he framed what he called the categories, which indicated the different ways in which a predicate term might define a subject. Phrased differently, this means the different senses in which a thing may be said to *be*. Thus, let us start with an object, which I designate as "this." I can make a great many statements about it. I can say, this *is* brown; it *is* square; it *is* three feet across; it *is* in the kitchen. All these statements can be true and each of them tells us something about this object. But still more important is the statement this *is* a table. When we know this, we know its essential property.

Although we started with the individual object, the property of being a table or "tableness" is not an individual object but rather a universal. We can speak of it as the essence which, present in this object, relates it to an entire class. From the standpoint of science the important aspect is the class, the general term, that is, the essence.

Once we know that this-here-object *is* a table, that it embodies tableness as its essence, we know the most important thing about it. This essence contrasts with what the logicians call accidents. If the table were grey instead of brown, oblong instead of square, eight feet across instead of three, and in the living room instead of the kitchen, these facts would not affect its essential property, namely, that it is a table. These other features are designated as accidents, and the distinction between essence and accident is fundamental.

These various properties of an object, both the essential and the accidental, Aristotle classified as categories and he identified ten different ones. For our purposes the most significant are substance (or essence), quantity, quality, place, and time. The other categories are less important. For any given object, any particular predicate may indicate the essential character, or something quantitative, or some quality of a spatial property, or something temporal. In the first category, the word translated as *essence* is the same *ousia* — the Latin *substantia* — translated previously as substance.

We are now in a position to appreciate the two widely different senses of this term substance. One refers to a grammatical subject, the other to a grammatical predicate; one is ontological, the other logical; one stands in contrast to unreal or less real, the other contrasts with accidents.

Substance, as the category that conveys essence, refers to what a thing is in itself; accident refers to properties that affect the quantity or quality or place, or any of the other categories, without affecting the thing's essence. The term substantial form involves the opposition between substance (that is, essence) and accident.

There is here a question of value, that the substance or essence is important, the accident much less so. The medieval philosophers paid a great deal of attention to determining the essential attributes of a thing — that is, how to define it and how to identify its essential nature. The philosophers wanted to know whether any given attribute is an *accident* or part of the *essence*. Disputes on these questions might get quite heated, but we must not think such controversy is restricted to medievalists. Today we have exactly the same problem. For example, we try to find out what features (or properties) are essential to a disease; what characteristics are constant and truly constitutive; what is pathognomonic and what is only accidental or occasional, inconstant, or unimportant. However, today we use different modes of proof, different kinds of evidence, different criteria. But the basic problems, I maintain, are the same.

We cannot dismiss the search for the essential as unimportant. No more can we dismiss the concern with categories as "merely" a question of grammar, bearing no relation to reality. Aristotelian logic has fallen from its once proud estate, yet the modern conceptions of logic are quite irrelevant to eighteenth century medicine. That topic we must approach in its own context, wherein substance and accident are problems of vital import.[13]

For the neo-Galenists of the seventeenth century the important meaning of substance had to do with the essence as contrasted with the accident. The substantial form is the essential or significant form. Certain other forms, however, might have an accidental relation to a given object rather than an essential one. For example, if we have a wooden table which is attacked by termites, the termites and their forms are in the table but only as an accident and not as an essence. Similarly with, say, the rust on a knife or a pimple on a man's face.

The essence of an object, that which defines it and provides its characteristics, is the form of that object. But the two words, form and essence, although having much the same meaning, are used in rather different contexts. Essence, or more properly, substance, is a category that has correlative standing with other categories such as quantity and quality and also contrasts with the concept of accident. However, when we talk of form we mean not only that it represents an essence, that it conveys and bestows qualities and controls functions, but we also mean that it contrasts with matter. At this point we should study matter in greater detail.

Matter

The concept of matter is one of the most confusing in late seventeenth century thought. Like the word substance it conveys an aura of solidity in the naive modern sense. We think of a material object as having dimensions and thus falling into the realm of sense perception. But to understand the neo-Galenic usage we must go back to the original Aristotelian sense. This I will approach by indirection, through the Aristotelian notion of principles.

In the analysis of nature, Aristotle had to explain process and change, the coming into being and the passing away. The concrete object was the ultimately real, but the concrete object was constantly changing. To understand this process Aristotle sought the ultimate conditions of existence, that is, the irreducible aspects under which the objects and entities of nature can exist, and the irreducible concepts that can serve to explain the real world. These conditions he formulated as *principles*. These are not *things*. Instead, they are conceptual tools that permit us to understand and explain things in all their process and change.

To formulate principles Aristotle laid down strict criteria in his *Physics*.[14] "First principles must not be derived from one another nor from anything else, while everything has to be derived from them." The neo-

Galenic writers all emphasized this.[15] The principles of Aristotle are comparable to the postulates of a modern deductive system such as a system of geometry. Postulates must be irreducible. No one can be derived from another, nor from any other term, nor should they overlap one with the other. On the other hand, all postulates of the system must be sufficient and adequate, so that all terms in that system derive from these elementary concepts. Principles thus comprise the logical foundation on which the entire system rests.

Ordinarily a set of principles concerns one particular system only, and each system may have its own logical foundation. Aristotle was dealing with nothing less than nature, the most comprehensive of all systems, and hence his principles were the most general of all. He enunciated three principles or conditions of existence, and these he called privation, form, and matter.

These terms are not arbitrary but relate to an underlying belief, that all change involves an opposition between contraries. This Greek concept is most widely known in relation to the four elements and their qualities of hot and cold, moist and dry, existing in definite oppositions. In accordance with this background tenet, Aristotle sought contrariety on the most general level, and this he found in the two terms form and privation, considered as opposites. "Everything that comes to be or passes away comes from, or passes into, its contrary." And everything "that comes to be by a natural process is either a contrary or a product of contrary."[16]

In change, one entity passes into its opposite: in a particular object the absence of form may pass into the presence of that form. Privation, the absence of the form, is the *terminus a quo,* the form is the *terminus ad quem.* The sequence from privation to form does not occur at random but only within a context of potentiality. As Aristotle pointed out, "white" does not pass into "musical," but into "non-white";[17] and not merely any property that is not-white, but specifically into a color, such as black or some intermediate color. "Musical" can pass into "nonmusical," not into "any chance thing other than musical." Context is important. Form and privation, then, represent contraries in opposition, so that we start with one and end up with the other. Matter, the third principle, is the subject. It is that which lacks form at one moment, acquires form at another.

As Sennert indicated for these three principles, "Matter is that which is suitable for receiving all forms. All three of these principles are necessary for generation [that is, change], which is nothing else than the progression from the privation of form in matter to the acquiring of new form. The form is the *terminus ad quem;* privation is the *teminus a quo.* Matter is the subject of the change."[18]

Aristotelian matter, then, is the subject of change. In any process or change, matter lacks a particular form and this is privation, but it has the specific power to acquire that form. Privation thus involves not only the absence of a form but the potentiality of acquiring that form.[19]

Matter is that-out-of-which change occurs. All objects already have their own form, but they undergo *transformation* in the literal sense — that is, an object gives up one form and acquires another. The block of marble, rough hewn, and irregular, becomes a polished statue; a tree becomes a table; a measure of wheat becomes a loaf of bread. The marble, the tree, the wheat are, respectively, the matter of the statue, the table, or the bread, as the privation gives way to the new form.

The neo-Galenists, although they all discussed the Aristotelian principles, did not have much use for the concept of privation. Indeed, it does seem quite an artificial distinction, useful chiefly to preserve the Aristotelian doctrine of opposites. Consequently, privation tends to disappear from sight, and form and matter remain as the significant principles.

Prime Matter

The concept of matter, holding as it does such an important place in early seventeenth century thought, must be considered in two different modes. First we have matter in conjunction with form, constituting an aspect of the object. Yet when we talk of an object we ordinarily mean a three-dimensional body, a corporeal object, and considerable difficulty may arise from confusing corporeal with material. They are not synonymous, nor are their negatives, incorporeal and immaterial.

A body fills space — in Cartesian terms it has extension. Matter as such does not fill space. Body exists as the independently real; matter exists only in conjunction with form. However, in a different sense matter is independent of form when it is the so-called prime matter. We can arrive at the concept of prime matter in the following fashion. If we subdivide actual bodies into smaller and smaller particles, we get down to the ultimate body that cannot be further divided. Yet each ultimate particle has both matter and form. But if we *could* divide the ultimate still further — and we can do so in thought — we would find that they too are combinations. They contain form and matter — the ultimate matter, independent of form. This, the so-called first or prime matter, has no association with form. Samuel Butler indicated this in his poem *Hudibras,* (Part 1, Canto 1, 560)

> He had First Matter seen undressed;
> He took her naked all alone
> Before one rag of Form was on.

Let us examine this concept. In all three-dimensional objects matter exists not separately but only in conjunction with form. We can speak of prime matter *as if* it could exist separately — which it does not. Yet we can make the separation in thought. Although we cannot take hold of prime matter in any corporeal fashion, we can appreciate what it does—we can provide it with a sort of functional definition or circumscription.

I suggest that prime matter serves three distinct functions. Matter provides each thing with *potentiality,* that is, a capability of becoming something other than what it is. Actuality comes about through the presence of form, but the capacity of a thing for becoming something else depends on its matter.[20] Wheat becomes bread, the tree becomes a table. Wheat and bread, objects in themselves, have the capacity to change, and this capacity comes from prime matter. Prime matter, itself *completely undetermined, is that which permits determination.*

In its second function prime matter provides *individuality.* When we speak of "this table" there is a dual reference. We have the "tableness" that is the universal or the form. But whence come the "thisness"—this table in contrast to that one? The same form is present in this table as well as in that one. But the two are different individuals. Individuality depends on matter, not form. The bestowing of individuality, that is, spatial separation, is a property of prime or first matter. The quiddity through which it is an individual different from other individuals, comes from matter.[21]

There is a third function which I attribute to prime matter. Although it has no corporeal existence, in the sense of three-dimensionality, prime matter permits objects to come into the category of quantity, that is, extension, measure, number. Matter is, so to speak, that which allows for *quantification.* In concrete objects the quantitative aspects—spatial relations, position, number, divisibility—derive from prime matter.

Only things exist in the corporeal sense, but things are composites of matter and form, neither of which exists in a corporeal sense. Neither can exist without the other, yet they are both real. We might reduce all this to simple terms by calling form and matter abstractions or constructs of reason. But this is precisely what Sennert and others explicity denied.[22] Matter and form are real and not constructs of reason, and to understand seventeenth and eighteenth century medical thought we must adapt our notions of reality to include matter.

Quantity

If my interpretation is correct, prime matter allows objects to share in the category quantity, while form brings objects or bodies into relation with the category quality. Let us examine this category of quantity and its connection with matter. Again Sennert provides the clearest and most detailed exposition and he can serve as the spokesman for other neo-Galenists.

Quantity depends on prime matter, which is the basis of extension and of mass. Extension, representing quantity, involves the three dimensions of length, width, and depth. Thus, a surface is *quantitas longa et lata,* while body (*corpus*) is *quantitas longa, lata, et profunda.* Through quantity and dimension bodies are divisible and occupy space. Then Sennert makes a distinction of extreme importance. Two bodies, he said, cannot occupy the same space at the same time, not because they are substance, for many incorporeal substances can be in the same place at the same time; but because bodies have matter, provided with three dimensions, where penetration is not possible.[23] This clearly shows the basic distinction between corporeal and incorporeal. Both may be substance but one occupies space, the other does not. Incorporeal substance is best exemplified by the substantial form. It is without dimensions, for dimensions pertain only to matter, yet form is real.

We can better understand the opposition between corporeal and incorporeal, if we examine the famous query, how many angels can dance on the point of a pin? This problem, to which the scholastics devoted much thought, is often regarded as the height of futility, and hence, like the *virtus dormativa,* became the butt for satire. But the problem is important. It concerns the question, how corporeal are angels? Angels are real and they are substance, but if incorporeal then an infinite number can dance in the smallest imaginable space. If, however, angels have even the smallest quantity of matter, then only a finite number of angels can occupy space. And this question becomes significant in medicine when we consider the problems of spirit and spirits, central to neurophysiology and psychology. How material is spirit? This problem I will discuss later.

We must note Sennert's distinction in regard to space. He distinguished occupy from fill. To occupy is a property of bodies that refers to extension, and two bodies cannot occupy the same space at the same time. It is quite different with entities that have no dimensions, that is, that do not fall into the category of quantity, such as forms, whether substantial or accidental. Yet whatever has no dimensions may fill (*replere*) space just as the soul fills the whole body or light fills the sky. So, too, God is free of dimensions and matter, yet he fills all things to infinity. An unlimited number of forms can fill any given space without hindering one another.[24] Sennert thus preserved and amplified the difference between corporeal and incorporeal, and allowed the incorporeal to have spatial reference while still remaining incorporeal.

Qualities

Quantity is a category that permits description in terms of dimension and size, limit, number, extension, impenetrability, and the like, all of which depend on matter. Totally different is the category of quality, which relates to form. Said Sennert, all natural bodies are *quanta* because of their matter, they are *qualia* because of their form.[25]

The subject of qualities is confusing, for the neo-Galenists used the term in two quite distinct ways, one of which deals with perception, the other with activity. Let us take as a concrete example the quality hot—or heat. Fire is hot and heat is a quality immediately manifest to the senses. Sennert spoke of it as a manifest quality. But then, fire is highly active; it burns, destroys, or otherwise alters numerous objects. When it does so the action takes place through heat. Hence, heat is the agent through which fire accomplishes its activities. Heat, therefore, is not only perceived as a sensory quality but it also is something that burns and brings about various complex results. And since heat is a quality, we say that the quality produces the activity. Heat as perceived and heat as agent are both considered manifest, and when Sennert used the term manifest quality, he was referring to both aspects at the same time.

However, activity derives from the form of an object. Through its form a thing is what it is and does what it does, a generalization that applies to the simplest bodies as well as the most complex. An essential premise of neo-Galenism holds that forms act through their qualities. "The forms, in their activity, use the qualities as instruments."[26] Or again, "that forms produce their effect through the qualities is a commonplace among philosophers, and is conceded by all as an axiom."[27] The quality, then, is perceptible; it is also an active agent that serves as the instrument or tool of the form.

Let us look for a moment at the four elements, the familiar earth, air, fire, and water. Elements are the simplest bodies, and as bodies they have their forms in which inhere their activities and directing forces. Fire, therefore, has its form. On this the heat of the fire depends.[28] But the form of the fire—its intrinsic character—involves properties other than heat, properties all too often ignored. For example, fire rises up and causes to rise up anything that it attacks. It is generated in large quantities and whatever it meets it destroys and converts to its own substance without itself being diminished.[29] The form of fire includes many properties or qualities other than heat, but since fire is so familiar, we tend to ignore the complexities of its action.

A manifest quality, then, must be understood in three related ways: something directly perceptible by the senses; an active agent that *does* something; and an instrument controlled by form. Once we accept these assumptions, that forms act by means of their qualities, and once we realize the ambiguity attached to the word quality, we have passed the main barrier for appreciating the neo-Galenic position.

Sennert, following the entire Galenic tradition, distinguished two kinds of qualities, the manifest, immediately and directly recognized by the senses, and the occult, not immediately known by the senses but appreciated only mediately by their effects.[30] At first glance this sounds formidable and the term occult quality has probably done more to alienate modern writers than has any other aspect of seventeenth century thought. The very word occult conjures up mysticism and woolly thinking, or else imbecility, or perhaps something in between. This reaction may block any effort to understand the worth of that term, which has its own empirical basis and its own logic. To be sure, his thoroughly straightforward analysis rests on certain assumptions. But if we grant these, or at least regard them sympathetically for the sake of better understanding, we can see the merits of the concept.

The favorite example of an occult quality is the action of a magnet, which attracts iron. When we say that a magnet attracts iron we make a statement that is entirely comparable to the statement, fire burns wood. Fire has its form and this possesses a quality "hot" as an instrument, which in turn is the active agent that achieves the combustion. This quality is also directly perceptible to the senses. Similarly the magnet has its own form, which possesses qualities as its instruments. One of these qualities is the property of drawing iron to itself. But this property, unlike "hot," is not directly perceptible to the senses. All we see is the result, namely the movement of the iron. The property, that is, the quality, that brings this about does not directly affect the senses. As something hidden from our senses it is by definition occult.

To appreciate occult qualities we must be aware of the rather confused terminology—a wide range of terms often used synonymously or at least shading the one into the other. We have *qualitas,* which today connotes some sort of elementary perception like red or hot or loud. But for Sennert this merges into the word *vis,* ordinarily translated as force or power; and *virtus,* which in the seventeenth and eighteenth centuries had a quite similar meaning. In both these words the essence lies in activity and production of change. Then there is *proprietas,* suitably translated as property or characteristic, and today connoting a term of description applicable to both *qualitas* and *virtus,* and often used synonymously for both.[31] Sennert did not keep these terms distinct and while these may not be completely synonymous, each of them includes components of all the others.

Before discussing occult qualities in greater detail and their relationship to the primary or manifest qualities, I would mention the connection between primary and secondary qualities. The four elements are characterized by the four primary (or elemental) qualities, hot, cold, moist, and dry. These are manifest as well as primary. Said Sennert, "It is beyond all doubt that there are in nature four elements, and that they exert their effects through their qualities, the so-called primary ones, manifest and obvious to the senses."[32]

But the term primary immediately calls up the term secondary, and in this connection we think of the primary and secondary qualities of Boyle and Locke and Berkeley. Unfortunately, this usage is totally at variance with the tradition of neo-Galenism and serious confusion may result unless we keep in mind the appropriate distinctions. In the classical tradition, to which Sennert and the neo-Galenists adhered, the four primary qualities — the hot, the cold, the moist, and the dry — exist in certain modifications. One modification is the concept of gradation. Qualities exist in four degrees, and "hot" in the first degree was quite different from "hot" in the fourth degree.[33] But more important for our present purposes are the modifications that yield the secondary qualities.

Obviously, hot and cold, moist and dry, do not exhaust the range of manifest qualities. Since these four are by definition primary, various other qualities derived from them, whether by combination or alteration, may be designated secondary. We find a good enumeration of secondary qualities in Riverius, who distinguished fourteen different ones: "rarity and density, gravity and levity, hardness and softness, subtility and crassity, aridity and lubricity, friability and clamminess, asperity and levity."[34] Rarity, for example, arises from strong heat through which an object becomes more tenuous. Density is a property arising from cold, through which objects become more compact. Heaviness (*gravitas*) arises from cold and density, hardness from dryness, softness from moisture. Sennert gave a somewhat smaller list without making any claim to completeness.[35] These secondary qualities, derived from the primaries, are also directly perceptible by the senses. From the list of secondary qualities Riverius expressly excluded colors, smells, and tastes, for these, he said, "are not the immediate effects" of the primary qualities, "but more remotely and obscurely depend upon them."[36] Sennert made them directly dependent on the form and not on the primary qualities.

Occult Qualities

Occult qualities are in a quite different category. Since they are hidden, we cannot identify them directly and immediately: we can only point to what they do. We observe the concrete objects that manifest an occult quality. A magnet is such an object. So, too, are various drugs such as opium or rhubarb; or poisons like snake venom; or the saliva of a rabid dog. In all these we see the action but we do not see the qualities by which these actions are mediated. Each of these substances has its own occult quality, and certain differences from the manifest or primary qualities are immediately apparent. Occult qualities, like poisons, can act suddenly and in very minute amounts. Manifest qualities, however, when applied in small amounts, have no significant effect and certainly are never lethal.[37] The poison transmitted by a rabid dog differs remarkably from the elementary qualities, for the poison may lie latent for a long time, completely invisible and imperceptible, and yet it can kill.

All occult qualities have a specificity in regard to their actions. Sennert, trying to understand the phenomena, adopted a more or less empirical approach, that is, he observed different examples and tried to classify them. In so doing he identified six different groups, each having certain distinct relationships and properties.[38] Of these six, only one group dealt with inorganic objects; the others all had to do with living creatures — plants or animals. In his categorization, however, he did not consider life as such; he did not include properties that characterized all living creatures and separate them from all nonliving objects. Instead he sought only particular properties within the completely general class of living bodies.

In his first category he placed occult qualities that were species specific, that is, found in all members of a given species but not in any other species. Among his examples was the torpedo fish, which gives off an electric shock — a phenomenon that had particularly intrigued Pliny and many naturalists since then. Sennert also mentioned the remora, the sucking fish that could attach themselves to the hulls of ships and impede their progress. The properties in question are present only when the animals are alive and disappear when the animals die. They are highly specific and clearly different from any of the manifest qualities. Indeed, the electric shock from the torpedo fish is one of the most splendid examples of an occult quality.

A second category also pertained to living creatures but here Sennert referred to phenomena found in some individuals of a given species but not in all. The examples hold special interest for us today, for he described what we call allergy or hypersensitivity. Some persons, he pointed out, cannot eat cheese; if they do they vomit. Other persons are troubled by certain specific kinds of fish but not by other kinds. He also mentioned aversion to cats, so strong that even if the animal is enclosed in a box and cannot be seen, the persons in question may react and break out in cold sweats.[39] Such individuals manifest sympathies and antipathies.

The specific reactions depend on the peculiar constitution of those individuals. The antipathies — the occult qualities — may change with age. Some food that might have been intolerable or dangerous in youth might become tolerable or even pleasing in maturity or old age.

In regard to these idiosyncracies Sennert made some significant distinctions. These reactions do not derive from any organic disease or any disproportion of qualities (*intemperie*) but "from an occult and inexplicable disposition."[40] A difficulty in digesting *all* foods can arise from a disturbance of the stomach — a "manifest disproportion," but when a person can digest all other foods except cheese or a particular kind of fish, this phenomenon derives from an occult quality. Such a particular disposition may be hereditary; or, if not in the parent, may have been implanted in the fetus through the imagination of the mother when pregnant. Sennert also referred to what we call immunization. He mentioned the case of Mithradates who, by taking very small doses of many poisions, so accustomed his body to these that larger amounts were not able to harm him. This resistance was a change in the special disposition or property of his body and did not relate to the human *anima*.[41]

These two categories deal with occult qualities found only in living creatures. The first, completely generic, is found in all members of the species; the second, idiosyncratic, involves some individuals but not all others. In a third class Sennert placed those occult qualities that inhere in inanimate objects. The prime example is the magnet. The peculiar properties of the magnet that enables it to attract iron represent an occult quality deriving from its own specific form.

The fourth class of occult properties has to do with dead creatures — plants or animals that in their entirety or in their parts have some medicinal properties. These virtues do not belong to the living plant or animal but emerge only when it is dead. Thus, said Sennert, a dried toad is effective in extracting poisons, or the ashes of river crabs as a remedy against the bite of a mad dog, or peony root against epilepsy. The medicinal virtues — the occult qualities — no longer have connection with the living creature, for the *anima* of the plant or animal is no longer present. Nor is this virtue due to a simple mixture of elements. Since every qualitiy presupposes form, any such occult quality must proceed from a particular form that existed in the living animal or plant but was subordinate to a higher form (the *anima*). The medicinal properties inhere in the subordinate form, to emerge when the animal dies but disappear if there is decay or putrefaction. Sennert also pointed to chemical operations, like coction or infusion, that can separate out those parts containing the occult qualities, (for example, the purgative forces), while the residue remains inert.[42]

In the fifth category Sennert placed the occult qualities found in products generated naturally within animals and plants. These products are separable from the animal or plant — for example, the poison produced by the scorpion or asp or tarantula; or the bezoar stone found in the stomach of some animals; or the castoreum from the beaver. He also included secretions, gums, resins, and juices. Opium would be in this class. In regard to these substances each has its own distinct form, retaining its powers when separated from the *anima* under which it arose. However, Sennert admitted that it was not easy to explain just how these separate forms arose. Just as the *anima* has a chyle-producing power, so also, in certain species, the *anima* has, say, a poison-producing power. This poison is separable and endowed with its own form, its own occult qualities.[43]

Finally, in a sixth category he placed those substances produced in living creatures, especially animals, but through abnormal processes and hence related to disease. Examples are the deadly matter in the saliva of a rabid dog, or the humors producing dysentery or scurvy.[44]

The many different kinds of occult qualities indicated to Sennert that they derive from different causes, had different origins. The occult qualities in the first class, for example, might have been implanted directly by the Creator; those in the second class might arise from adventitial or environmental circumstances. In inanimate nature the occult qualities flow directly from the original form of the substance. In the fourth class the occult qualities have their own form, once subordinate to the *anima* of the original animal, but they become active only when death has supervened. Quite different is the fifth class, where the occult qualities appear in some specific natural product generated within the living creature. The product is separable and then has its independent form. And finally there is the last category, analogous to the preceding, but involving an abnormal pathological product of a living creature.

Sennert derived the qualities, both manifest and occult, from the forms; and forms existed in hierarchies, the higher (or "nobler") controlling the lower. But there was a contrary view, that the occult qualities, with their complexity, derived from a mixture or compounding of the elements. Each element has its own quality and if we mix the elements in various proportions, we get new qualities, some of which would be those called occult.

Galen seemed to favor this latter view, although he used a somewhat different nomenclature. Galen recognized the simple or primary qualities, derived from the elements. The more complex properties, such as were manifest in the Galenic faculties, he attributed to the "whole substance" rather than to separate elements. The four great faculties — attraction, retention, alteration, and explusion — are the effects of the whole substance, and this in turn represents a mixture of the hot, the cold, the moist, and the dry, in a particular proportion (*temperamentum*).[45]

The key word here is *temperamentum,* with its cognate *temperies.* There is no precise English equivalent, but the concepts of proportion, of arrangement, of suitable and appropriate mixture, are the essence. For Sennert the Galenic whole substance was the equivalent of the form, since they served equally as the source of the occult qualities.[46] But regardless of what Galen said, Sennert denied that the form could be construed as merely a compound of elements or their qualities. *The form was separate and distinct from a mixture of elements.*

Sennert was wrestling with a problem, how do new qualities come about? We cannot, he felt, get new properties merely by mixing the old. From a mixture of colors, for example, you can get another color, to be sure, but you cannot get a new property such as the specific virtues of opium or scammony. "Nothing can act beyond the powers of its own class." He denied flatly that from elements, however mixed, and from their qualities, however proportioned, there could arise occult qualities with powers above and beyond the forces of the elementary qualities. In whatever way the elements might be mixed and mixed again, nothing except elements would emerge, and he repeated this concept in many different variations.[47]

Where then do new qualities rise, qualities above and beyond the separate powers of the separate components? Sennert's answer is from the form, a coordinating and directing force in addition to the elements that compose a given body. He was dealing with a problem that has continued to exercise philosophers and scientists, namely, the problem of *emergence*. This was especially troublesome earlier in the twentieth century, with its discussions of evolution, and more recently with concepts of organism and holism, and levels of organization, and the view that the whole is more than the sum of its parts. These problems, I believe, are implicit in Sennert's discussions, although his terminology may appear antiquated.

To the question of the relationship between form and primary qualities, Sennert replied with an analogy.[48] The qualities are the instruments of form, and he compares this to the activity of a sculptor who, to achieve a given end, uses not one but several instruments — a divider for measuring, a saw for cutting, an ax for cleaving, a chisel for scraping, a hammer for pounding. And from all these activities a statue emerges. Yet a saw, for example, regardless of who uses it, does nothing but saw. What it accomplishes depends on the person who uses it.

Sennert applied this metaphor to the bodily activities. Heat, for example, may be used for many different activities. It takes part in chylification, formation of blood, generation of seed. These actions are to be ascribed not primarily to the heat itself but to the *anima*. *The principle that acts is the form; the principle by which it acts is the quality.* The action is not to be attributed to the instrument but to the efficient agent. Although the substantial form operates only through its qualities, these cannot act to bring about "noble" activities beyond their powers and condition. Thus, when directed by the form of fire, heat burns; but when it is the instrument of the *anima* it can bring about results that far exceed its natural state — it is responsible for life, it generates, it produces spirits and chyle, and is even to be considered the source and preserver of life. Not by accident does the heat bring about an act that is "more sublime than its own nature." The perfection of an effect does not exceed the perfection of the active agent. Those actions which surpass the power of the primary qualities arise by virtue of the form.

And just as a saw has no other action than sawing, so heat has no other action than that of warming. For other actions nature must use other qualities. From the form arise more noble qualities, and the form uses qualities *sui generis* for the particular actions. The magnet does not attract iron through the hot, the cold, the moist, and the dry, or any mixture thereof, but through an occult quality.[49]

The use of the word noble deserves comment. For Sennert it seems correlated with complexity — the more complex, the more noble. In any hierarchy the upper levels, exerting control over the lower, are obviously the more complex — and consequently the more noble. This term introduces value judgments in regard to forms and serves to emphasize the holistic background of the doctrine. But in all of Sennert's voluminous discussion we perceive a great similarity. He keeps on repeating his basic assertions, that the form is dominant over the qualities and that occult qualities take their origins directly from the form and not from the elements.

The doctrine of substantial forms and occult qualities has logical force if we understand the premises on which it was founded. We can see the significance of Sennert's views, but only when we study them sympathetically within the limiting context that he established.

FOUR

IATROCHEMISTRY

Historians of medicine who discuss the seventeenth century customarily make a sharp distinction between two schools of thought. One,
with the label iatrochemistry, supposedly began with Paracelsus and includes van Helmont, Sylvius, and Willis as the chief exemplars, together
with several lesser figures. These men all relied on chemistry to provide the
basis for their theory and practice. The other school, called iatromechanism, supposedly based its doctrines on the principles of mechanics. By
general consent, Borelli is considered the founder of this school, although
some historians would see Sanctorius as the precursor. Other important
figures in the school include Bellini, Baglivi, and Pitcairn, together with
several lesser physicians.

I believe that any sharp separation into two schools and the resulting
opposition between chemistry and mechanics obscures rather than clarifies
the profound intellectual movements of the seventeenth century. We can
better understand the relations of iatrochemistry and iatrophysics if we regard them both as assaults on the prevailing Aristotelian philosophy. Indeed, the attack took place along several fronts that included not merely
medicine but physics and astronomy and other branches of science.
Involved was the whole area of natural philosophy, and natural philosophy
was intimately connected with speculative philosophy, so that the whole
intellectual world was in turmoil. The end result was the decline of Aristotelian thought in all modalities. We must, however, restrict ourselves to the
medical sphere.

In the first half of the seventeenth century certain key figures demand
particular attention. Harvey's discovery of the circulation did much more
than destroy some basic Galenic teachings. When scientists regarded the
heart as a pump, they opened the door to what would eventually be a
mechanical interpretation of physiological processes. The action of a
pump readily involves certain concepts of hydrodynamics—the movement
of different kinds of fluids through tubes of varying sizes, with analogies to
mechanical models. Other mechanical principles such as elasticity and
friction fitted admirably into a mechanical schema, while this whole aspect
of physiology harmonized with the atomistic philosophy that Gassendi was
introducing. The billiard ball model of the mechanical philosophy gained
a more ready acceptance when applied to the concept of circulation than
could ever have been the case with the Galenic schema of humors.

Of course, the concept of the circulation did not gain immediate acceptance, and not until the second half of the century did it triumph unequivocally. Only at that time did physiology and mechanics, and the atomistic
and Cartesian philosophies combine to virtually topple neo-Galenism and
its Aristotelian heritage. The full force of the attack came in the second
half of the century, while in the first half the science of mechanics had only
a modest effect on orthodox medicine. To be sure, atomism as a philosophical doctrine was gaining favor over Aristotelian formulations, as the
writings of Francis Bacon testified, but this influence was making relatively
slow progress in medicine. The more profound effects, and the great influence of Descartes, became important medically only after mid-century.

In the first half of the century chemistry had far greater impact on
medicine than did mechanics. Paracelsus (1493-1541), the first truly
important chemical physician, was a rebel who shared in the rebellious era
we call the Renaissance. Elsewhere I have presented my own views of his
teachings in some detail and here I would stress only a few features.[1]

When we study Paracelsus we cannot extract any purely medical doctrine. His medical teachings entail a mixture of philosophy, astronomy,
and alchemy, all interconnected. The cure of disease involves not merely
the care of the patient but the study of earth and heavens and the search
for essences through fire, that is, alchemy. In this search, Paracelsus condemned the study of books and recommended the study of nature in all her
manifestations. His philosophy was dynamic, concerned with function and
activity rather than with structure. He studied powers, forces, spirits, influences, and sympathies in nature.

Activity is hidden below the surface of things. One way of penetrating
below the surface is through alchemy, and here we find the famous doctrine of the three principles, mercury, sulfur, and salt. These represent not
material substances but functional and dynamic components of things. The
classic example is combustion. When wood burns, for example, what
actually burns represents a sulfur; what comes off in smoke—what is
volatile—is mercury; what remains as ash is salt.[2] This represents a generalized account applicable to all objects. It is only sulfur that burns, only
mercury that sublimes, only salt that comprises the residue; and conversely,
whatever burns is a sulfur; whatever is vaporous or "spirituous" is mercury; and whatever is solid is a salt. Pagel phrases this particularly well: the
sulfur, salt, and mercury, he stressed, are not the same in each object.
"They are not comparable to the elements of the ancients or of modern
chemistry, for each object has its own sulfur, its own salt, its own mercury.
In fact, there are as many sulfurs, salts and mercuries as there are objects
. . . the innumerable individual and species differences in nature are thus
derived from the differences between innumerable sulfurs, salts, and mercuries." In this sense, he went on, "sulfur, salt, and mercury were simul-

taneously capable of material, functional, quantitative and qualitative interpretations."[3]

Paracelsus was concerned with tying together different kinds of activity so that, for example, the volatility or the inflammability of one substance would relate to the volatility or inflammability of another substance. The concepts of mercury, sulfur, and salt could bring together metallurgy, chemistry, biology, and the treatment of disease.[4]

Paracelsus violently rejected the Galenic notions of form. Nevertheless, in my interpretation, he disguised many of the properties of the forms and reintroduced them under the terminology of mercury, sulfur, and salt. These "principles" were not *objects,* in the sense of discrete building blocks like the earth, air, fire, and water of the Greeks. Rather the mercury, sulfur, and salt combine material or corporeal aspects with functional dynamic components, thus uniting in one term some of the properties of both forms and elements. For Paracelsus the mercury, sulfur, and salt accounted for the qualitative differences found in *things,* whereas in neo-Galenism it was the forms that accounted for the major qualitative differences. I do not mean that the *prima tria* are the precise equivalent of the forms, but they do preserve certain characteristics of the Galenic account.

Principles and Elements

There is a distinct conflict between the concepts of element and of principle. Originally, in seventeenth and eighteenth century medicine, elements referred specifically to the classical earth, air, fire, and water, although certain subsidiary meanings also developed. The term principle had great significance in Aristotelian philosophy, but the chemists used the same word while giving it a quite different meaning. We must clarify the different usages of these terms.

The concept of principles, deriving especially from Aristotle, represents what in traditional geometry were called axioms—the ultimate and irreducible terms, independent of each other, not derived from elsewhere, capable of explaining all else in that system.[5] Sennert expressed the concept in the widely used definition *neque ex se mutuo sunt neque ex aliis, sed ex quibus omnia.*[6] Gassendi offered the formulation *Principia neque ex se invicem esse, neque ex aliis, ex ipsis vero esse omnia.*[7] In translation we may offer the rendition, "Principles do not derive from each other nor from anything else, but all things derive from them."

For Aristotle, Galen, and their followers, the basic principles were form, matter, and privation. These were considered the most general terms, through which the phenomena of nature and the process of change could be understood. The concept of privation soon disappeared and we are left with form and matter as the principles of nature.

To appreciate these terms we must carefully distinguish between material and corporeal. Too often they have been regarded as synonymous, as if they both involved three dimensionality. In the strict sense this is not the case. Form and matter, as principles, are both conceptual. This is quite obvious in regard to form. Matter, however, is used in two senses. Prime matter, devoid of all qualities by definition, has no dimensions and no corporeal existence. But when prime matter receives form, then we have body, corporality, dimensionality. If we fail to distinguish between material and corporeal, then we have the apparent paradox, that matter is incorporeal. We avoid this paradox if we are more precise in our terms. Prime matter is incorporeal by definition; body (*corpus*) comes into existence only when prime matter combines with forms.

The elements or primary building blocks are the elemental bodies out of which all material objects—all corporeal things—are composed, namely, the familiar earth, air, fire, and water. In these inhere the primary qualities of hot, cold, moist, and dry. What, then, is the relation of form and matter to the elements? Sennert gave an unequivocal answer: the elements, as simple bodies, are themselves composed of form and matter. They have their own specific qualities. Since qualities proceed from forms, the qualities characterizing the elements derive from the forms of the elements.[8] In any absolute sense the elements are compounds and not principles; in the ultimate scheme of things they are not "primary."

But if we shift our point of view, and if, instead of looking at ultimate philosophical concepts, we regard only the world of tangible and visible objects (the world of compounds), then the elements, the most simple bodies, are indeed primary. In regard to elements Sennert declared, "Insofar as they consist of matter and form, they can be called composite: but in regard to compound bodies they are called simple."[9] In the context of corporeal objects, and only in that context, the elements can be construed as principles, as irreducible components.

Elements are principles only in relation to compounds and the corporeal world of generation and change but not in relation to ultimate philosophical analysis. The elements thus can be construed as compounds or as principles, depending on the context.

Every neo-Galenist might not agree with Sennert, but it is not feasible here to trace the variations in thought. The important features, for our purposes, may be expressed as follows: form and matter as basic concepts must be distinguished from elements or building blocks. Within a limited universe of discourse the elements as building blocks were sometimes called principles. But this is a limited usage and must not confuse the basic distinction between building blocks, which by themselves are inert, and the forms, which provide dynamic activity, goals, and, of course, qualities. The substantial forms, incorporeal, combine with matter to comprise bodies (*corpora*). The simplest bodies, the elements, aggregate into complex bodies. All tangible and visible objects are compounds of these elements.

The chemists, rejecting the substantial forms and the four elements, could not offer any equally neat substitute, any equally well-tailored schema. Yet the *tria prima,* albeit vague and confused, opened the way to a new kind of analysis.

The *tria prima* — mercury, sulfur, and salt, generally designated as principles — introduced further complication. We can overcome any confusion if we regard principle as a term completely irreducible within its own universe of discourse but not necessarily irreducible when used in a different context. What served as a principle in one philosophical system might be reducible to simpler ideas in a different system.

Mercury, sulfur, and salt combined some features of the elements and some features of the forms, and in this combination the dynamic aspect seemed to predominate over the structural characteristics. The *tria prima* accounted for certain functional properties and certain particular qualities but did so in a quasi-material fashion. Unlike the substantial forms which were entirely incorporeal, the *tria prima* served as a sort of qualitative atomism.

Mercury, sulfur, and salt were not things or bodies, but neither were they pure qualities or immaterial essences. They were entities that accounted for some particular properties and qualities and yet were not immaterial. In the doctrines of Paracelsus it would be difficult to identify the exact ontological status of the *tria prima,* yet in the confusion we can perceive certain aspects that Galenists assigned to forms, and certain others that show kinship to the elements. Debus, discussing the early chemists, declared, "Varying between spiritual and material interpretations, the elements and principles were often pictured as almost indefinable aspects of a primal stuff that had to exist as a basis for the more complex things of the world." In the sixteenth century chemists had discordant and often contradictory ideas and Debus pointed to the "ever growing anarchy over the elements," an anarchy contrasting markedly with the earlier views when the four elements were universally accepted in a neat schema.[10]

Sennert

Daniel Sennert held firmly to the Aristotelian principles of form and matter, but he was also sympathetic to the atomism that was being revived and to the doctrines of the chemists. He tried to bring about an accommodation between the traditional views of the four elements and the newer concepts that the chemists offered. He thus tried to harmonize the explanations involving mercury, sulfur, and salt with the classical doctrines of elements, without doing violence to either. His important text, *De Consen-su . . .*, first published in 1619, dealt with the problem.[11] Among the more recent commentators on this work I can mention particularly Rambert Ramsauer, Robert Kargon, and Allen Debus, as well as the older writings of Kurd Lasswitz.[12] The *De Consensu . . .* has never been fully translated. There is a markedly abbreviated translation by Culpepper and Cole, from 1662, bearing the title *Chymistry Made Easie and Useful.*[13] This work translates only certain passages and sometimes inserts transitional sentences and phrases that are not in the original. The translation is often unclear. To reach the meanings that Sennert intended, the original Latin text must be studied.

Sennert, although sympathetic to the *tria prima,* emphasized that the elements and principles of Aristotle were not to be rejected. He specifically denied the Paracelsian claim that the three principles were primary or existed prior to the elements.[14] Principles, that is, the chemical principles, are to be accepted as explanatory terms *in addition to* the elements.

To establish his assertion he engaged in a logical analysis. How can we explain certain simple qualities? The four elements can account for the properties — the manifest qualities — that involve the hot, the cold, the moist, and the dry, and their combinations and degrees. But how to explain the qualities of color, odor, and taste? The four elements had no power to produce such qualities and therefore other principles must be sought as their source.[15]

Sennert did not fall back on occult qualities or forms as explanatory concepts. Instead, he attributed color, odor, and taste to the chemical principles — the qualification chemical is necessary, since he is referring to mercury, sulfur, and salt, to be sharply distinguished from the Aristotelian principles.

In all compounds or "mixed bodies" he recognized that both the traditional elements and the chemical principles might coexist as discrete entities. In explaining the properties in such compounds, any heat, cold, moisture and dryness are to be derived from the elements, while "odors, tastes, and other qualities of this kind" are derived from the chemical principles.[16] Just as a compound might be hot or cold, depending on the predominant element, so from the chemical principles derive the qualities we identify as acid, salt, odorous, or inflammable.

In regard to the nature and character of these chemical principles, we find a clear line of reasoning in Sennert. He considered them to be not simple bodies prior to the elements, but rather *the first of compound bodies (prima mista).* God created the elements and also the chemical principles subsequent to them. And these, perfect in their kind, have their forms through which they are what they are.[17] Sennert thus firmly announced his adherence to the basic Aristotelian schema of form and matter. The elements have their forms combined with matter. The chemical principles are the first and simplest compounds, made up of elements as their matter but having their own characteristic forms.

Compounds can exist in hierarchies, each with its form and matter. The chemical principles are themselves compounds. They can serve as matter for other "more perfect" compounds. In present-day terms we would say that the "more perfect" had a higher degree of organization. In a hierarchy of compounds the lower serve as matter for the higher, and the form of the lower would be subordinate to the form of the higher. But we have a knotty problem when compounds break down, which might take place either "naturally" or by art (by chemical means). When this happens some components pass off as fire or earth or water; still others as salt or sulfur. The specific form of the compound passes away; and forms which had previously been subordinate in a more complex compound now resume their own function. But the resumption of independence occurs only within limits. Thus, bone and flesh are composed of blood which gives up its own nature and assumes another form. But flesh or bone cannot be resolved back into blood. The relationship of components to the compound and the resolution that may take place represent "a most difficult problem."[18]

Let us regard for a moment the earlier explanatory framework. The elements earth, air, fire, and water embodied the qualities of hot, cold, moist, and dry. These, the primary qualities, could seem to explain a limited number of manifest properties of things. To expand the scope of explanation we must have a corresponding expansion in explanatory terms. This the philosophers of the schools accomplished not by introducing additional elements but by enlarging the range of their characteristic qualities. Thus, each of the four primary qualities was judged to have four degrees. "Hot in the third degree" might explain something that "hot in the first degree" failed to do. Another mode of expansion was to increase the number of qualities from the four primary ones: various combinations of primary qualities could produce secondary qualities, of which Riverius enumerated fourteen, such as rare or dense, hard or soft. But even so, many observed properties did not fit comfortably into this schema. Riverius had pointed to color, smell, and taste, which certainly did not represent the immediate effects of the primary qualities nor even of the secondary qualities. But we can still keep color and taste in the same explanatory framework if we "place them in subordination by the term of third qualities."[19] However, we must realize that this particular explanatory maneuver did not by any means find complete acceptance.

In the study of nature, those properties which could be satisfactorily explained by the primary or secondary (or even tertiary) qualities were called "manifest." Those properties that could not be readily correlated with the primary qualities or their derivatives, for example, the activity of a magnet, were called occult and were attributed to the action of the form. The form thus served as a sort of explanatory buffer accounting for complex properties that could not, without excessive strain, come under the rubric of the qualities.

The chemists, dissatisfied with all this, offered an alternative with some merits and some drawbacks. Sennert sought to improve the explanatory force of the traditional doctrines by expanding its base. This he did by adopting the *tria prima,* with their own characteristic properties and qualities, and adding them to the four elements. If we have seven qualitatively different building blocks instead of four, and each of the seven has its own special qualities, then we have a vastly increased explanatory power applicable to a much larger range of phenomena.

However, Sennert carefully preserved the formal purity of the Aristotelian framework, for he kept the traditional four elements as "really" primary, while the *tria prima* had a nominally subordinate status as first compounds. It was, so to speak, a relationship of father and son. Yet from the functional standpoint the elements and the *tria prima* enjoyed coordinate status.

With this maneuver Sennert did not in any way give up his allegiance to neo-Galenism; he merely expanded the doctrines to deal more effectively with current science. He fully retained the key doctrine of forms, which explained the properties of complex phenomena, such as magnetism, selective action of drugs, physiological functions, and the like.

The Five Elements

Sennert tried to make traditional doctrines more consonant with the progress of science, but in retrospect his attempt appears as only a stopgap. The road to further progress lay in a different direction. This involved not a simple addition of one set of concepts to another, but a real amalgamation whereby the four elements and the three principles were fused into a new set of five elements, namely, mercury, sulfur, salt, earth, and water, each with complex properties. In this new grouping of elements the characteristic qualities were not limited to hot, cold, moist, and dry and their combinations but included functional activities and properties that reflected chemical behavior and could be experimentally studied. Chemists had the task of identifying the properties of the elements. This was a totally new departure from neo-Galenism.

So far as we can tell, the first man to make this new grouping of elements was Joseph Du Chesne, who in 1584 added the two traditional elements, water and earth, to salt, sulfur, and mercury, resulting in five components for all natural bodies. The detailed story recounting the triumph of the five-element system is properly part of the history of chemistry.[20] Of more immediate concern to the study is the conflict between this new schema and the traditional or neo-Galenic view. A dramatic episode in this conflict took place in Paris in 1624 — only a few years after Sennert published his attempted compromise.

Marin Mersenne, describing the event, told about certain alchemical theses that were condemned because they conflicted with the orthodox doctrines.[21] The first three theses expressed opposition to the principles of Aristotle — to form, matter, and privation. The fourth and fifth maintained that mixtures or compounds were composed of five simple bodies — earth, water, salt, sulfur (or oil), and mercury (or acid spirit). The sixth struck at the very foundation of Aristotelian philosophy by maintaining that these simple bodies were of the same character in all individuals and that diversity arose only from different mixtures of these principles. The eighth thesis held that these principles were the cause of all actions and all movements in the world and that these movements did not arise from the world-soul. The other theses hold less concern for us, except for the twelfth, which denied the "virtual qualities." The effects ordinarily attributed thereto were assigned to the five substances comprising all bodies.

This dispute indicates several features important for the history of medicine. The five-element theory emerges as a major doctrine; it rejects the Aristotelian formulation and adopts instead an atomistic philosophy, which, influenced by Democritus, was exerting increasing appeal. A specific date, 1624, provides a perspective for the conflicts between the traditional neo-Galenists and the chemical and alchemical teachings, between the Aristotelian principles and the revival of atomism. Of special interest is the relation between this reference point and Harvey's discovery of the circulation (1628). Furthermore, the dispute calls attention to the strength of the establishment, against which these heretical doctrines seemed to bounce harmlessly. But the establishment was being undermined and within the next thirty to forty years it was disintregrating on all fronts. Nevertheless, as we shall see, many doctrines of the establishment persisted in a somewhat transformed state.

Van Helmont

In the first half of the seventeenth century the rejection of Aristotle characterized the progressive wing among philosophers, and chemists as a class were certainly among the avant garde. The most important chemist of the period, in relation to medicine, was van Helmont (1577-1644). He too expressly denied the teachings of Aristotle and the schools and expounded his own influential philosophy.[22]

Some chemists inclined toward atomistic philosophy well before Gassendi brought new light and force to the teachings of Democritus. While van Helmont did not adopt Democritean atomism, he strongly attacked Aristotle. But as is the case with so many rebels, his own doctrines bore an inner resemblance to those of the man he condemned. We might characterize van Helmont as a disguised Aristotelian tinged with Neoplatonism.

In the study of nature innumerable features demanded explanation from the philosophers. For our purposes I suggest some especially insistent problems. How can we account for the specific qualities that we perceive in the world around us? Or, differently phrased, what is the origin of specificity in things? To what can we attribute the process of orderly and predictable change? How can we account for the activity and dynamism that we constantly see in nature? What sort of structural components does the world exhibit, that is, what are the building blocks of which the world is made?

The neo-Galenic formulations provide coherent and elegant explanations, in terms of form and matter as principles, and the four elements with their special qualities as building blocks. Matter has a dual role. In one sense it has a conceptual and metaphysical aspect, but in its empirical and concrete sense it is corporeal. Aggregates of elements serve as corporeal matter. Yet matter exists not by itself but under the direction of forms as the organizing and dynamic factors that supply specificity and complex properties.

Van Helmont condemned all these aspects of Aristotelian philosophy and in his long, rambling, and obscure writings he developed his own philosophy. In a previous book I discussed major aspects of van Helmont's doctrines as they concerned medicine, and I refer the reader there for a general survey.[23] His terminology is indeed formidable and usually far from clear, for he used a varying terminology, derived from the schools, from Paracelsus, and from more contemporary chemists; and to all this he added his own special terms. I will discuss here only those aspects of van Helmont's philosophy that bear on the immediate problem.

Van Helmont indicated two sources for all corporeal objects. One is the *initium ex quo,* the matrix out of which everything arose. This source he considered to be the element water. And then there is the differentiating character, the *initium seminale per quod,* the agent that accounted for specificity. This he identified as a ferment.[24] The sulfur, salt, and mercury of the chemists, he declared, cannot be dignified as the beginning of all things, for they cannot all be found in all things, and furthermore they themselves have arisen from the primitive water. A ferment or, as he sometimes says, a seed, acting on water, produces a material entity.

Water, obviously, bears a close relationship to the prime matter of Aristotle, while the ferments correspond in many ways to forms. Van Helmont refers to water and ferments in a double sense, metaphysical and empirical. In the empirical sense they are subject to direct observation and experimental study as part of the scientist's concrete experience; in the metaphysical sense they transcend all experience and play a purely conceptual role as the principles of explanation. Van Helmont intermingled these two roles.

He studied the element water in an experimental fashion. The most famous example, perhaps, is his study on the growth of a tree.[25] He planted a small tree in 200 pounds of earth, to which he added only distilled water or rain water. After five years the tree gained 164 pounds, but the earth had not lost any weight — it still weighed 200 pounds. He drew the not unreasonable conclusion that the increase in the weight of the tree derived from the water only. He provided many other relevant observations. From his studies he drew the conclusion that water was the prime source of material objects. His conclusions were perhaps logical relative to the data at his command, and his generalizations, although faulty, were by no means unreasonable.

Ferments were also entities of observation, capable of experimental study. The fermentation of beer, bread, and other substances were quite apparent and well known. That ferments played a part in bodily processes van Helmont demonstrated through a series of brilliant observations and experiments. Best known are his studies on the digestive process, wherein he showed that there was a digestive ferment closely related to acid but having a specific vital property. This he identified as "a certain vital acidity, powerful in bringing about transformations, and possessed of a specific property."[26]

Again, van Helmont generalized and considered ferments the agents that provided the specific properties of things. He presented this doctrine at length in his tract "The Image of the Ferment" and in various other tracts. I have discussed this problem elsewhere and indicated the central role that ferments played in his system. Ferments, associated with the irreducible qualitative aspect of things, exert their activity in both living and nonliving objects. In living beings the fermental action generally expressed itself in a seed. The relationship between ferment and seed is not entirely clear. Sometimes van Helmont used the terms interchangeably, sometimes he seemed to indicate that seed has a special connection to living creatures, as if ferments were the more general term and seed the more specifically vital agent. But this was not consistent. At other times he declared that a seed, acting on water, can produce a specific substance that is not alive. For example, in speaking of combustion — a property of sulfur — he declared that every oil, in regard to its matter, is simple water which a minute quantity of seed transforms into a combustible mass, and "plays the part of a sulfur."[27]

The concept of ferment (or seed) has a strong empirical and experimental basis, but van Helmont generalized far beyond the evidence. He created a vast hypothetical superstructure and used the seed as a metaphysical principle to account for the world. *Water and seed (or ferment) are directly analogous to the matter and form Aristotle established as principles of nature.* On the more empirical level chemical reactions are brought about through actions of ferments, especially with the help of fire. "Chemistry digests, and brings putrefaction; and when a ferment is received, the parts split asunder into their smallest components."[28]

Seeds and ferments not only provide specificity but also have a certain dynamic quality. They make things happen in a limited fashion. A certain propulsive driving force is implied in the concept of the seed but on a relatively simple level. On a higher level, where animal life is involved, the dynamic force is the archeus.

In the neo-Galenic philosophy, based on that of the schools, the substantial form accounted for the appearance and qualities of a thing as well as the dynamic properties concerned with its function. This is readily seen for living creatures, which exhibit a life span over a time course, and we can readily translate the concept into the more familiar terms of the Aristotelian four causes. The indwelling form combined into a single entity the formal and final causes of Aristotle, and also the efficient cause, so far as this is *internal.* For example, in an oak tree the propulsive force, active from the earliest stages of the acorn to full maturity and decline and death, is indwelling within the acorn and determines the shape and size and properties of the tree. This is quite different from the external efficient cause, as in the relation between a blacksmith and a horseshoe.

Van Helmont framed his philosophy around living creatures. He did not distinguish too sharply between the living and the nonliving but combined them both into a single broad unity. Van Helmont analyzed, although in a somewhat obscure fashion, the meanings of form, emphasizing the aspects of end or goal, and potentiality. He identified an internal efficient agent, which he called archeus. "Whatsoever Aristotle hath attributed to the form, or to the last perfection, in the scene or stage of things, that, properly, directively, and executively belongeth to the Agent, or seminal Chief Workman." The archeus, or chief workman, is thus the internal efficient cause and includes aspects of the final and formal causes.[29] The relationships between the archeus, the seed, and the ferment and the "chemical principles" are intimate indeed but cannot be phrased clearly and unequivocally. For our purposes we may consider the archeus the vital agent, very close to the substantial form of the schools.

As a chemist van Helmont emphasized ferments and seeds, acting on water and, in living creatures, intimately related to the archei. The mercury, sulfur, and salt, in my interpretation, he regarded as products, as combinations of seeds and water, having special properties and entering into the composition of things. His great contributions in regard to the concept of gas are not relevant here and may be studied in histories of chemistry. However, his emphasis on ferments and the process of fermentation were important for later physiological doctrines, as well as for chemisty in its own right.

In the first half of the seventeenth century the three dominant philosophical systems were the neo-Galenic, the chemical, and the corpuscularian. Representatives of the first two of these we have already discussed. Sennert was a neo-Galenist who, however, came to terms with some of the chemical formulations. He died in 1637. Van Helmont, the leading chemist in the first half of the century, died in 1644. For the third major system, the corpuscularian philosophy, the outstanding proponents were Descartes (d. 1650) and Gassendi (d. 1655). Gassendi we have already discussed at some length; the relevant teachings of Descartes I will take up not in any separate section but only as they appear in relation to later physicians and scientists.

When we come to the third quarter of the seventeenth century we find some of the problems so far discussed showing signs of resolution and new problems coming to the fore. To illustrate the changes and trends in this third quarter I will present four individuals: Franciscus Sylvius and Thomas Willis, who were physicians; Nicolas (Nicasius) LeFebvre, who was a chemist; and Robert Boyle, whom we can call a natural philosopher. They all played a prominent part in the so-called iatrochemical movement and the relation between chemistry and medicine.

Sylvius

Franciscus Sylvius, as I have indicated elsewhere, was not really a natural philosopher.[30] Instead, he was a practicing physician, an outstanding clinician, with a strong interest in chemistry. His interest, however, stemmed not from any significant original experimental investigations but derived mostly at second-hand from the work of others. He seized upon the concepts of fermentation, the opposition between acid and alkali, and the properties of salts. These concepts he elaborated to account for physiological processes and the functions of various organs playing a part therein — for example, digestion (with special reference to salivary glands, stomach, pancreas, liver); circulation and respiration; the production and function of the various humors; and certain pathological processes. He made chemistry the basis not only of his physiological and pathological explanations but also of his therapeutics.

His interest in chemistry, however, was limited quite sharply to medicine, with no metaphysical extension. Unlike most natural philosophers, he showed no interest in the fundamental structure of the world in any larger sense. For him physiology—the study of the *physis*—had to do with the functions of the body and not with nature in its wider meaning. He rejected philosophy in any broader context. He also claimed to reject speculation, authority, and dogmatism, and to adhere to experience as the basis of medicine. And in his writings he indicated some views on the proper methodology of science. To explain the data of experience, he provided hypotheses but he did not indulge in higher levels of abstraction. However, his bent toward positivism was verbal rather than actual. Instead of following his own methodological principles, he indulged in dogmatic statements, made uncritical inferences, and relied on feeble evidence.

Sylvius had considerable influence. His academic prominence and his outstanding reputation as a clinician enhanced the status of chemistry for explaining physiology and pathology. While his own special doctrines of fermentation and of acid and alkali did not hold up under more critical examination, nevertheless his emphasis on salts, and their "acrid" properties, played an important part in later medical theory. Sylvius thus helped promote chemical explanations for bodily processes. And he also encouraged—by words more than by deeds—positivistic attitudes in medicine and better lip service to empiricism, in contrast to rationalism.

Chemical Physicians

Despite the outstanding stature of Helmont and Sylvius and of a few others, most medical practitioners who embraced chemical doctrines were looked down on by their orthodox colleagues. It is entirely misleading to study iatrochemistry merely from the standpoint of intellectual history. The chemists, beginning with Paracelsus, had challenged the Galenists. While the challenge seemed to involve primarily theoretical considerations and points of doctrine, the actual battles were fought along at least three different yet related fronts: the concrete practice of medicine, that is, the efforts to cure sick patients; the struggle for social recognition and the economic benefits; and the search for scientific validity, for theoretical supremacy. An essay in the history of ideas must necessarily concentrate on the last but must also appreciate the relevance of the others. The acceptance or rejection of theories does not take place in intellectual seclusion but in the world of social and economic and political struggles. Doctrinal disputes, supposedly dependent only on science, also reflect social and economic rivalries. In this book I stress ideas and concepts but, especially in the realm of iatrochemistry, I must note the importance of socioeconomic and practical factors.

In treating disease the chemists offered new medications involving especially the heavy metals and various artificial products of the "fur-

nace" — chemical substances entirely foreign to the traditional remedies of
the learned Galenists. We might think that whoever cures most effectively
would clearly stand out as the better physician, and that the superiority of
one medicine, in comparison with another, might be quite easy to settle.
We need only to answer the question: in point of fact, did these new remedies cure? Yet this question, apparently so straightforward, was at that
time impossible to answer in any clear-cut fashion. There were no acceptable ways of proving an alleged fact. For the most part there were merely
assertions and counterassertions, with reference to this or that particular
case. But how much conviction would a simple assertion convey, or the
exhibition of a concrete instance? Even today, with all our methodological
refinements, our double-blind studies, and our statistical sophistication,
one group of investigators may find it impossible to convince a rival group.
How much more difficult it was in the seventeenth century when there were
no canons of validity. We must not be surprised if seventeenth century
physicians could not agree on a simple question of "fact." There was tradition and if tradition failed in a particular instance, there were always innumerable avenues of excuse. We can appreciate the bite in Molière's
satire, that physicians preferred to have a patient die while following the
rules, than to have him recover by breaking the rules.[31]

Yet in certain instances experience left no doubt that the chemists had
the better modes of treatment. Boerhaave described this graphically while
giving a historical overview of chemistry and the progress of alchemy. He
declared that the physicians — the traditional Galenists who represented
the schools — "were unable, by their bleeding, purging, and the few effi-
cacious medicines in use, to cure the venereal disease, which had then
lately made its appearance. But the chemists attacking it with more powerful medicines . . . in particular with *mercury,* discovered the cure; it increased the triumph of chemistry and utterly baffled the schools."[32]

Such success, Boerhaave continued, was of course quite disconcerting to
the physicians "who, after infinite pains employed in enquiring into the
nature of the human body, and thence tracing the rise and cure of disease;
had the mortification to find all their laborious writings on ætiologics,
diagnostics, prognostics, diaetetics and therapeutics exploded, as idle and
useless, by the arrogance of alchemists; who, without regarding diet, or
attending to the cause and nature of disease, cured all by the mere application of one single medicine."

Chemistry had indeed scored a triumph over traditional medicine. The
use of metals, especially mercury and antimony, formed an important part
of the new therapeutics. And some of the remedies, in some instances, undoubtedly worked.

The history of therapeutics, especially in the seventeenth century, is a
fascinating topic.[33] It emphasizes the struggle between the new and the

old, between the forces of change and the forces of conservatism, a struggle waged on many fronts. The conservatives, with their long and expensive education and their high social status, resented the upstart chemists who not only propounded heterodox theories (and often achieved success) but who usually had little education and little social standing.

Despite exceptions — some few chemists were highly regarded — the adherents of chemical practice included all gradations of undesirable characters, down to the most ignorant quack — to "the rabble of coal-burners with so-called laboratories . . . the empirics, quacks, imposters and cheats, false impudent men." These opponents and rivals of orthodox physicians were deemed "illiterate, and their ignorance of learned languages a measure of their incompetence in medicine; their writings were the work of empty and dishonest scribblers, whose object is self-advertisement."[34] The orthodox physicians possessed status and material well-being and intended to retain them. But the unorthodox — among them the chemists were prominent — craved these goods and tried to achieve them. The conflicts between the various levels of medical practitioners form an essential part of medical history.[35]

The practitioners of medicine who were less well educated and who sought fame and economic competence could very easily adopt chemical orientation, especially since this claimed substantial therapeutic successes and did not require the long period of preliminary education. The new remedies would attract an increasing following among the less learned who objected to the privileges of the orthodox and who tried, through the newer trends, to achieve their own place in the sun. Thus, the problems regarding medicinal chemistry became entangled in currents involving social and economic aspects of medicine. Theory must take account of socioeconomic tensions.

LeFebvre

Chemical medicine was merely one branch of science that flourished vigorously in the seventeenth century. There is a vast literature on the history of chemistry as an independent science. In its medical aspects, the reader can get good orientation from the books by Hélène Metzger, J.R. Partington, Robert P. Multauf, and Allen Debus.[36] The seventeenth century chemistry textbooks provide important information for understanding iatrochemistry. These texts have considerable similarity one to the other. I choose the writings of Nicasius LeFebvre (1615-1669). This French chemist, a son of an apothecary, became a demonstrator in chemistry in the Jardin du Roi in Paris and gave courses there. In 1660 he went to England as "professor of chemistry and Apothecary in Ordinary to the King."[37] In 1660 he published an important text with the title *A Compleat Body of*

Chymistry. The informative subtitle reads in part "wherein is contained whatsoever is necessary for the attaining to the curious knowledge of this art . . . teaching the most exact preparation of animals, vegetables, and minerals, so as to preserve their essential vertues."

While the book is in large part a series of chemical directions, it also contains some theoretical and methodological aspects highly relevant for our purpose. Chemistry as a whole, he said, is "nothing else but the art and knowledge of nature it self," and it has to do with the "principles, out of which natural bodies do consist and are compounded."[38] Although this concept derives from traditional alchemy, I would emphasize its connection with the natural philosophy that developed in the seventeenth century.

LeFebvre indicated three different aspects of chemistry, each directed toward a separate goal.[39] The first is to be "wholly scientifical and given to contemplation, and may very well be termed *philosophical*, having only its end in the knowledge of nature"—the knowledge of heaven and earth, of minerals, plants and animals. This view of science follows the distinction that Aristotle established, that the goal of science is contemplation; and the attainment of knowledge through contemplation is directed not toward practical affairs but toward such things as are not in our power to change. However, the chemist achieved his knowledge not by armchair contemplation but by experiment and inferences.

The other two divisions of chemistry that LeFebvre mentioned are practical. The first of them, which he calls iatrochymy, has to do not merely with knowledge but also with applying that knowledge. The physician, learned in the theory of chemistry, can cure disease when he applies his knowledge. This aspect uses chemical theory in the practice of medicine. He knows chemical theory and he uses it to cure his patients. The other division LeFebvre called pharmaceutical chymistry, concerned not with theory at all but only with the practical work of carrying out "the precepts and orders of iatrochymists." It is technical only and does not imply a knowledge of theory.

Of the three divisions the first we might call pure science; the second, the application of science to the practice of medicine; and the third, the practical work of the technician who need only have manual skill but not any theoretical knowledge. We can still see this division in modern medicine— we distinguish the basic scientist from the clinician and the clinician from the technician.

Iatrochymistry indicates an opposition not to iatromechanics but to iatropharmacy. The iatropharmacist is merely the technician who prepares the medicines and carries out the orders of chemical physicians. The contrast between iatrochemistry and iatromechanism came much later, as the result of other complex influences, as we shall see in the next chapter. For the present we must keep in mind the distinction between the learned physician who knew chemical theory and applied it to the care of the patient; and the empiric, the technician who learned from experience, without benefit of theory, and who had no right to treat patients.

LeFebvre pointed to the methodological advantage of his own discipline. Chemistry was science, but empirically grounded, in contrast to speculation and uncontrolled rationalist elaborations. Chemistry, he said, was the science of nature but a science "reduced to operation, and examining all its propositions by reasons grounded upon the evidence and testimony of the senses, and not relying upon bare and naked contemplation." If, he declared, you ask the chemist, "What parts do constitute a body, he will not give you a naked answer, and satisfy by words and mere discourse your curiosity, but he will endeavor to bring his demonstrations under your sight, and satisfy also your other senses, by making you to touch, smell and taste the very parts which entered in the composition of the body."[40]

For LeFebvre the philosophy of the schools offered mere verbal quibblings. This philosophy rested on a high degree of abstraction. The chemists wanted to remain closer to concrete experience. "Chymistry doth reject such airy and notional arguments, to stick close to visible and palpable things . . . for if we affirm, that such a body is compounded of an acid spirit, a bitter or pontick salt, and a sweet earth; we can make manifest by the touch, smell, taste, those parts which we extract."[41]

This manifesto cannot be taken too literally but it does indicate a substantial point of difference between the Galenists and the chemists. The chemists paid particular attention to observations and the results of experiment, and they tried to bring their explanations into a *proximate* relationship with the observations. The neo-Galenists were content with explanations whose terms were quite remote from the immediate phenomena, and the hiatus between the sense data and the explanatory terms did not bother them.

LeFebvre did not go deeply enough into methodological principles. Granted that the analyses of the chemists *did* reveal certain acid or watery substances, what did this prove? To what general conclusions could such empirical results lead? We can sympathize with the chemists, who, dissatisfied with the traditional explanations through earth, air, fire, and water, sought new explanatory principles. But while the experiments of the furnace did indeed disclose substances palpable or odorous or visible, what right did the chemists have to proclaim these as elements or ultimate principles? LeFebvre did not tell us.

The problem involves the questions, what are the limits of natural philosophy? What are the ultimate principles? How do we know? Are ultimate principles beyond sensory experience? If so, what right do we have to bring in metaphysical "airy and notional arguments"? Or are they unavoidable in natural philosophy? Answers were slow in coming, and when they did come they were not necessarily very firm. But these questions and their concern with rationalism, empiricism, and critical evaluation, mark a change in the direction of medicine in the latter half of the seventeenth century.

Thomas Willis

At this point we can leave LeFebvre and proceed to our third figure, Thomas Willis (1621-1675). Unlike Sennert, who tried to harmonize neo-Galenic doctrine and Paracelsian chemistry, Willis rejected Aristotelian philosophy and its scholastic modification. For our present purposes his most relevant work is the extremely influential *De Fermentatione,* first published in 1659.[42]

Willis briefly considered the three main schools of thought and indicated the structural elements proclaimed by each. The peripatetics considered that all objects were composed of the four elements, earth, air, fire, and water. The atomism of Democritus and Epicurus, "lately . . . revived in our age," relied on the "conflux of atoms diversely figured," whose combinations accounted for the "figure, work, or efficacy" of an object. The third doctrine, chemistry, analyzed objects through fire, and "resolves all bodies into particles of spirit, sulphur, salt, water, and earth" and of these all bodies consisted.[43] Willis adhered to the third view, although he expressed sympathy with the atomistic view.

Atomism was much preferable to the peripatetic views. Atomism, he declared, explains phenomena mechanically, without involving "occult qualities, sympathy, and other refuges of ignorance," and does "very ingeniously disentangle some difficult knots of the sciences." This is all fine, but nevertheless atomism is too hypothetical — "it rather supposes than demonstrates its principles." This, of course, is the same argument that LeFebvre used against Galenism. Said Willis, in regard to atomism, its "notions are remote from sense and . . . do not sufficiently quadrate with the phenomena of nature, when we descend to particulars." That is, atomism expresses itself in vague generalities and has little explanatory power when dealing with particular and concrete phenomena. Chemistry, however, avoids this reliance on hypothesis, for its principles are empirically grounded. The spagyric principles, by which he meant the five elements, are not merely conceptual but real, and by this he meant corporeal. The principles with which the chemists deal are not the ultimate simple bodies but rather the "kind of substances into which physical objects are resolved, as their ultimate perceptible parts."[44]

Here Willis emphasizes the empirical aspect of chemistry. The five elements of the chemists are demonstrable and thus are subjects for experimentation and empirical analysis. Their ultimate metaphysical status was not a problem of great concern for Willis. Of course, despite his brave words he did depend largely on speculation, but he had a much firmer empirical basis than did the rival theories. The chemists could point to their principles and demonstrate their properties empirically, while for the atomists the properties were purely conceptual and hypothetical.

Like his predecessors, Willis had to provide explanations for the various aspects of nature, for the variety and specificity of things, for their change, generation, and corruption. The five elements were the building blocks whose "diverse motion, and proportions" might account for many properties, even though the quantitative values remained hypothetical.[45]

Of particular importance was Willis' conception of fermentation. Van Helmont, as we have seen, paid special attention to the doctrine of ferments, around which his philosophy centered. Isler points out that while van Helmont spoke very often of ferments, he seldom used the term fermentation and gave no hint of the way the ferments might work.[46] For van Helmont the ferments were metaphysical principles, akin to the Aristotelian forms (with an admixture of the Stoic *logoi spermatikoi*) which provided specificity of qualities and also the principles of functional activity. However, for van Helmont ferments and water were not only metaphysical concepts but also material objects subject to experimentation; but unfortunately, he did not adequately distinguish between these two aspects.

Van Helmont embodied many features of the idealistic tradition including facets of Platonism, Aristotelianism, and Neoplatonism. Ferments had ideal status. Willis, on the other hand, was philosophically an atomist, with his own modifications of the classical doctrines. He believed in material agents having certain specific properties—it was the function of the chemists to define these properties. His concern with properties and dynamic activity led him to emphasize process in relation to ferments, rather than any metaphysical status.

Fermentation had to do with heat formation. It represents "whatsoever effervency or turgency that is raised up in a natural body, by particles of that body variously agitated."[47] Later he defined fermentation as the "intestine motion of particles, or of the principles of every body. The motion tends to the perfection of that body, or its change into some other body."[48] The perfection of a process recalls the entelechy of Aristotle. It implies process and development and the change from a less developed state to one that is more developed. The process of change requires some specific directing force, which for the scholastics lay in the substantial form, but for Willis in the "intestine motion" of fermentation. This intestine motion of particles will "either frame the due perfections in the subject, or complete the alterations and mutations designed by nature."[49]

Fermentation, especially in relation to "spirit," thus had a functional relationship to the substantial form as a directing principle. In plants "the architect spirit, with its ministers salt and sulphur, still stretching forth it self like a snail, frames for it self an house, whose inhabitant it is . . . until it hath wrought the plant into the due bulk and figure designed by nature." Again, in animals "the first beginnings of life proceed from the spirit fermenting in the heart."[50] The spirit, by virtue of its intestine motion accomplished the specific activities that, in scholastic terms, would have been attributed to the form.

Besides the ferments in the "chimney of the heart" on which depends the motion of the heart, there are other ferments in the viscera. Some "serve for the perfecting of the blood, transmuting it into other liquors, and freeing it from excrementitious matter."[51] In the stomach there is an acid ferment and various ferments in different organs. He was indicating what we might call metabolism. All things, he said, "appointed for human use," acquire a "greater perfection and vigor, by fermentation." He referred specifically to foods and medicines.[52]

Through the process of fermentation Willis attempted to explain specificity, especially in function. A specific change or series of changes implies some specific agent or efficient cause. This Willis attributed to the fermentative process. This, in turn, he related to the "intestine motion" of the elementary particles, and somehow there resulted the highly specific activity that characterized fermentation. We must thus postulate two different kinds of motion, one general, relatively coarse and mechanical, correlated with physics and mechanics; and the other much more subtle and "intestine," correlated with chemical activities. The real specificity lies in the intestine motion of the particular elements, especially of spirit and sulfur.

Willis thus depended on a qualitative atomism. The elements differed one from the other not merely in quantitative aspects like size and shape but in characteristic and intrinsic qualities. This differentiation provided considerable explanatory power, vastly increased if we assume special kinds of intestine motion, applicable to some elements or aggregates but not to others. The specific intestine motion of Willis—fermentation—had the same role in his system that the textures—patterns of atoms—had for Boyle.

The major interest of Willis lay in process, change, and their explanations. He emphasized the way bodies "tend from crudity and confusion toward perfection." There is an "exaltation," to use the alchemical term. Matter is brought to a state of perfection. God (*parens naturae*) placed a stock of spirit, salt, and sulfur in the "primogeneous seed" of each object, sufficient to bring it to the ultimate characteristics.[53] I would emphasize again the relation between this process and the entelechy of the scholastics, the notion of orderly development, which constitutes the essence of substantial form.

Obviously, Willis had trouble explaining specificity. Fermentation was the intestine motion of the elements and these motions, he believed, exerted a directive function formerly called entelechy. For the most part he expounded his doctrine only in vague generalities. We see this in his Chapter 8 and in his discussion of the special fermentation noted in putrefaction. Thus, when an animal, dies, "presently the spirits, with salt and sulphur . . . cease from their regular motion, and are moved into confusion: then they partly exhale from the pores . . . and partly being shut up within in the cavities, inordinately ferment with heat . . . The active principles . . . do often mutually take hold of one another, and . . . produce worms." He continued, "Active particles are loosened, and begin to be in motion, tending to exhalation" (that is, the most active ones flying off).[54] This whole process he called fermentation without trying to pinpoint specific agents that deserve the name of ferment.

Rather different, however, is his analysis of the process involving mold or must, noted especially in damp places. To explain this phenomenon he spoke of a "tincture or impression of a stink," which is widely pervasive. This is "as if it were a certain ferment," present in a vessel, and capable of infecting "whatever liquors are put into it." He conjectured that this mustiness involves a moist inanimate body; that it derives from surrounding air stagnating, "whereby the elementary particles of that mixture, being combined together with those sent in by the air, are exalted into the nature of a ferment." The bodies so produced "retain their own nature" and can infect other bodies.[55] Ferment in this sense represents a concretion of elements, forming a specific body with specific properites and activities, capable of infecting other bodies and transforming them into its own specific and characteristic nature. Ferment in this specific context is clearly different from the more general and nonspecific intestine motion.

We find other examples where external circumstances may either hinder or promote fermentation. Thus, in the southern air there are "hot and humid particles" which easily enter into bodies, "obtain the force and place of a ferment," and "impress a notable motion of fermentation in very many different things."[56] Here again we see a distinction between the general process of fermentation (whose specificity is more verbal than actual) and the definite particular body—here carried by a south wind— that promotes the process of fermentation and can be designated as a truly specific ferment.

Robert Boyle

The vagueness in Willis became clarified in later authors, after Robert Boyle exerted his harmonizing influence. To appreciate Boyle's position we must realize the relatively low estate of chemistry. In one passage he described why he felt impelled to apologize for getting himself concerned with this subject. He realized that those who had no first-hand knowledge of the topic might, in accordance with the popular view, condemn chemists for their "illiterateness, the arrogance and the impostures of those who profess skill therein." Even "many learned men" would look askance "when they see any person, capable of succeeding in the study of solid philosophy, addict themselves to an art they judge so much below philosophy." It was distressing, apparently, "when they see a man, acquainted with other learning, countenance by his example sooty empirics."[57]

These passages tell us a great deal about chemistry in the late seventeenth century, emphasizing the sharp separation between the "learned," who perform intellectual tasks, and the "sooty empirics," who work with their hands. While Boyle did not direct these remarks specifically to medicine, his ideas were definitely applicable to that discipline. The medical hierarchy at that time rested on a distinction between the knowers and the doers, between those who used their minds and those who got their hands dirty. The learned physician, well educated, had a high status; the apothecary, less well educated, performed the more menial tasks and was not deemed fully qualified to engage in the more intellectual aspects of medicine, such as diagnosis and the determination of the proper remedies.

Boyle was referring to the snobbishness that distinguished "the study of solid philosophy" from the study of chemistry. The practitioners of the latter subject, who analyzed by fire, traced their lineage to the alchemists. Prejudice against the alchemists ran deep. In the revolt against the Aristotelian tradition the chemists had indeed played an important role, perhaps not as profound as that achieved by the corpuscular philosophers but effective nevertheless. Yet the corpuscularians represented "solid philosophy," eminently respectable (even though suspect to religious orthodoxy); while the chemists, wearing the rather soiled mantle of Paracelsus, remained in much lower repute.

Boyle combatted this social and intellectual prejudice against the chemists. As a student of nature he welcomed every activity that contributed to knowledge. Referring to medicine, he encouraged physicians to take seriously all manner of observations, even if made by the unlearned. Boyle declared that physicians would do well "to collect and digest all the approved experiments and practices of the farriers, graziers, butchers, and the like," despite "their ignorance and credulousness."[58] He had a comparable attitude toward science generally and he rejected the view that chemistry was a "study not fit for any but such, as are unfit for the rational and useful parts of physiology."[59] Boyle, devoting much effort to breaking down these prejudices, succeeded in making chemistry intellectually respectable, even though many of its practitioners were crude empirics.

Boyle shows us the tensions and disagreements between the chemists on the one hand and the corpuscular philosophers on the other. He was trying "to beget a good understanding betwixt the chymists and the mechanical philosophers" and regretted the "general misunderstanding" between the two groups. Most of the philosophers looked on the spagyrists "as a company of mere and irrational operators, whose experiments may indeed be serviceable to apothecaries, and perhaps to physicians, but are useless to a philosopher that aims at curing no disease but that of ignorance." The chemist, however, could regard the corpuscularians "as a sort of empty and extravagant speculators, who pretend to explicate the great book of nature, without having so much as looked upon the chiefest and the difficultest part of all; namely, the phaenomena."[60] Here we have the distinction between the pursuit of theory, which involved thinking, and the collection of observations, which involved getting the hands dirty.

We see this problem satirized in the brilliant Restoration comedy, *The Virtuoso*, by Thomas Shadwell, first published in 1676. The play makes fun of the science of the day and seems aimed at the virtuosi members of the Royal Society. In one scene Sir Nicholas Gimrack, the caricature of a virtuoso, is trying to learn to swim. First he observes the movements of a frog, and then he imitates these while lying on a table. He declares, "I content myself with the speculative part of swimming, I care not for the practick. I seldom bring anything to use; 'tis not my way. Knowledge is my ultimate end."[61]

Shadwell might have been supporting the views of the philosophers against the chemists, but the opposition goes far deeper, namely, that between the rational and the empirical. Each had its extreme proponents, who made a sharp contrast between contemplation and activity, between theory and practice. In a given situation, should we be reflective or active? The corpuscularians—the "philosophers"—condemned the chemists for inadequate theory while the chemists condemned their opponents for inadequate attention to experience.

Boyle did more than any other man to resolve the conflict between the philosophers and the chemists. He was able to harmonize the theories of the one and the practice of the other and weld them both into a unity. He showed that the practical activity of the chemists was valuable in the extreme—that it had already achieved much and promised even more. On the other hand, the theories of the chemists were defective, while the theoretical foundation of the corpuscularian philosophy was far superior. Furthermore, the experimental data of the chemists furnished sound confirmation of the corpuscular philosophy, but the latter could explain the data of chemistry far better than could the theories of the chemists themselves.

Boyle examined the criticisms that the chemists and the corpuscularians hurled at each other and he appreciated some validity on each side. The corpuscularians needed the data of the chemists to shore up their own theories, and without those chemical data the philosophers might be subject to legitimate criticism for having too much airy speculation. On the other hand, the chemists were under a handicap if they relied on their own traditional principles to explain the data. The corpuscularian concepts were far better suited to providing a sound explanation. As Boyle said later, in regard to acids and alkalis, the principles of the chemists are far too narrow "to afford any satisfactory explication of the phenomena."[62] The experiments of the chemists could be "happily explicated by corpuscular notions," and the latter in turn could be "either illustrated or confirmed by chemical experiments."[63]

One of Boyle's most important works bears the title "On the Usefulness of Natural Philosophy." This is in two parts. The first, composed probably about 1650, indicates that the knowledge of nature not only provides practical power but promotes the glory of God and of religion and is a bulwark against atheism.[64] The second part, written over a decade later — probably only a short time before its publication in 1663 — bears directly on medicine and makes us realize the kinds of problems that were moot and some of the possibilities envisaged for their solution.

Boyle is pleading for a careful and detailed study of nature. Of course, in all this he was continuing the tradition of Hippocrates, of Aristotle and Galen, as well as Paracelsus, Bacon, and van Helmont. But by the second half of the seventeenth century the students of nature were beginning to acquire tools for investigation and experimentation. Various technical advances permitted greater precision and sharper discrimination. New anatomical techniques, such as injection studies, enlarged the intellectual horizon, while the primitive microscopes vastly extended the range of direct vision and contributed to the analytic capacities of investigators.

Rather different were the techniques that chemistry was forging. A microscope was extending the senses and provided data that could fit into an orthodox conceptual framework. Chemical studies, however, gave data often at variance with ordinary sense expectation, data that, to be meaningful, seemed to require a new conceptual framework. Otherwise the results of chemistry might remain on a purely empiric or practical basis quite distinct from rational or theoretical implications. In LeFebvre's terms this would be merely the realm of the iatropharmacists — technicians innocent of theory. And as we have seen, many of the educated men of the time regarded chemists as "sooty empirics" or else as rash and fanciful theorists.

Boyle's insights led to harmony. He saw that chemical techniques, crude and inexact as they were, nevertheless held out vast promise for the future. Devoted as he was to "natural philosophy," he could see that many problems in the animal economy could be approached with the new chemistry. "If chymical experiments, and mechanical contrivances, were industriously and judiciously associated by a naturalist profoundly skilled in both," then great advantage would result. The physician should know both the mechanical and the chemical philosophy. He should be naturalist enough "as to know, how heat and cold, and fluidity, and compactness, and fermentation, and putrefaction, and viscosity, and coagulation, and dissolution, and such like qualities, are generated and destroyed in the generality of bodies." All this would have special importance in studying the normal functioning of the body. In reference to physiology Boyle spoke of "that handmaid to it, which is Chymistry," and declared that the juices and humours and liquors of the body could be better studied by one versed in chemistry than by one "the hath never had *Vulcan* for his instructor."[65] On this point of view he rang the changes many times.

However, Boyle was under no illusions that the chemists had discovered the secrets of the body. Instead he emphasized his *faith* that the pursuit of chemical studies could and probably would in time lead to great advances in knowledge. He expressed himself in hypothetical terms, in conditional statements and subjunctives. "If the juices of the body were more chymically examined . . . it is not improbable, that both new things related to the nature of the humours, and other ways of sweetening, actuating, and otherwise altering them, may be detected, and the importance of such discoveries discerned."[66]

Boyle was emphasizing the importance of chemistry not only for its practical value, but for its contribution to theory and to knowledge. He made a sharp distinction between "vulgar chymists" and the proponents of "true chymistry." The former were the traditional spagyrists; the latter those who would assimilate chemistry to the corpuscular philosophy and to the other branches of learning, thus inducing a better understanding and better control of nature. He indicated what he considered the naturalist of the future—one "well versed both in chymical experiments, and in anatomy, and the history of diseases, without being too much addicted either to the chymists notions, or the received opinions of physicians."[67]

Boyle described many areas of medicine where chemistry could be of value.[68] He went much further than did LeFebvre, who indicated three categories where chemistry would be useful, the first having to do with knowledge as such, the second with the cure of disease, and the third with technical procedures. Boyle pointed out advantages not only for achieving practical goals but also for achieving greater understanding and theoretical knowledge. But the great contribution that chemistry might make toward understanding nature would come to pass only when the traditional chemical theory was altered. The "vulgar or Spagyric chymistry" rested on faulty theory and would never lead to sound knowledge. Boyle directed a great deal of time to criticizing the theories of the chemists, particularly in *The Sceptical Chymist* (1661), "The Imperfection of the Chymist's Doctrines of Qualities," and "Reflections upon the Hypothesis of Alcali and Acidum."[69]

In these studies he indicated a high degree of critical judgment in regard to hypothesis. He demanded precision instead of vagueness, and the spagyric teachings could not measure up. The doctrine of the three principles he found lacking, and the substitution of five principles instead of three did not offer any advantage.[70] Boyle paid special attention to the concept of elements and the composition of mixed bodies. He pointed out that fire, the important tool of the chemists, was not equal to the task of identifying components, since the action of fire and its results depended on the conditions under which it acted.

Even more important, the chemical principles could not satisfactorily explain the observed qualities of things. "The Spagyrical doctrine of qualities is insufficient, and too narrow to reach to all the phenomena, or even to the notable ones; that ought to be explicable by them."[71] Thus, the *tria prima* cannot satisfactorily explain qualities such as, among others, "gravity, fixedness, colour, transparency and fluidity" as well as magnetism. The chemist who, with the help of the *tria prima,* tried "to interpret that book of nature, of which the qualities of bodies make a great part" is acting like one who, "seeing a great book written in a cypher, whereof he were acquainted but with three letters, should undertake to decypher the whole piece."[72] Three chemical principles, or even five, were insufficient to provide a sound explanation of the observed phenomena. The proper way to understand nature and the concepts proper for a sound natural philosophy lay with the corpuscular philosophy.

The corpuscular philosophy could completely absorb the specifically chemical doctrines. Once we accept the notion of minute particles differing in size and shape and position and entering into combinations that differed one from the other in their pattern, we have an explanatory tool of great power. If, in trying to understand the constituents of a material object, we say that it is composed of mercury and sulphur, we might indeed account for certain observed properties and qualities, but we are offering only a "proximal" explanation. If we want constituents that provide comprehensive or ultimate explanations, we must fall back on the "catholick affections of matter" — the size, shape, position, and "texture" or pattern of the component atoms. That is, we must fall back on the details of the corpuscular philosophy. The ultimate simple bodies are the atoms, and differences in bodies arise from differences in size, shape, position, and "texture."

Boyle's contribution to our immediate problems can be summarized in two propositions. First, the corpuscular philosophy can explain qualities and change better than can the principles of the chemists. A complete natural philosophy can be deduced from matter and motion, but not from salt, sulfur, and mercury.[73] And second, the experiments and data of chemistry provide a sound experimental foundation for the corpuscular philosophy. In a sense Boyle simply absorbed chemistry into the mainstream of natural philosophy. The five elements that Willis, for example, dealt with, might form objects of study but they were not the true elements. They were merely the first compounds. The true principles—in the Aristotelian sense—were matter and motion.

Deidier and Lemery

Let us now go forward almost half a century and consider one of the French iatrochemists, Antoine Deidier. His date of birth is not precisely known but he received his doctor's degree in 1691 and in 1697 succeeded to the chair of chemistry at the University of Montpellier. Here he remained until his death in 1746. He wrote extensively on a wide range of subjects, such as chemistry, anatomy, institutes of medicine, and various clinical topics, including plague, venereal disease, tumors, gout. Nevertheless he is either ignored or barely mentioned in most histories of medicine or histories of chemistry. A moderately detailed account in Bayle and Thillaye is highly critical, declaring that he pursued novelty much more than truth and that he exhibited more imagination than judgment.[74]

I have studied only his *Institutes*. The full title is *Institutiones Medicinae Theoricae Physiologiam & Pathologiam complectentes*. Bayle and Thillaye list the first edition of this work as 1716, as does Hirsch, but my copy bears the date 1711.[75] The book does not deserve the strictures that Bayle and Thillaye imposed on Deidier's writings. While I have not studied his clinical texts, his *Institutiones* seems reasonably cautious when compared with other seventeenth and eighteenth century writers, and although his conclusions far transcend his evidence, we cannot consider him unique in this respect nor condemn him for it. In regard to chemistry he does not present novel doctrines; rather, he gives a fairly traditional account of the theoretical aspects before he indicates its relationship to medicine.

We might profitably make a brief comparison with Nicholas Lemery (1645-1715), who, although he did eventually get an M.D. degree in 1684, was primarily a chemist. He gave courses in chemistry, wrote his vastly successful textbook, and won substantial fame before he took his medical degree in Caen. Partington devotes considerable space to his place in the development of chemistry.[76] For our purposes he is important not for his theoretical contributions but rather for the role that he played in introducing and popularizing chemistry in medical education and practice. Deidier, on the other hand, was a scientifically oriented clinician who based his doctrines on the chemical philosophy. We can see the difference between the two men by comparing the titles of their respective books.

Lemery wrote *A Course of Chemistry;* Deidier, *Institutiones Medicinae Theoricae,* that is, *Institutes of Theoretical Medicine.*

It is worthwhile comparing the two works. For Lemery I have consulted the first English edition of 1677 (translated from the French of 1675), and also the fourth English edition of 1720, translated from the eleventh French edition "which has been revised, corrected, and much enlarged . . . by the author."[77] Lemery enumerated the five principles of chemistry, of which spirit, oil, and salt were "active," water and earth "passive." In the 1720 edition (although not in the first edition) he indicated that the term principle "must not be understood in too nice a sense," and what he designated thereby might still be divided "into abundance of other parts," which might more appropriately be called principles. However, the traditional five principles are those that "are separated and divided, so far as we are capable of doing it by our weak and imperfect powers." This capability of being empirically demonstrated, of being pointed at, was an important argument for the chemists, who prided themselves on avoiding empty speculation. Lemery criticized "the fond conceits" of other philosophers, who, in regard to "natural principles", would "puff up the mind with grand ideas, but they prove or demonstrate nothing."[78] He thus is rejecting speculation — the same type of rejection that we found discussed by Boyle.

Lemery admitted that the chemical division into five substances "may seem a little gross" but could serve as a "ladder" to the "true principles of nature" and could give some idea of the "figure of the first small particles which have entered into the composition of mixt bodies."[79] He also considered the vexing problem (that Boyle had mentioned) regarding the validity of analysis by fire and the preexistence of the substances thereby disclosed. This aspect need not concern us here. Then in the following pages he briefly discussed the nature, characteristics, and diversity of these principles, the different kinds of salts, the acids and alkalis, fermentation, and the like. After describing technical procedures he devoted the remainder of the book to the main divisions of nature — the chemistry of the mineral, the vegetable, and the animal kingdoms.

Deidier had a rather different orientation. As befits the concept of *Institutes of Medicine,* he was concerned with theoretical explanation — with the way the body functions in health and disease. And for his explanations he relied chiefly on chemistry. A volume of *Institutes* traditionally began with a consideration of physiology. Deidier's concept of this subject differed from that of the earlier writers. The ancients had established seven divisions of physiology — elements, temperaments, humors, spirits, parts, faculties, and generation, a division, said Deidier, that rested on the old concept of the four elements (air, fire, water, and earth). However, since in recent times physics, chemistry and anatomy "have led to the more perfect knowledge of the nature and structure of the human body, the modern

writers consider the body under two divisions — the liquids and the solids."
And since the inner knowledge of these cannot be known "unless their intrinsic and proximal principles are distinguished," the subject of physiology is now divided into three parts — the principles, the fluids, and the
solids. By "principles" he understood "those essential parts that intrinsi-
cally constitute the fluids and the solids and give rise to their properties."
The fluids are the humors, and the solids are only the vessels containing the
humors.[80]

In accordance with this analysis Deidier divided his treatise on physiology into three separate parts. The first, which deals with the principles, is
the most significant. By principles he meant those essential parts of a compound "from which their proximate properties immediately derive."[81]
"Properties" apparently refers to what the neo-Galenists had called the
qualities. The word proximate I interpret in the sense of manifest, so that
the proximate properties are the equivalent of the neo-Galenic manifest
qualities. Traditionally these are opposed to the occult qualities, that is,
the properties that lie hidden within the inner composition. The
"immediately derive" implies a minimum of logical elaboration. No chains
of reasoning are needed. Instead, the derivation of the qualities follows
simply and directly from the character of the principles.

The word principle, Deidier recognized, has several meanings. He mentioned the Aristotelian definition — what does not arise from itself nor from
anything else, but that from which all else derives.[82] Curiously, Deidier,
instead of describing all the Aristotelian principles, mentioned only
matter, completely ignoring form and privation. The Aristotelian notion
of form had completely dropped out of the picture and Deidier dealt
exclusively with matter.

In this regard he followed quite precisely the philosophy of Descartes.
The essence of matter is extension. There is no void, but the universe is a
plenum in motion, with vortices. Matter exists in a threefold division — with
three elements. The first is extremely subtle matter, extremely active and
filling all interstices; the second comprises larger particles, globular in configuration; while the third is still larger and irregular. Each of these elements is responsible for particular properties. But Deidier did not concern
himself with ultimate constituents. Instead, he attended to the three manifest components of the world, that is, the mineral, the vegetable, and the
animal kingdoms. These are subjects for investigation.[83]

They are all composites and must be divided into proximal parts which
account for their characteristics. These proximal parts are reducible to
five — the familiar spirit or mercury, salt, water or phlegm, oil or sulfur,
and residual earth.[84] It is these that the chemists investigate — the substances that can provide proximal explanations — while the ultimate components are left for the philosophers. Metaphysics no longer exerts any

pressure, but study of the five elements and their properties can take up all the efforts of the chemists. Interest now centered on the empirical, on what can be directly perceived or else inferred by a modest amount of reasoning that stays relatively close to the data. There was little concern with internal dynamics, or with functional components that had to do with a *terminus ad quem* and with goals, or with organism-acting-as-a-whole rather than as parts. All this became unimportant when the Aristotelian form dropped out of sight.

Deidier devoted much space to describing the characteristics and properties of different principles. The nature of a principle—for example, whether it was rigid or smooth or pointed—could be inferred from its properties and its behavior. These features, however, are more relevant to the history of chemistry in the stricter sense.

The term principle in Deidier's usage is a far cry from the definition of Aristotle. Deidier and his fellow chemists had in mind the components that could be handled and dealt with in a proximal fashion. The terms elements and principles had exchanged meanings. For the neo-Galenists principle was primary, and the elements were derived from them. For Deidier, however, principles were compounds derived from the Cartesian subdivisions of matter, which he called elements and regarded as primary. When these early spagyric concepts of the *tria prima* were absorbed into the corpuscular philosophy, the term principle was retained for the chemical substances, but these were regarded as derivative from the elements of Descartes.

We have an interesting sequence of metaphysical systems. Sennert, Boyle, and Deidier all refused to accept the three (or five) chemical principles as ultimately primary. For Sennert these chemical principles derived from the classical four elements (earth, fire, air, and water), which in turn derived from the true Aristotelian principles of form and matter. For Boyle the chemical principles represented compounds of atoms, whose true principles (in the Aristotelian sense) would be matter, motion, and the void. Deidier, in contrast to Boyle, was a Cartesian who referred the chemical principles to the three elements of Descartes. But these in turn might be considered derivative from the more fundamental thought and extension (*ex quibus omnia*, according to Descartes). We might note here that Boyle stressed the similarities between the Cartesian and the atomistic metaphysics, rather than their differences. [85]

Thus the word principle, widely used in the seventeenth and eighteenth centuries, exhibited rather different shades of meaning, parallel to different systems of philosophy. The whole topic of iatrochemistry, centering as it does on elements and principles, is indissolubly linked to contemporary metaphysics.

FIVE

IATROMECHANISM

Labels, although often useful, can be quite tyrannical. We see this, for example, with the term iatromechanism, through which historians of medicine and science try to bring order into seventeenth and eighteenth century doctrines. A fine symmetry seems to emerge: iatromechanism contrasts with iatrochemistry; a contrast provides opposition; opposition suggests an either . . . or disjunction, and this enables us to categorize individuals in a neat fashion.

But the world of ideas is not really neat. A dependence on labels illustrates what I would call the "box approach" to history. Historians provide iatromechanism with distinct characteristics, which in our metaphor would serve as the walls of the box. These have some degree of elasticity. Into this box we place this or that individual, who thereafter bears the label on the box: "So-and-so is an iatromechanist." Sometimes, of course, we are not quite sure whether a given person really fits, and there may be a certain amount of pushing and squeezing before we make up our minds. Thus, into the box called iatromechanism all historians place Borelli, Bellini, Baglivi, Pitcairn but are not quite sure about, say, Santorini.

Now there are two great advantages to a box. First, it provides a definite location, so that whatever is inside is there and not someplace else. Second, whatever is inside can be evaluated by the characteristics of the box, and these in turn may be neatly epitomized by a label. Iatrochemistry and iatromechanism offered two such nicely labeled boxes which, apparently, simplified the task of the historian.

Unfortunately, the box approach to history has a severe drawback: it isolates individuals and thereby destroys the intricate web of relationships that comprise the past. If we want to reconstruct the past, we should try to restore some of these intricacies and thereby we complicate the situation instead of simplifying it.

The origin of the terms is not clear. Iatrochemistry was used in the seventeenth century but in a special context. LeFebvre, as we have seen, distinguished philosophical chemistry from iatrochemistry and these, in turn, from pharmaceutical chemistry. The first was the domain of the natural philosopher who sought to understand nature; the second involved the physician who applied chemical knowledge to the theory and practice of medicine; and the third was purely technical, quite divorced from theory.

Iatromechanist and iatromathematician became current considerably later. Haller used these terms quite freely in his *Bibliotheca Medicinae Practicae,* when referring to various physicians of the late seventeenth and early eighteenth centuries. Haller would often introduce his bibliographic comments with some biographical data or with brief characterizations — sometimes only a few words, sometimes an entire paragraph. Thus, he used the word *Jatromechanicus* in reference to Bellini, and Pitcairn he designated as *Jatromathematicus.* Haller used other descriptive words. Thus, Freind was *vir doctus medicus;* Kerkring was *chemicus;* Morton was *medicus & clinicus;* Ramazzini was *medicus & philosophicus;* and Deidier he identified as *professor & clinicus monspeliensis. Fermentationibus deditus.* Of Hoffman he said, *mechanicae se sectae addixit.*[1]

Haller was not writing medical history and his characterizations were casual indeed — perhaps on this account all the more valuable, as indicating a looseness of the descriptive categories. Incidentally, I did not find the term iatrochemist.

Sprengel, writing only a few years after Haller, used definite categories. In 1799 he wrote a long chapter entitled "History of the Chemical Schools of the Seventeenth Century," in which he used the term *chymiatrie* — best translated, perhaps, as medical chemistry or iatrochemistry but in its adjectival form best rendered as chemiatric.[2] This chapter, quite long and detailed, takes up the Rosicrucians and the eclectics; and then the systems of van Helmont, Descartes, and Sylvius; and then there is a section "Further Development of the Chemiatric Systems" in which Sprengel dealt with various medical chemists in the major Western countries, predominantly of the seventeenth century. We may, perhaps, raise a questioning eyebrow at finding Descartes discussed, in part, in a chapter entitled "Iatrochemistry," but perhaps this merely shows how vague were the categories at the end of the eighteenth century.

Sprengel entitled his next chapter "History of the Iatromathematical School," with iatromechanism as a synonym. This doctrine, he said, compared artificial machines to the human body, and the functioning of the body he attributed to statics and hydraulics.[3] In this system the solids played the predominant role, as lifeless canals or machines composed of nonliving conduits, and exhibited no forces beyond cohesion, gravity, and attraction, as found in hydraulic machines.

As features responsible for the rise of this school, he invoked the discovery of the circulation of the blood, and the Cartesian philosophy that connected mathematics and medicine. If all changes in the body are to be explained by the configuration and movement of the smallest particles, then physiology is only a branch of applied mathematics. The laws governing the movement of the particles — of whatever configuration — can be defined as for any other machine. Italy, said Sprengel, led the world in the rise of science and experimental physics, and he selected Galileo and the Academia del Cimento for special mention. He also gave detailed attention to Sanctorius as a sort of forerunner of the iatromechanical school. Then Sprengel discussed relatively briefly a large number of investigators, starting with Borelli and proceeding to others in Italy, France, Germany, and England. He included Sauvages, Boerhaave, Hoffmann, Hamberger, Pitcairn, Cheyne, Robinson, Martine, among a great many others. The teachings of Newton were, of course, extremely significant, and in this connection Sprengel mentioned specifically the two types of force, the one involving contact and the other *attractio electrica*.[4]

In his exposition Sprengel remained rather critical of the entire school. He pointed out that in the body there are no straight lines and flat planes and that the Cartesian method was just as arbitrary as the "dreams of the chemiatrists" on the fermentations, distillations, and precipitations in the body. And he commented how few physicians in this school knew the spirit of the Newtonian philosophy, how few followed the path of induction and the analytical method. Most of the writers merely preened themselves with fine sounding words like attraction, and centrifugal or centripetal forces, and made display of higher mathematics, producing a deceptive appearance of certainty and truth.[5]

For comparison with Sprengel, who wrote in 1799, we may refer to Daremberg, whose *Histoire des sciences médicales* dates from 1870.[6] While showing occasional additional insights, Daremberg generally followed Sprengel's approach. Iatromechanism (synonymous with iatromathematics) explains organic movement, that is, physiology, by the laws of mechanics, statics, and hydraulics, and the help of mathematical formulae. Disease is similarly explained. All this, Daremberg felt, was a reaction against the natural faculties and archeus-doctrine and, in pathology, against the excesses of humoralism. Galenism was rejected yet Hippocrates still had strong defenders. Daremberg took up in detail numerous physicians of Italy, France, England, Holland, and Germany, and included Boerhaave and Sauvages among his examples.

In his exposition Daremberg did give passing acknowledgment to the alterations and mixtures of concepts. He mentioned the way that Boerhaave and Hoffmann, for example, modified the doctrines of mechanical explanations. Iatromechanism, he declared, led to solidism and solidism dominated the second half of the eighteenth century, leading in turn to Brown and Broussais.[7] Daremberg thus distinguished sharply between iatromechanism and solidism.

Nothing could be more futile than to discuss whether Sanctorius was or was not an iatromechanist or whether Hoffmann should be called a solidist.[8] Let us rather study some sequences of ideas and their remarkable complexity at the turn of the century.

The early historians—and following them the later ones too—distinguished quite sharply between the chemists and the mechanists, but in what does the difference really consist? We note a temporal factor—iatrochemistry as a school seems to concentrate in the two middle quarters of the seventeenth century, with a diminution in importance thereafter. The iatromechanists became significant in the third quarter of the seventeenth century, much more important in the fourth quarter, and entirely dominant the first third of the eighteenth century. There seems to be relatively little overlap and we may fairly ask how much direct conflict there was.

Iatrochemistry, as a distinct entity, seemed to come to an end, but chemistry, as such, did not; instead, it shared in the massive growth of knowledge, became increasingly important in the development of science, as well as medicine. The leading physicians who spanned the turn of the century—Boerhaave, Stahl, Hoffmann—were all prominent chemists, and this subject played a significant role in medical education, with professorships established in medical schools. How does it happen, then, that the concept of iatrochemist went into eclipse?

To find the reasons for this we should, I believe, attend to certain aspects of the intellectual background. In that complex web we can attend to only a few strands which intermingle in the total fabric but which can at least be identified and partially traced.

Quantity and Precision

One major thread represents the age-old conflict between quality and quantity, which is essentially a problem in reductionism. In the competing philosophies does the qualitative aspect maintain some sort of primacy, as we find in the Platonic ideas, the Aristotelian forms, the Neoplatonic emanations, and, in medicine, in the doctrines of the substantial forms? Or are qualitative aspects reducible to the configuration of particles, as we find in the various corpuscularian philosophies? Or can we find some sort of compromise, wherein certain qualities or qualitative properties are irreducible, although corpuscularian explanations dominate?

Cognate to this problem is the question of specificity, especially important in medicine. Physiology studies a great many different processes, which it first identifies and describes and then explains. The various functions seem quite specific—muscular contraction is quite distinct from bodily growth; the functions of the kidney are distinct from those of the liver. How to account for the specificity? Will it have an irreducible qualitative basis? To what extent will we find quality as a primary feature?

Similar considerations apply to disease. There are a great many distinctive diseases. Certain fevers, for example, are quite characteristic—smallpox will not be confused with intermittent fever, and both are readily distinguishable from gout. Wherein lies the specificity? Does it involve a basic and irreducible qualitative aspect, like a form or an archeus? Or can specificity be reduced to factors amenable to quantitative study, such as size, shape, number and pattern of particles, and forces that activate them? For the present I would merely point to the need for explaining specificity and the alternate ways of doing so—through qualities or through quantity. Chemistry, I suggest, tended toward qualitative specificity as a major tenet, while the mechanical philosophy embraced quantity.

A vast increase in knowledge took place in the seventeenth century, in such widely different aspects as physiology, physics, chemistry, astronomy. Knowledge was expanding not only in extent but also in what might be called precision, that is, in possibilities for careful measurement and quantification. In anatomy, for example, the drive to greater knowledge led to abundant discoveries and the identification of structures previously unknown. But these discoveries we may regard as purely qualitative. The microscope provided a powerful tool for new observations and furnished abundant new data but again of a purely qualitative nature. Other anatomical studies, such as those involving vascular injections and the discrimination of blood vessel patterns, also disclosed qualitative differences but in addition opened up an opportunity for counting and measuring or, in the most general terms, estimation of "more" or "less." Precision increased when better tools became available.

In physiology the situation was comparable. The study of bodily functions in health and disease yielded primarily qualitative observations yet could provide scope for actual measurements. Sanctorius (1561-1636), who discovered the "insensible perspiration," also devised a thermometer, a "pulsilogium," and a hydrometer and made other quantitative investigations. He is important not because he was (or was not) an iatromechanist but because he used quantitative methods. He developed techniques for carefully weighing and counting and measuring physiological changes. He provided new observations, provided them in a quantitative form and made a great advance in the ongoing search for precision.

This search for precision was, I suggest, an important factor in seventeenth century intellectual life, going hand in hand with the general expansion of knowledge. Toward the end of the century chemistry, although it did perform approximate measurements in its *in vitro* experiments, did not have the tools whereby it could compete in precision with the mechanicians. This was especially true when physicians tried to apply chemical reasoning and chemical methods to physiological processes.

Let us examine a different thread in the pattern. Observations alone, whether qualitative or quantitative, remain incomplete by themselves. They must fit into a framework of explanation which, as a result, may suffer considerable strain. For example, we may speak about ultimate explanation, which deals with completely general first principles. On the other hand, we may also deal with more proximal explanations, closer to experience, less hypothetical, and applying to only a limited field of discourse. The doctrine of acids and alkalis in disease applies at a level we might call proximal, the atomic hypothesis at a level more profound, and the metaphysical concepts of form and matter would be ultimate.

With this distinction in mind, we note that the iatrochemists offered explanations that were progressively more limited, that is, remained close to the phenomena. Van Helmont, an exception, offered a completely general philosophical position with basic principles of water and ferments applying to the entire universe, but later chemists worked in a far more limited sphere. They dealt not with the ultimate constituents of the universe but with compounds, not with completely first principles or even with true elements, but with aggregates (*misti* or *mixti*).

In the early seventeenth century medicine sought to be a total philosophy, to integrate the data of health and disease into a closely knit picture of the universe. Physiology was the study of nature and nature had unlimited extent. By the late seventeenth century chemical medicine could no longer serve as a philosophy of nature. It was no longer sufficiently general in its theories. Generality was being recognized as a function of physics, and chemistry, in its theoretical aspects, was merging into physics.

LeFebvre, as we have seen, distinguished those chemical activities aiming at pure knowledge—science or natural philosophy—from those having practical goals, such as pharmaceutical or industrial application. By the late seventeenth century the original spagyric principles could no longer support their own natural philosophy. With Boyle, chemical theory merged into the corpuscularian philosophy. As Crosland declared, referring to the end of the seventeenth century, if chemistry "is to be considered as a science at all, it must be by reference to the corpuscular theory of Boyle and Lemery or (rather later) to the phlogiston theory of Becher and Stahl." Boyle considered matter as corpuscular. Chemical reactions took place because "the size and shape of the particles of one substance happened to correspond to the size and shape of another."[9]

For their basic concepts of matter, for their notions of the ultimate and simplest substances, the chemists relied on corpuscularian doctrines. But in their own activities they concerned themselves not with the ultimately simple but with compounds. If we think of the distinction between atoms and molecules, the chemists dealt with molecules and their combinations and reactions. Particles and forces more primitive than these were the domain of the corpuscularian philosophers and the physicists. The chemists thus worked at a level that I call more proximal to experience than did the mechanists, and of more limited generality.

Those physicians who sought after maximum generality, who, in the older tradition, wanted to make medicine virtually coterminous with all knowledge, would find much more appeal in physics than in chemistry. An inclination of this sort—undoubtedly a matter of temperament—usually went together with a rationalist frame of mind. Chemistry was more limited, more empirical, more wedded to the laboratory.

Newton dominated all of science, including chemistry. Carrying on the tradition of Kepler, Galileo, and Descartes, that the world was mathematical in essence, he brought this doctrine to what seemed its ultimate pinnacle. He provided a unified theory of matter based on accurate experiments and elegant mathematics. Careful observation and precise mathematical elaboration, together, led to an all-embracing generalization, extending from the smallest particle of matter to the largest corporeal aggregate in the heavens. The nature of the effective forces, the transmission of force by contact, the problems of action at a distance, of the ether, of attraction, of the relationship between the earlier and the later Newtonian ideas, all these are special topics of Newtonian physics taken up by various scholars, and I will not go into these aspects.[10] Let me merely emphasize that Newton presented a universe of particles in motion, acted on by forces about which there might be some dispute, to be sure, but which are amenable to mathematical treatment.

Physics dealt with the basic structure of the universe; chemistry, at the turn of the century, did not. For their concepts regarding the simplest bodies and their properties the chemists were already captive to the theories of Boyle. He, however, dealt frankly with conjecture and his formulations lacked rigor. Newtonian physics superseded the cruder formulations and provided a much firmer theoretical basis for chemistry as a science. In this connection the writings of Freind are especially important. In 1709, under the direct personal influence of Newton, he wrote a chemistry text that rested explicitly on the doctrine of particles and forces that Newton had discussed in his *Optics*.[11] The Newtonian concepts grew in influence and for Boerhaave, as Crosland declared, chemistry was a branch of Newtonian physics.[12]

We might try to analyze some of the characteristics of chemistry in relation to medicine in the late seventeenth century. I suggest the following features as significant.

For the chemists practical activity played a major role. For example, they had long been involved with "experiments of the furnace," using fire as an analytic tool. Chemistry studied certain special processes such as calcination, distillation, sublimation, fermentation, digestion, and the like. These studies, performed *in vitro,* were carried over to the living body by the process of analogy. The chemists dealt with certain characteristic substances such as acids and alkalis and salts, oils and sulfurs. As we have seen, these were regarded as compounds, made up of more elementary constituents. But ultimate composition was not a topic of any great practical concern. The chemists were closer to what today we might call a phenomenological approach, and their experiments and observations tended to emphasize the qualitative differences and the specificity of various reactions.

Certain practical activities such as preparing or purifying drugs need not detain us. We need consider only the relations of chemistry to physiology and to disease states. Only to a slight degree could chemists perform relevant experiments directly on living bodies. To be sure, body fluids could be subjected to various procedures in the chemical laboratory but the transference to *in vivo* status remained problematic. At this time theorizing about vital processes depended principally on analogy, on some similarity between *in vitro* or other artificial situations and the actual living body. The use of analogy was the core of biological inference in the seventeenth and eighteenth centuries and was not restricted to chemists. The mechanists were equally adept at finding similarities between *in vivo* and *in vitro* processes. The great difference between the chemists and their opponents lay in the terms of the analogy. Whereas the chemists found similarities between experiments of the furnace and the living body, or between fermentation and human physiology, the mechanists ridiculed these asserted similarities. The analogies of the mechanists rested on experiments or observations that had to do with statics and kinetics, with particles differing in size, shape, and motion, and with mathematical calculation. Indeed, what distinguished the chemists from their opponents was not the use of analogies but the particular kinds of analogies that were accepted as cogent.

Mathematics, enjoying a major role in physics, played an increasingly important part in biological theory. The Newtonian method had twin components: experience — careful and controlled observation; and reasoning — mathematical elaboration. And these two components, although their importance had been recognized since Greek times, now took on a canonical significance, while a definite self-conscious methodology of science developed regarding the place of reasoning and the whole status of rationalism.

Borelli

With this brief preamble we can study the writings of a few investigators commonly accepted as iatromechanists. We will start with Giovanni Alfonso Borelli (1608-1679), whose *De Motu Animalium,* published posthumously in 1680, is a landmark in physiology.[13] Borelli was a mathematician and not a medical man, but he developed a strong interest in physiology and he applied the principles of mechanics to the workings of the animal body.

Borelli's book is in two parts, of which the first deals mainly with gross muscular movements. This he entitled "On the External Movements of Animals," and in it he related bodily motion to the principles of mechanics. He had performed much anatomical dissection in many animal species, including mammals, birds, and fish, and his studies involved mathematical calculations as well as the principles of statics and kinetics. In all this he provided a mechanico-mathematical analysis of gross or external movements. The second part, however, "On the Internal Movements of Animals," is a true text of physiology, albeit only a partial coverage. He discussed many aspects of "animal economy" such as muscular contraction, including the role of muscle, blood, and nerve components; kidney function; secretion of bile; many aspects of digestion and nutrition; together with some pathologic states, such as fever. For our purposes the first part holds little interest, while the second part, even though only a partial text, is a splendid exposition of an influential point of view. Yet, the more we study this text, the more we can see how invalid is any sharp distinction between iatromechanism and iatrochemistry.

Borelli dedicated the book to Christina, the enigmatic one-time queen of Sweden, whose generosity helped support his researches and who, after his death, was responsible for the posthumous publication of the book. In the dedicatory preface, dated December 1679, he echoed the Platonic concept that God was a geometer. The animal body and its operations, said Borelli, are understood in terms of motion, and body and motion are the subject of mathematics. Animal functions take place through mechanical causes — the balance, the lever, the pulley, the wheel, the wedge — and the knowledge of these is wholly mathematical. God works through geometry, through which alone can we perceive the divine plan.[14]

This outspoken preface, together with the first part of the book, has given rise to what I consider a distorted interpretation. When in the second part Borelli devoted himself to studying the minute structure and function of the animal body, he showed an eclecticism, a breadth of approach, a critical evaluation of the available data that compel our admiration. He ignored most of his own flowery declamation and presented concrete evidence and the reasoning and interpretations deriving therefrom. He showed a sound respect for certain chemical principles, adapted them in some of his explanations, but rejected them in others.

When we read the first part we must keep in mind certain features. First, Borelli was not a physician but a mathematician and savant, who had studied animals and, as a natural philosopher, tried to explain the phenomena. Since at that time technology was crude, any explanations necessarily involved analogical reasoning rather than direct demonstration, and the search for logical consistency took the place of that verification of inference we demand today. To be sure, Borelli did start with observations but he built a large superstructure of hypothetics upon a small basis of fact. This, however, was the methodology of his era, and when we compare his exposition and reasoning with those of some of his followers, we are impressed by his sobriety and restraint. This will become apparent when we consider, for example, Pitcairn.

Borelli had a high regard for chemistry. He accepted certain chemical concepts and appreciated their role — admittedly to a limited degree — in explaining bodily activity. The most renowned chemists of that period were Willis, who stressed fermentation, and Sylvius, who emphasized acids and alkalis, with the ebullition that seemed related to fermentation. Borelli had great respect for the role of fermentation, and this phenomenon I will consider as the signpost, so to speak, of chemical thinking.

Borelli, under the influence of Galileo, Toricelli, and other Italian scientists, had primary interest in physics, that is, the inorganic. As a product of the new learning, he maintained an anti-Aristotelian and, where relevant, an anti-Galenic posture. In the late seventeenth century Aristotle and Galen still exerted a profound, even a dominant influence, and Adelmann's study of Malpighi vividly shows the power of the reactionaries in the 1670s and 1680s, and even later.[15] The chemists were also anti-Aristotelian and anti-Galenic. The significant intellectual battle lines were drawn not between chemists and physicists but between the pro- and the anti-Aristotelians. In this battle Borelli used the weapons of mathematics and mechanics, in which he was expert; but he did not disdain the chemical weapons as well. Where chemistry could flesh out his system of explanation, he was not adverse to such an ally.

Let us examine some of his doctrines. Muscular contraction played an important part in his overall formulations. After considering various phenomena of muscular contraction and showing that these could not be due simply to the blood, he paid attention to the structure and function of the nerves, particularly where muscular contraction attended on the will — the action of voluntary muscles. A nerve was a hair-like bundle of fine threads compacted into a membrane, and each fiber was hollow, even though it seemed solid to the eye. That the cavity is not visible proves nothing, for we cannot see the fine cavities and pores that exist in our skin, for example, or in minute insects, but we know they are there. The nerve transmits the *succus nerveus,* that very fine and subtle animal fluid. This juice or spirit, acting in the brain, stimulates the nerve. This convulsive action in the brain is transmitted through the entire length of the nerve, and squeezes out a minute quantity of the juice. But the nerve juice alone is not capable of producing muscular contractions. This requires other elements, as a sort of substrate. The combination that produces the contraction is a "fermentation & ebullition" arising from the mixture of the nerve juice with the lymph or the blood. This, he said, is similar to what is observed in chemical laboratories, and only in this way can we explain contraction.[16]

In Borelli's discussion of muscular contraction there are some important features. He claimed that he was propounding mechanics, presenting a *modus mechanicus*. He accepted chemical concepts but tried to explain them in mechanical terms, that is, in terms of particles in motion. But this, of course, is nothing more than the corpuscular philosophy. As we have seen, the corpuscular philosophy was the alternative to neo-Galenism. The real opposition lay between an explanatory schema involving forms and faculties, and the alternative involving particles in motion. There might be dispute over the precise nature of the corpuscles, the locus and ontological status of qualities, and over the character and kind of forces at work, but the progressive scientists were all dealing in corpuscular terms.

So-called chemical forces were not clearly understood and chemists tried to explain chemical action in mechanical terminology. Chemistry made progress when it attended more to discovering new phenomena and less to propounding explanation. But once a wider data base was achieved, new explanations soon came to the fore. Of course, Borelli had to use the data base then available, and we would be guilty of severe presentism if we tried to evaluate him through the concepts of a later century. He used all available data, including the phenomena of fermentation, the special domain of the chemists.

Since technical methods were often not available for direct demonstration of assertions, indirect proof — analogy — was the only available method. Borelli relied on chemical analogies.

He recognized that the inner phenomena of contraction could not be directly perceived and could be understood only through the similarity to certain chemical operations.[17] We cannot doubt, he said, that the nerve juice had a "spirituous, saline, and volatile nature" and that the blood had abundant alkaline salts. And therefore from the entrance of the nerve juice into the warm blood there must necessarily result a heat and ebullition. This momentary ebullition occurs in the fibers — the spongy tubes of the muscle fibers — and this effervescence is no different from what takes place in ordinary fermentation.

Effervescence and ebullition have great motive force. The blood within the muscles is abundantly impregnated with alkaline salts, and when the nerve juice acts on these, there takes place a sort of breaking of the bonds of the salts. The liberated particles, when the bonds have been ruptured, are able to freely exert their motive power and thus the "porosities" are instantly rendered turgid and inflated. All this Borelli called mechanical action to explain the way in which the act of will produces muscular contraction.

He realized that the explanation as offered was open to extensive objections. He enumerated five of these and then provided responses. For our purposes only three are relevant.[18] First, that this ebullition depends on the imagination, not on perception; second, that the effervescence in chemistry lasts a long time but muscular contraction can cease in a moment; and third, that contraction can take place in avulsed muscle, free of nerve impulses. The way he handled these objections is quite illuminating for the scientific methodology of that time.

To the first objection he admitted that although we do not perceive the ebullition, it can be necessarily deduced from the effect. And he referred us to a long analysis, previously given, that demonstrates the way that swelling and hardening necessarily take place when there is a violent breaking up (*incuneatione*) of other bodies. Such an ebullition occurs in the muscle even though not visually apparent.

The second objection he met by offering another chemical analogy. He pointed to gunpowder, where all ingredients catch fire and are consumed in a moment. This analogy he admitted was not exact, and then he went on to show how it could be adapted to the special case of muscular fibers and nerve, if we hold to a successive or sequential mixture of very minute amounts of the ingredients.

To answer the last objection he pointed to the nerve juice previously sent from the brain into the nerve and claimed that this acted on the residue of the blood within the pores of the muscles. In this way we can have posthumous effervescence. And to the objection, how could such minute amounts remaining in a nerve account for successive contractions over a period of hours, he fell back on a further analogy. He pointed to odoriferous substances such as musk, where extremely minute quantities can be given off, exerting an effect over large areas for many months, without any sensible diminution of the original amount.

His actual refutations are much more detailed, but this brief account provides an insight into the modes of reasoning. He ended his chapter with a proposition entitled "the necessity and the mechanical reasons [*ratio mechanica*] why that weak ebullition taking place in the muscles is able to exert an immense force." For our purposes the important term is *ratio mechanica*—he is using chemical concepts and explaining them by the action of particles in motion, obeying the laws of mechanics.

Borelli's analysis of kidney function offered broad insight into his concepts of fermentation and its role in physiology. The kidneys control the excretion of the watery humors which play an essential part relative to the solids. For example, in digestion the watery humors "mixed with the dry foods received into the stomach, aid in their maceration and fermentation."[19] Thus, the humors provide fluidity. The solid particles, he said, could not flow through narrow tubes without abundant fluid to provide lubricity. Then, watery fluids are essential for the movement of the alkaline and tartaric salts from the serum. Furthermore, the fixed salts, firmly and tenaciously bound to the fibers and porosities of the flesh, can be moved only by means of moisture.

Borelli combined mechanical and chemical thinking when he declared that "by a mechanical necessity water avidly embraces salts and retains them." By the agitation attending on the circulation, the fluids can suck out and retain the "hidden" salts. When the fluids become heavy with salts, they can be harmful. They can, by their very sharp character, irritate the membranes and sensitive nerves; and by long continued fermentation can undergo a harmful corruption inimical to nature. It is, therefore, necessary to eliminate these harmful substances. This takes place through mechanical separation in the kidneys.[20]

Here we have an important feature in Borelli's system. In the actual excretion by the kidneys fermentation does not play a part, and he demonstrated this by a detailed course of reasoning. By fermentation he understood "the internal motion of the particles comprising mixed bodies," that is, compounds, whereby the particles are moved "by either their own motive power or that of some adventitious body."[21] In the original Latin he used the same term, *motus intestinus,* so important for Willis.

He indicated two kinds of mixture—one where the components are bonded together and the other where they are merely in contact without any uniting force. Where there is a firm connection to be split, separation must take place through local motion. This, however, is not necessary when dealing with a mere aggregate, such as a mixture of millet and wheat. In chemical operations the bonds are dissolved by the motive force of fire or of an added ferment. When this has occurred, then the compounds, "the enclosed fire particles, spirits, and other self-moving parts, can freely exert their [own] motive character." The simple action of a ferment can, by its own internal motion, break up the firm bonds of "etherogenic particles, so that they are united by no other bond than simple contact."[22] Once the bonds have been broken, separation can take place, by causes such as the natural motion of gravity.

Different kinds of particles "swimming" in water would have greater or less specific gravity than the water. Borelli thought there could be a differential separation through specific gravity, which could be altered in many ways—by adding or removing igneous particles, by attenuating the saline particles, or condensing the fluid medium, or by dissolving the connections of the contained particles. Dissolution, as we have seen, may take place through internal motion or fermentation. And once the division has occurred, that is, once a chemical action has taken place, the particles spontaneously regain their proper place by virtue of their own specific gravity, and may be separated from the fluid.[23]

Clearly, Borelli had no quarrel with the chemists, for the concept of fermentation and the *motus intestinus* of particles are indeed central in his theories. There is, however, the problem whether, in any given physiological process, fermentation does in fact take place. Borelli indicated that in some actions it does, and in others it does not. Specific investigations are necessary to determine what sequence actually occurs in any given activity.

In regard to kidney function Borelli denied any fermentation, and he based his conclusions on careful reasoning. For example, fermentation cannot take place in very narrow channels but requires relatively broad ones to allow for the agitation and ebullition involved in the process.[24] This, he said, cannot occur in restricted places, such as the very narrow vascular channels found in the kidney.

Borelli made reference to a mixture of fine droplets of oil and water, where the molecules mix by simple contact, comparable to the heaping together of millet and wheat. Then he offered analogies of selective separation by physical means through pores, just as a mixture of grains can be separated through a sieve. Certain solids, such as leather or wood, permit the passage of water and oil, but not of air. Mercury can penetrate pores of gold, while water, oil, and air cannot. The fluids he mentioned can be separated from other fluids with which they are mixed and this takes place through the character of the filter or sieve. If the molecules of the fluids have a shape congruent with the small pores of the sieve, they will pass through; otherwise they will not.

Mixtures of fluids, however, can have very diverse composition, far more complex than that of simple contact. Such compounds can be broken up by fermentation, but they also can be broken up through mechanical action, without any fermentation. The molecules forcibly driven through the pores of a sieve or through funnel-like capillaries, are acted on as by a wedge, but in a sort of reverse fashion. Whereas very sharp and hard particles dilate and lacerate fragile pores, soft particles undergo contusion in passing through a narrow opening. He spoke of a fluid wedge. The particles, however much bound together, are thus separated and broken up by the force driving them through the narrow channels they must traverse.[25] Under certain circumstances, therefore, mechanical action can exert the same effect as does fermentation, in breaking down the bonds that join particles together.

In regard to kidney function, Borelli showed that there was no fermentative action in the renal glands.[26] He was not rejecting fermentation as such but only its occurrence in the kidney. First of all, the urinous material, although dispersed in the serum and contained within its very minute "vesicles," is held not by any firm bonds but only by simple contact and hence is easily separated. Since a ferment acts to dissolve firm bonds, and there are no firm bonds, a ferment would be unnecessary in the kidneys.

The separation of urinous fluid from the serum takes place through mechanical means, by way of the wedge-like action of the blood within the narrow vascular channels. Furthermore, as indicated above, ferments could not act within the extremely narrow and convoluted vessels. And then, even in wider channels, the rapid motion of the blood is inconsistent with the action of a ferment. Since blood does not halt in the "glands" but is continuously moving, the turbulent activity of a ferment cannot take place during the momentary transit. The fermentation that occurs in the stomach and in abscesses does not take place in the kidneys.

In the kidneys nature employs mechanical means.[27] The efficient cause of the separation is the vigorous movement of the blood. The more rapidly the blood flows and the more vigorous the action of the "blood wedges," the more the blood is broken up into minute particles; the urinary portions, separated from the other parts of the blood and having only a simple contact, can pass through the pores of the renal glands.

Pitcairn

Although Bellini (1643-1703) ordinarily occupies an important place in the history of iatromechanism, I will not specifically discuss his somewhat confused doctrines, of which there is an adequate exposition in Daremberg and in Brown's dissertation.[28] As a theorist Bellini stands midway between Borelli and Pitcairn (1652-1713) and for our purposes it is more illuminating to study the latter.

Pitcairn had a wide range of interests.[29] Originally he intended to enter the ministry, then he turned to law and pursued his studies in Paris. While there he became interested in medicine, and when he returned to Edinburgh he studied both medicine and mathematics. In 1675 he went back to Paris to study medicine in a more formal fashion, and in 1680 he graduated M.D. at Rheims. Returning to Edinburgh to practice, he soon became one of the leading physicians. He also established a reputation as a mathematician and became acquainted with Newton, under whose influence he remained. In 1692 he was called to Leiden as Professor of Medicine. There he remained for a year, during which time he propounded his own system of medicine, which exerted considerable influence. Returning to Edinburgh the next year, he continued practice and wrote several essays. Perhaps the most significant was his address of 1692, given at Leiden to inaugurate his professorship and bearing the title "Oratio qua ostenditur medicinam ab omni philosophorum secta esse liberam,"[30] a title which Sewell translated as "An oration proving the profession of physic free from the tyranny of any sect of philosophers." All Pitcairn's significant writings were originally published before 1700. He died in 1713.

In his dissertation Brown devoted a large portion of his study to Pitcairn, his predecessors, and his followers. This presents a large amount of valuable data but neglects the role of the chemists and the Galenists and the way they molded medical thought. Because of this limitation, Brown's conclusions must be regarded cautiously.

We may fairly ask, why did Pitcairn play such an important role at the turn of the century and for the first twenty or so years thereafter? Today we find dogmatism and arrogance in his works and a lack of critical judgment toward his own works or those of others. But these findings reflect a point of view more than 250 years removed from the events we are judging. If a physician highly esteemed in his own time seems to us rather puerile in his approach, then we are not taking into account the setting in which he found himself. We must not fall into the morass that entrapped Daremberg, for example, who judged all previous physicians by the parochial values of his own era.

Let us begin, rather, with a contemporary view, written shortly after Pitcairn's death. His posthumous *Elementa medicinae physico-mathematica* was published in 1718 and translated into English the same year. The translator provided an introduction that offers a contemporary evaluation.[31] He made the following points: that Pitcairn was the first physician "this side of the Alps acquainted with the true method of reasoning in the art of physick." Formerly there was only "a confused jargon" so that the theory of medicine was more of "a mystery than a science." To the Italians "we are obligated for the first certain light we had in the true philosophy." Galileo gets particular credit for indicating "the only sure means of arriving at the knowledge of nature and her operations; which were founded on experiment, and a mathematical way of argumentation." He thus was able "to shew the falsehood of the peripatetick principles."

In regard to England the translator praised Bacon, Boyle, the Royal Society, and especially Sir Isaac Newton, who showed "the usefulness both of all experiments and the mathematicks, in discovering the laws of things." Yet no one before Pitcairn applied "this way of inquiry" to medicine. Harvey and Lower had laid a foundation but other "theorists"—he named Charleton, Willis, and Morton—"have only abused us with new words, without any ideas," and their doctrines "have no relation to the animal oeconomy." A harsh judgment indeed.

Among the Italians Borelli was lightly dismissed but Bellini received considerable praise, especially for his *De Urinis et Pulsibus*. Pitcairn had been vastly impressed by this work and had become a staunch admirer of Bellini, an admiration that was reciprocated.

In Leiden, Pitcairn created his own system, comprehending both the theory and the practice of medicine. In his practice Pitcairn "followed the method of Riverius, one of the best of the practical physicians." For the clinical aspects he depended on Riverius, but for "the causes and methods of cure" Pitcairn "built on the Bellinian principles and the improvements he had himself raised on that sure foundation."

Pitcairn's *Elementa,* published posthumously, represents the lectures at Leiden, put together from student notes with the help of Pitcairn's own manuscripts. We must consider it, therefore, as expressing the views principally of 1692 or the years immediately following. The translator admits that in some places "the doctor might have found reason to alter his opinion, if he would have given himself the trouble of making a revisal of what he had formerly written." Nevertheless, "whatever defects or errors there may be . . . will in time be supplied and amended" by those who follow "in the same rational method of inquiry." Yet caution is urged, "since the animal system is the most complicated of any part of the universe." Hence workers should not be too hasty in forming conclusions but should imitate Sir Isaac Newton, as one who from "appearances [that is, the phenomena] investigates the laws of motion and then from those thus discovered, determines the reason of the phenomena."

These prefatory comments represent the critical valuation of 1718, several years after Pitcairn's death. The medical doctrines in the actual text, however, seem to date from 1691 and 1692. In this preface of 1718 there is emphasis on methodology, as distinct from content. Pitcairn had made errors but these, it is implied, could readily be corrected by others who would be following the same method. Mathematical analysis is highly praised, as is Sir Isaac Newton. The laws of motion were deemed the touchstone for explaining the animal economy, yet there is the caution that the animal body is complex and hasty conclusions should be avoided.

The praise for Pitcairn refers to his doctrines of the 1690s, preserved with negligible change. Ignored are later writers, particularly on the Continent, who were exerting an equal or greater influence. By 1718 the views that Pitcairn was opposing in 1692 had pretty much succumbed, and his own doctrines were being recognized as needing repairs. All this renders more significant the emphasis on method rather than on fact.

Pitcairn's methodology had several components. First there were the Baconian principles that received lip-service from the Royal Society — emphasis on empirical observation, with careful inductive reasoning and avoidance of rash hypotheses. Second, there was the specific application of quantitative methods to the study of living organisms. Although quantitative study, as such, was not new — Harvey had provided a striking example of quantitative reasoning, while Santorini showed a passion for measure-

ments—the application of more precise mathematics to physiology marked
an important departure. In this connection the work of Borelli, especially
his first part, provided a tremendous impetus, and the general acceptance
of the corpuscular philosophy in the late seventeenth century supplied the
substrate for quantitative approach.

Mathematical analysis, however, applied especially to particles in motion
and neglected the qualitative differences among bodies. Qualities savored
too much of the peripatetic philosophy and, as this declined in prestige,
qualities tended to be ignored. We must, therefore, include among the
methodological aspects a neglect of qualitative differences. And we must
appreciate the vast influence of Sir Isaac Newton, who emphasized not
only mathematical expression but the need for experiment; and for limiting conclusions to those inferences that can be directly derived from the
phenomena themselves.

Since we can take up only a few features of Pitcairn's thought, I want to
stress two aspects that, while separate, nevertheless impinge on each other:
first his views on the proper way of conducting an inquiry; and then his
concepts of digestion, which indicate his attitude toward chemistry and
illustrate his own mechanistic doctrines.

The key to his thinking lies in his inaugural address of 1692, delivered
when he took up his professorial duties.[32] I used four separate versions of
this lecture: the complete text in the *Opuscula Medica* (1714) and the
translation by Sewell and Desaguliers (1727); the *Auctoris Praeloquium* of
the *Elementa Medicinae* (1718), wherein the first twelve and a half sections
of the lecture are republished; and the translation of 1718. There are quite
insignificant differences between the two Latin versions. The two translations, however, show considerable divergence. All direct quotations of this
oration are my own translation, unless otherwise indicated.

For his general background Pitcairn depended heavily on the conjectures and data offered by others, and he chose only such aspects as fitted in
with his preconceived theories. He insinuated his own prejudices in a manner quite fascinating to follow. He wanted to demonstrate that medicine
must be mathematical and as a basis for this idea he made sweeping assertions about the dawn of medicine. The ancient physicians, he said, attributed diseases to the gods and cultivated the "science of the stars." In the
beginning the ancient physicians probably examined diseases attending the
changes of the seasons. "Consequently in the judgment of the most ancient
physicians and philosophers, medical thought ought to rest on those principles of which the astronomers make use."[33] At this time philosophers
were all of one sect, philosophical dispute had not arisen, and medicine in
its origin was not tied to any one system.

Pitcairn vigorously attacked philosophers, their doctrines, and their
quarrels, but with much obliquity in his reasoning. In the practice and

teaching of medicine, he said, nothing should be asserted as true of which we are uncertain. He seemed to demand complete assurance, with an implication that only in mathematics can this be attained. Nothing, he said, should be offered as a principle — a fundamental concept — that can induce dispute among men both learned in mathematics and free of prejudice, that is, among the only persons qualified to have an opinion. He is obviously implying that mathematical reasoning and demonstration lead to agreement, unless the persons involved are entrapped in prejudices. I would interpret this passage as praising Newton and Newtonian methodology and as making a contrast to the verbal disputes of the philosophical sects.

He continued his attack on the philosophers. Ignoring any gap in his own reasoning, he declared "from all this I conclude that the investigation of physical causes, such as philosophers are accustomed to propound, are neither necessary nor useful for medicine."[34] Indeed, the philosophers have disputed about these since earliest times until the very present.

This concept of physical causes is a principal object of his attack against traditional philosophy. "The founders of sects sought at the very outset the absolute natures and inmost causes of things, and neglected the study of properties; they used many postulates and few data," and so inevitably they propounded many different opinions. The characteristics of bodies are to be learned only by observing their actions and reactions. In contrast to the methods of the philosphers who sought the inner causes, anyone versed in mathematics, or engaged in the practice of medicine, realizes that we know nothing about things other than their relations to one another and the laws and properties of their appearances. He thus is pleading for a sort of positivist approach.

He used the word *virium,* whose meaning must be precisely understood if we want to avoid confusion. The word *vires,* in the eighteenth century translations, is usually rendered as powers, but this is utterly misleading to the modern reader. Actually, the word has a definite phenomenological sense. Pitcairn spoke of *leges virium* and the *proprietates virium,* by which he seems to mean the observed sequences of events and their characteristics. These he contrasted with *caussa physica* and *rerum natura* that the philosophers sought — the unknown something from which the *vires* derived.[35] We cannot know the *caussa* unless first the properties of the *vires* and their laws have been found out. "It follows that so long as the manifestations are unknown there is no knowledge [of the inner *caussa*], and if the manifestations are known, then that [inner *caussa*] is of no use." Physicians, therefore, should devote themselves only to discovering and evaluating the *vires* of medications and of disease and reduce these to laws and not bother about hunting for physical causes.

Pitcairn's methodology centered around these terms. Instead of the literal translation of *vires* as forces, the sense that fits into his thought should be phenomena or manifest properties or even data of observation. These contrast with *caussa,* which are not data of observation and should be rendered as inner essence or even internal force.

This distinction is significant through its reference to the neo-Galenic concepts discussed previously. The substantial form, for example, an inner essence, was thought to be the cause, the indwelling and formal cause of the phenomena attending any event or process. Pitcairn wanted to study the phenomena, their interrelations, their properties and laws, and to ignore any inner force "responsible" for the observations. There is a Newtonian ring about all this but couched in an earlier terminology. Pitcairn is attacking anything occult, anything not subject to direct observation. Hence his scorn for the "philosophers" and "leaders of sects," who inferred inner causes and principles, yet disagreed violently about them all and who wasted their efforts in idle disputes.

All this sounds quite enlightened in the empirical tradition, which in England received such an impetus from Francis Bacon. But Pitcairn, despite his lip service to empiricism, was highly rationalistic. He was constantly praising mathematics and held the astronomers as the model for physicians — again, I believe, a covert endorsement of Newton. Astronomers, said Pitcairn, in explaining the motions of the heavenly bodies, pay no attention to mere opinions and fables, however popular, but depend on observations and the phenomena of the celestial movements. Physicians should do likewise. They also should collect observations concerning diseases and their remedies and have no regard for "opinions." Opinions have less certainty than sensory perceptions.[36]

In this passage Pitcairn seems to praise the empirical approach as did Sydenham. But actually he was merely trying to eliminate what he called the fables and the popular opinions, that is, the concepts of the philosophers, from medical theory and practice. Astronomy — his model — does not rely on substantial forms, subtle matter, or fortuitous concourse of atoms. The astronomers have no concern with the opinions of the philosophical sects and do not concern themselves whether substantial forms do or do not exist, nor whether there is or is not a subtle matter.[37] He wanted to carry this over into medicine. In medicine there are the same laws as in astronomy. The nature of all bodies is the same, he said, and all bodies, of whatever size, are subject to the same concepts of motion or change. The laws governing the fluids and the canals of the human body may also be defined, after we have gathered enough observations or properly related those we have already collected.

Pitcairn provided methodological guidelines. He insisted on sensory evidence and not taking for granted what has been a matter of dispute, or what depends on evidence less certain than that of the senses.[38] He con-

demned the passion for system and the adoption of concepts resting only on
conjecture. He also criticized other viewpoints. Thus, while learned men
have eliminated occult qualities and substantial forms, they have brought
in occult ferments and pores, and this is no improvement. He could see no
real difference between unknown configurations and occult qualities, between subtle matter and astral influences. He condemned subtle matter
just as much as fear of a vacuum. In other words, he felt that the prevailing
physical concepts of the late seventeenth century were no improvement on
the concepts of the ancients and he condemned various rival theories, particularly those of the chemists and the Cartesians. He denied any ferments
in the glands of the human body, asserted that all the pores and the orifices
of vessels share the same configuration, and that the diversity of configurations and of ferments, as propounded by various sects, are useful neither in
theory nor in the practice of medicine.[39]

This early text, from 1692, written under the influence of early Newtonian thought, expressed the philosophy that Pitcairn's other writings amplified. He wanted to eliminate qualities and to reduce medical theory to a
quantitative basis as much as possible. He condemned quite impartially
the Aristotelian-Galenic doctrines and those of the iatrochemists and the
Cartesian teachings as well. Since in this lecture Pitcairn drew his analogies
largely from astronomy, he achieved an extraordinarily high degree of
abstraction.

We must examine a few concrete examples of his medical thinking. Particularly instructive is his analysis of fermentation. For Pitcairn the denial
of fermentation as a physiological process represents a key feature. In a
sense, the distinction between iatrochemistry and iatromechanism may be
epitomized by this single doctrinal feature. Pitcairn attacked the whole
concept of fermentation in several essays and from several different directions. I will discuss the subject as it relates to the stomach and digestion.

The major sources are the various studies published separately in the
1690s and collected in his *Opuscula Medica*; and also, the *Elementa Medicinae*, published posthumously in 1718 but apparently representing his
thinking of the 1690s. That ferments exist was not in dispute. The problem
was whether or not they acted in the living body. Pitcairn denied that they
did. He said bluntly, "There are no peculiar receptacles of ferments, and
no ferments at all in an animal body," a conclusion he arrived at by a process of logical reasoning.[40]

A living body is composed of canals of various kinds — the containing
parts — and the different sorts of fluids — the contained parts.[41] The functioning of the parts takes place by mechanical principles only. This is a
concept that he cannot prove. Indeed, it is a gigantic *petitio principii,* that
assumes what it has to prove.

Pitcairn's analysis of fermentation has a certain scholastic quality to it.

The food we ingest is changed into a form so that it can mix with the blood. This process takes place in the stomach and the intestines. He wanted to know what "is the most simple and natural force which can convert those parts contained in the stomach into fluids fit to circulate with the blood." How does the change come about? What is the cause? The cause, whatever it is, must not dissolve the stomach itself, nor the tissues of the animal itself. Therefore, the cause cannot be a fluid containing any ferment, for "a fluid that abounds with a ferment, or can by any means dissolve the solid ingested parts of another animal, must by the same action necessarily dissolve the parts of the vessels in the animal and the stomach in which it inheres," that is, if there were a digestive ferment, it necessarily would act on the stomach as well as the food. And since animals are nourished by ingested food, with no injury to their stomachs, it follows that such animals do not contain in their stomach any liquid which "can dissolve, digest, and convert into chyle" the ingested food. He went on, "And indeed it were miraculous if a liquid dissolving and digesting the food of the stomach, should not dissolve those parts which are not more solid than the food itself." Therefore, digestion is not performed by any ferment.[42]

Digestion requires only that the masses and particles of food be separated one from the other, so that they can serve for "nutrition of the parts." Since this is not done by any ferment, "it follows that it is only the motion of the stomach working and comminuting the food." This comminution is performed by mechanical action. Chyle is produced in the stomach and intestine but the particles of the chyle are larger than the particles in the blood, and so there is a further comminution in the lungs.[43]

The comminution in the stomach, or concoction, divided the food into parts "not differing from what they were before," except for lesser bulk — just as when coral is ground and reduced to a powder, the parts are simply small pieces of coral and "not any principle into which coral is resolved." He "proves" this by pointing to the gastric content of fish which had devoured other fish — the chyle is only "a liquor filled with the fibers of the flesh of the fish devoured." This is easily seen with the microscope which, he claimed, shows that the small parts of the fibers do not differ from the undigested parts of the fish, except perhaps in magnitude.[44]

This comminution is achieved solely by mechanical forces which do not dissolve the coats of the stomach. Worms, for example, can live in the stomach for, being alive, they can "withdraw themselves from the strokes of the stomach," which dead substances cannot do.[45]

Pitcairn considered numerous subsidiary points that, to his mind, proved the mechanical forces in digestion and militated against the concept of ferments, but it would be tedious to examine these in detail. Suffice it to point out the rationalistic approach, the reasoning from fixed premises, the dependence on fragmentary evidence, the lack of detailed empirical study or critical evaluation of evidence. The key to the method lies, perhaps, in Pitcairn's phrase with which he introduced his comments on the microscopic examination of the fish stomach. Pitcairn said, "For the proof of this matter there is no need of any other argument than . . . "[46] He would choose what fitted into his concepts and ignore everything else. This cavalier attitude toward evidence is remarkable indeed and is the key to understanding Pitcairn.

In his inaugural address of 1692 he made a bold show of praising empirical evidence and of condemning sects. But his own system represents rationalism at its very worst — as a low point from which the only direction was upward. Many of his precepts and recommendations are excellent indeed, but in his own theorizing he did not follow them. He attended only to the evidence that fitted into his preconceived ideas and this he formulated into a system buttressed with mathematical elaboration that had only a pseudo-relevance.

Before leaving Pitcairn we must examine briefly his views regarding ferments in the blood. He defined fermentation as "a mutual action of an alkali and an acid upon one another with ebullition." And with this definition it was quite apparent that there was "no real fermentation in the blood."[47] Or again, "There is no fermentation of the blood in the human body, since Mr. Boyle has shewn that there is no acid in it."[48] Furthermore, he denied Willis' basic concepts regarding "intestine motion" of particles in the blood and "proved" its absence by reasoning. There was only one type of motion, provided by the circulation and powered by the cardiac muscle. "Intestine motion," the alleged source of fermentation, did not exist.

Since the body consisted only of vessels and fluids, there was no locus for ferments to act. In a body made up only of tubes and fluids, any ferment in an organ would necessarily be washed out by the flow of blood during the circulation. There are no "receptacles of ferments," no spaces intermediate between artery and vein where ferments might act.[49]

Hostility to ferments is part of Pitcairn's hostility to any qualitative type of explanation. Ferments differ qualitatively one from the other, and Pitcairn wanted to reduce all differences to a quantitative basis. He attacked the concept of pores having different configurations. Differences in shape introduced an additional variable. He considered that all pores were circular and similar and accepted the inference that any gland could separate any humor, even those normally secreted elsewhere. In proof he pointed out that in jaundice the bile could be secreted through the glands of the skin; that excess salivation could be cured by inducing a sweat; that diarrhea could be checked by sudorifics.[50]

After reading Pitcairn's texts, we can sympathize with Haller's critique of Pitcairn as a person: "Eloquent, a man of great talent, harsh in disputations, skeptical [this seems a reasonable translation of *incredulus;* although perhaps hard to convince might be appropriate], a bitter Jacobite, trusting in his own hypotheses."[51] Haller's judgments were usually strongly biased and often malicious, but in this instance they seem accurate.

Pitcairn exerted considerable influence, even though perhaps not quite as much as Brown suggests. He represents what I would call a fanatic view, virtually a fixed idea. Remarkably lacking in critical judgment, he was perhaps the major exponent of an extreme reductionism in medicine. He wanted to reduce medicine to a mathematical science and ignore whatever did not fit into his doctrines. He did not deliberately manipulate evidence, he merely had a hugely hypertrophied blind spot.

The historian must account for his undoubtedly great influence. We can attribute this to the effective advances in physics and mathematics and also to the dissatisfaction with the qualitative viewpoint that had dominated Galenic medicine and, with different emphasis, much of chemistry. Ferments smacked of the substantial forms that were already anathema to progressive physicians. Mathematics and physics had made great progress and offered a bandwagon on which Pitcairn quickly took a leading position. But his inflexibility, his biased critical judgment indicate a great deal about the thought processes and methodology among medical leaders at that time.

Pitcairn represents one aspect of medicine in the 1690s. His views embodied the newer and progressive concepts: the ostensible rejection of Galenic qualities, especially those that were occult; the emphasis on particles in motion; the dependence of all bodily actions on the circulation; the concern with mathematics and the reliance on both experience and reason. On these, the common property of the "moderns," Pitcairn had no lien. His own special elaborations are traceable, perhaps, to his friendship with Newton, and Pitcairn represents one of the early examples of a specifically Newtonian influence on biology. But the mechanical philosophy was the common property of the learned world and not restricted to any one country or proponent.

Hoffmann

As a contrast to Pitcairn we can refer again to the early work of Friedrich Hoffmann, the *Fundamenta Medicinae,* published in 1695. This book, intended for students or, more accurately, in Hoffmann's own words, *in usum philiatrorum,* is an entire "Institutes" of medicine, with the characteristic five divisions: physiology, pathology, semiotics, hygiene, and therapeutics. He presented these in more or less aphoristic form. Hoffmann wrote in short paragraphs without elaborations—a dogmatic presentation that provides the essentials of a system but with no supporting evidence or detailed steps of reasoning. The *Fundamenta Medicinae,* almost contemporaneous with Pitcairn's *Oratio* of 1692, offers an epitome of the current medical thought as Hoffmann interpreted it. For our present purposes I will indicate some features especially relevant to the views of Pitcairn.

Medicine, said Hoffmann, is the art of "properly using physico-mechanical principles" in the interest of health. The first principles of mechanics are matter and motion and he dismissed the principles of the peripatetics and of the chemists as mere imaginings. Hoffmann adhered to the Cartesian concepts that matter existed in three forms, coarse, intermediate, and extremely subtle. Pitcairn had expressly repudiated the concept of subtle matter, but to Hoffmann this was basic. This subtle matter, on which God had impressed an immediate impulse, was the first cause of motion.[52]

Particularly important is the concept of fermentation. In this process "the finest particles moving violently in the pores of liquid bodies, do not find an outlet, and in their reaction break up the body into parts, loosen it and render it more fine." How relevant was this in physiology? Hoffmann's attitude was a little equivocal. He believed, as did Willis, that the blood had a twofold motion: one is that of the circulation; the other, "internal, is of the smallest particles reciprocally with each other." In the blood there was no fermentation "of the vinous sort that takes place in vegetable substances," but he did grant a fermentation in the sense of "the internal motion of particles which bring about the subtilization of the blood."[53]

Hoffmann thus combined chemical and mechanical concepts. He recognized different kinds of particles, with differing properties or qualities, such as spirituous, sulfurous, or saline. Moreover, the particles differed in physical characteristics such as fineness and degree of branching and also in activity.

His views on digestion contrasted markedly with those of Pitcairn. Hoffmann appreciated the chemical changes induced by saliva and pancreatic juice. He did not identify a separate gastric ferment but considered the saliva to be the source of the "gastric ferment" and the "real menstruum" of the stomach that serves for the "resolution of foods." The pancreatic juice, mixed with food, "disposes it to ready fermentation." Digestion takes place "by solution and extraction." The saliva and the pancreatic juice are the solvents that dissolve and extract the nutritious portions, but the actual separation of the chyle is due to "mechanical filtration in the intestines." Absorption, thus, is mechanical.[54]

Fermentation plays a role in digestion but not in excretion, that is, in the separation of the "excremental humors." There is no ferment that "precipitates the humors to be secreted, but all secretion of the bile, urine, sweat, phlegm, saliva, is accomplished by mechanical means and a particular manner of filtration." Hoffmann denied variation in the size and shape of pores, or any unique configuration. The pores of glands, like the orifices of vessels, are circular, differing only in width.[55]

The various humors and spirits, for example, the saliva, pancreatic juice, and nerve spirits, all come from the blood. Important here is the internal motion. Blood, said Hoffmann, has not only progressive and circulatory motion but also an internal one. "The internal motion is prior to the circulatory and on this internal motion depend the formation of spirits, strength, and energy itself." This motion is "maintained by subtle particles of elastic air."[56] And the natural heat of the body is also due to the "internal motion of the ethereal particles in the pores and interstices of the blood."[57]

The internal motion of particles in the blood, powered somehow by elastic air, was Hoffmann's version of what we today call metabolism and bodily heat.[58] The difference between circulatory and internal motions is of far-reaching import. Internal motion, which had special significance for Willis, was a means of dressing up chemical concepts in the guise of mechanics. Circulatory motion was readily observable and seemed a part of hydrodynamics. The behavior of fluids flowing through tubes of different diameters served as a model, and the laws of hydrodynamics, determined as a problem in physics, were judged to apply to the living body. Hydrodynamics was subject to quantitative formulation. It was far otherwise with intestine motion. This was not reducible to laws and quantification but remained on a qualitative basis. Intestine motion recognized some sort of qualitative specificity and postulated that certain characteristics of the blood — the production of spirits and bodily heat and energy — depended on this special kind of motion.

The concept of intestine motion revealed the defect in any simple reductionism. The primacy of motion as an explanatory principle was indeed maintained, but a special kind of motion had to be postulated, even though it could not be specifically demonstrated or measured. Since it was identifiable only by its effects, it might be compared to the occult qualities of the neo-Galenists.

This concept of intestine motion, I believe, is a crucial feature in the theories of that time. It renders untenable any rigid separation of iatromechanists and iatrochemists. Willis depended heavily on intestine motion; Pitcairn fanatically rejected it; Hoffmann, who expressly adhered to the "physico-mechanical principles," adopted it. The issue involved is much more significant than the mere application of labels or determining whether any given physician should or should not be designated as iatromechanist. The larger problem concerns the explanation of specificity, a topic basic in philosophy of medicine.

Boerhaave

Newton influenced the entire learned world, in all branches of natural philosophy, but this influence was far more intense in England (and Scotland) than on the Continent. Ideas diffuse slowly at best, even today, and at the turn of the eighteenth century the lag was vastly greater. Then, of course, on the Continent Newtonian ideas were competing with home-grown products, so to speak, such as those of Descartes and Leibniz. As we have seen, Hoffmann adhered to the Cartesian metaphysics, as did the French chemists of the seventeenth and early eighteenth centuries. In England the unassailable position of Newton and his overwhelming status had a special and not altogether wholesome effect on British medical theory. Pitcairn stands as the critical example. On the Continent a more balanced view eventually overcame the one-sidedness of the British extremists.

The major figure of continental medicine was Herman Boerhaave. His influence spread gradually and his mature views, elaborated and clarified by commentators, came to dominate medical thought during the first half of the century. At the turn of the century, however, his views had not yet become as fully articulated as they did later.

When we study intellectual currents at the turn of the century, a major document is an oration of Boerhaave, delivered in 1703 at the University of Leiden. At this time he was a man of vast promise rather than of concrete achievement. A lecturer in medicine since 1701, he was clearly destined for a professorship. Lindeboom, in his splendid biography, describes the circumstances in detail.[59] In 1703, at the beginning of his third year as lector, he delivered an oration entitled "On Mechanistic Reasoning in Medicine" (*"De usu ratiocinii mechanici in medicina"*), in which he discussed many aspects of the mechanical philosophy.[60]

He began with the significant sentence: "Mechanists are those who, by mathematical calculation based on rational premises or on observation, explain the operations [*vires*] of bodies from their mass, configuration, and velocity."[61] In this context I translate *vires* as operations, rather than properties or manifestations as I did in my discussion of Pitcairn. There is, however, the same phenomenological sense. I am emphasizing the distinction between the observations themselves and the explanation of those observations.

The science of mechanics, said Boerhaave, was recognized as useful in many areas, but only in medicine was it spurned. His thesis was that in medicine mechanics was of the utmost value and completely indispensable.[62] He developed this thesis by devoting his attention to "bodies" and their properties (*naturam corporis*) and the laws of physics that apply thereto. That is, he immediately sought utmost generality rather than remain on any proximal level or discuss the concrete properties of things.

He emphasized the validity of the mathematical method, which, starting with empirical data, can reach conclusions beyond the reach of mere observation. And, he stressed, the conclusions thus reached through reason are no less certain and no less useful than those the senses provide. Apart from these two modalities—sensation (sense data) and reason (mathematical inference)—there is no other key to reveal the special structure of the bodily machine.[63]

The same laws that explained the machines of the mathematician will also explain the human body. But for our data we must start not with products of willful imagination but with the special properties of things discovered by proper use of the senses. The body, continued Boerhaave in accordance with the accepted notions of that era, is composed of canals and the contained fluids. Then, again in accordance with the generally accepted views, Boerhaave noted those aspects of the body that revealed mechanical properties. Then he concluded from all these data that the human body is a machine whose solid parts are vessels suitable for containing, directing, changing, separating, and excreting the fluids; other solid parts served as framework and support.

After his presentation of the "modern" views based on mechanics, Boerhaave asked where was the need for the elements, qualities, forms, the chemical causes, the vital or metaphysical properties of attraction and repulsion. Where, he asked, was the need or locus or cause of so many fables? No school of thought has found any trace of such figments in the body.[64] In this passage Boerhaave indicated clearly the battle lines of doctrine. On the one side are the mechanists, who relied on reason and experience; who started with concrete sense data, not figments of the imagination; who employed mathematical reasoning, which yields complete assurance; who explained bodily activity by the laws of physics. On the opposing side are primarily the neo-Galenists, with their forms and qualities; but also the chemists, insofar as they relied on conjecture and speculation. He did not set up any special confrontation between iatromechanism and iatrochemistry as such. I suggest that his real concern was to establish a greater rigor in the methodology of medicine.

After discussing the solid parts of the body Boerhaave briefly attended to the fluids. But a fluid is only an aggregate of particles, which are solid, acting through mass, motion, and configuration. The effects produced by fluids can be studied only by the mechanician. Hydrostatics is a branch of physics. Yet this science of fluids, he admitted, had not yet been carried as far as it was capable of going, and he looked forward to the future. The phenomena of fluids, when studied by mathematics, may bring forth "better fruit in the medical garden" than anything hitherto achieved by other methods; and no one can know the vital actions of the humors who does not know the laws of hydrostatics.[65]

Chemistry is an auxiliary for medicine and can enlarge the field of observation, define certain limited conditions, and study particular phenomena. But it has only limited generality in explaining vital phenomena. The vital actions are due to the common or general action of fluids, as studied by mechanics, rather than to the individual properties of chemical studies. The essence of life lies in motion as studied by hydraulics and mechanics. However, Boerhaave did attribute a major role to ferments. If the free flow of fluids through the vessels is the cause of life, the primary reason for this motion is to be sought in the fluid itself, namely, in the "internal agitation" found only in fluids actuated by ferments. [66]

There seems to be a clear distinction between the more crude chemical activities like the reactions of acids and alkalis or of effervescence, and the more vague process of internal motion. Yet the causes of life and health (that involved internal motion) are less complex than we might think. If we had exact knowledge of the nature of the fluids, mechanics would show that they derive from very simple principles. [67]

Boerhaave had great faith that the knowledge of mechanics would unlock the mysteries of disease, and he considered specious the distinctions between theory and practice. Whoever knows the causes of perfect health will understand the origin of disease, and whoever knows the proximal causes of illness is in the best position to combat disease. Despite this close connection between theory and practice, Boerhaave admitted that the defects of the fluids had not yet been elucidated. But we must not expect that the mechanists who have applied themselves to medicine for only a short time should accomplish what all others have been unable to do in three thousand years. Boerhaave thus fell back on faith, rather than demonstration. He was cautious in predictions and looked hopefully to the future after pointing to the triumphs of the immediate past.

The whole oration is a plea for mechanics and mechanical reasoning in medicine, a forward-looking faith based on past achievements in explaining natural phenomena. With this in mind, Boerhaave gave a long description of the proper education for a physician. The student should study mathematics, confirm experiments in hydraulics and mechanics, but he also should clarify experiments in chemistry. He should regard the nature and actions of fire, water, air, salts, and other similar bodies. Chemistry was one of the important aids in acquiring a knowledge of the fluids, along with anatomy, hydrostatics, and even microscopy. [68] A physician should certainly know chemistry, even though its role in the bodily economy might be obscure, and the ultimate explanations would fall into the science of mechanics.

We must realize that Boerhaave later became one of the leading chemists of his era, and his textbook of chemistry had vast influence. When explaining health and disease in his mature medical works, he nevertheless relied chiefly on mechanical principles. This reliance appears as well in this early oration, written virtually at the turn of the century. Yet even then he kept open a door—and a fairly wide door—for chemistry.

Surely, to appreciate the history of medical thought at the turn of the eighteenth century we should avoid a sharp opposition between iatrochemistry and iatromechanism. We should think, rather, of the complex development of the corpuscular philosophy and its relation to preexisting doctrine and not be misled by the one-sidedness of Pitcairn's teachings. Above all, we should avoid the tyranny of labels.

SIX

SOUL, MIND, AND BODY

The soul has no part in modern medicine but its close relative, the mind, enjoys an honored status. Mind is definitely a part of science; soul, with its religious overtones, is not. Not too long ago, however, sacred and profane could mingle easily in the solvent of philosophy, where unity of knowledge was not an empty phrase.

By the late seventeenth century this unity tended to fragment as new knowledge developed, especially in the realm of natural philosophy. Yet despite the resulting specialization philosophers could agree that the living differed from the nonliving, that the domain of the living showed gradations from plants to animals to man, and that man differed from other living beings. Mind and matter, soul and body were distinct, yet somehow interconnected. Plotinus had described a continuum that extended from God to brute matter, a continuum that included mind, soul, angels, man, lower animals, the vegetable kingdom, and inanimate matter. Other philosophers rejected this continuum in favor of more or less discrete compartments. But the compartments refused to remain distinct, and various channels, even if poorly defined, led from one to the other.

These considerations affect any study of vitalism and the mind-body relationship as they relate to medical thought of the seventeenth and eighteenth centuries. For our present purposes I will take up in detail certain aspects of van Helmont (1579-1644) and his archeus concept, then proceed to Thomas Willis (1621-1675), and then to Georg Stahl (1660-1734). These men provided a wide range of views and were highly influential on later thought.

Van Helmont

Van Helmont was a learned physician, an original thinker, devout yet rebellious. Lacking literary skill, he enveloped himself in imagery and used a rather difficult vocabulary. As I have noted in Chapter 4, there are certain difficulties in studying van Helmont, because of the cloudy terminology and the obscurity of his concepts. The difficulties would be insuperable if we relied on Chandler's often barbarous translation of 1662, which, however, can provide the general drift of van Helmont's thought.[1] The Latin text is indispensable, even though it too is often quite opaque.

Van Helmont was an approximate contemporary of Sennert but they pursued quite different ways. Sennert, a staunch neo-Galenist, came to terms with the corpuscular philosophy, at least to a certain extent, and he served as a transitional figure for later seventeenth century chemistry. Van Helmont, however, had no sympathy with atomism. He explicitly rejected the dominant Aristotelian metaphysics, yet he disguised many Aristotelian notions in a new terminology.[2] In Chapter 4 I have discussed van Helmont as a chemist; in the present chapter I want to analyze his concepts of soul and the relationships of the living to the nonliving.

Despite his alleged opposition to Aristotle, van Helmont was a prisoner of scholastic terminology. Particularly important were the concepts of substance and accident. Substance indicated a primary existence in its own right; accident referred to what existed secondarily and dependently, through a relationship to something else. These terms had explanatory value in many contexts but led to difficulty when applied to certain physical phenomena, such as light and fire and heat. He might vary the meaning of a term according to the context, so that the sense might be idiosyncratic at one time, more conventional at another.

We find the same difficulty in regard to form and matter. Van Helmont could not avoid these terms even though he often combined them with his own special nomenclature—water, ferment, odor, seed. In his discussion of the soul and mind, he used form in various senses, for example, substantial form, essential form, and formal substance. Involved were the notions of specificity and of agency, as well as of substance and accident, mind and matter, dependence and independence.

All this is closely allied to the Aristotelian tradition. But van Helmont also had a major dependence on Neoplatonic concepts, especially in regard to hierarchy, gradation, and transition. To this we must add his nomenclature of light, seed, ferment, air, archeus. With this mixture of ideas and terms, we need not be surprised that his writings lack clarity and consistency.

Before we undertake specific exposition we must appreciate two other features that permeate his writings. Religion played a large part in his thinking.[3] Faith, based on revelation, conditioned many of his beliefs, and the glory of God was always prominent in his writings. Faith, however, had to harmonize with reason and the demands of logic. Furthermore, he was a physiologist, chemist, and above all a physician concerned not so much with the treatment of disease as with the explanation of its inner nature and its philosophic relationships. His approach differed markedly from ours. Where today a physician might discuss, say, the pathogenesis of disease within a limited framework, van Helmont mingled ontology and metaphysics with physiology, pathology, and physics. He was especially interested in the mind—its nature and functions, and its abnormalities such as "madness," delirium, rage, fever, and narcosis. Consequently, his discussion of mind has special interest for historians of psychology as well as of medicine and philosophy.

That man had a higher and a lower soul was a concept firmly rooted in Greek philosophy. Christianity had raised this view to a point of dogma, and van Helmont as a devout Christian clearly set forth this belief in an appropriate nomenclature. The higher part, immortal, comes directly from God; the lower aspect, a part of nature, comes from God but more indirectly. Van Helmont knew by faith that we have an immortal mind which surpasses all the powers of nature.[4] Mind, belonging directly and immediately to the realm of God, is not polluted by bodily contact.[5] God breathed the *mens* directly into Adam; and in the succession of Adam, God also inspired a *mens* into every fetus.

Van Helmont characterized the immortal mind as "a light-like substance, incorporeal, bearing the immediate image of its God." Here I would point to four important qualifying terms: the mind is incorporeal, it is immortal, it is "substance," and it has a light-like property. Coming directly from God, the mind is literally supernatural, above nature. In contrast there is another vivifying principle, the *anima* or bodily soul, a part of nature derived only mediately from God, existing in animals as well as man and performing vital functions. The relation between the *mens* and the *anima* requires explanation, which van Helmont furnished through reference to original sin and the fall of Adam. Before the Fall man had no lower soul, no *anima sensitiva*. It was unnecessary, for the mind performed all the vital functions. Not having a sensitive soul, man was immortal, and "animal-like darkness did not yet take possession of the intellect." However, after the Fall man became part of nature and subject to its laws; he entered the realm of the transitory and perishable. With this change in status he acquired a lower or sensitive soul that controlled the animal or natural functions, and thus there entered the death and corruption of our entire nature. After the Fall man still possessed his *mens* but this had become joined to the sensitive soul.[6]

I would emphasize the hierarchical aspect of his philosophy, its Neoplatonic heritage, and the awkward conjunction with Aristotelian concepts. A crucial passage occurs in the text, *Formarum Ortus,* where van Helmont offered a fourfold categorization of entities that include the three traditional kingdoms—the mineral, the vegetable, and the animal—and then, at the apex, man. Of the four grades the first comprises those things which have "scarcely" any manifestation of life (*vix ullam vitae manifestationem*). Here he placed stones, metals, salt, sulfur, earth, and he included decayed vegetables and dry bones. All these have their particular forms, and in all of them the form is characterized as "a certain material light preserving and imparting existence to things."[7]

This passage indicates some important ideas. Things are characterized by their forms, which provide specificity; the forms exist in a graded hierarchy, beginning with some minimal degree of life; and the forms are equated with light. The latter also exhibits degrees and gradations. Where there is "scarcely any manifestation of life," the light is also of the lowest grade.

The next highest stage of being involves nutrition and growth. Here we have the properties of plants which, while they seemed to contain the character of soul, were "vital" rather than "living." He drew a sharp distinction between the vital soul (*anima vitalis*) and a living soul (*anima vivens*). The third grade comprises animals — truly and unequivocally living and exhibiting both motion and sensitivity. Van Helmont characterized animals as having substantial forms which are substantial only in a derivative sense. Only the fourth and highest grade, which includes man, is truly substance, and to the form involved in this class van Helmont gave the name formal substance (*substantia formalis*). This never dies but has infinite duration. Angels, as well as the human mind (*mens*), the higher part of the soul, are formal substances and truly spiritual, wholly immaterial, and directly connected to God.

The concept of light enabled van Helmont to start with God, the source of light, inextinguishable, immaterial, spiritual, true substance, and eternal, and pass downward through various gradations to the world of nature. Of course, some sort of change necessarily took place in this passage, and van Helmont accounted for this through two variables. One was "luminosity" or "splendor" — that property of light providing illumination; and the other was the notion of materiality, whereby light, at first purely immaterial, acquired a certain material character — or perhaps we might say, an association with matter. The principle of life had its vital light, not true substance but only substantial form which recedes at death into nothingness, just as does the light of a candle. But the light of the mind, entirely spiritual and immaterial, is a luminous substance, a "gift of creation."[8]

In a somewhat mystical fashion van Helmont seemed to equate substance, spirit, form, and light, all of which derived from God. Each form had its own specificity and also a light. "Every form is created in its own kind by the Father of lights and is a sort of light of its own body." The forms, he went on, are distinguished among themselves not only by the degree of light but by their whole character (*tota specie*). That is, there is a qualitative specificity which somehow is related to light.[9]

In any monistic philosophy the great problem is to pass from the one to the many. Plotinus used the concepts of emanation or overflow, as well as light and radiation. Van Helmont did not use the term emanation, but he elaborated the notion of light as a means of passing from the higher to the lower, from the realm of God to the realm of nature. Van Helmont's expositions are usually fragmentary and discursive, rarely direct or comprehensive, and he leaves the reader with a sense of conjecture rather than of assurance.

The archeus involved both specificity and the internal efficient cause or indwelling source of activity. In the earlier Galenic tradition these had been included in the concept of substantial form. Van Helmont, however, as an opponent of Aristotelianism and scholastic doctrines, tried to escape their terminology wherever possible. For matter or *hyle*—the matrix of material objects in the earlier formulations—he substituted water and air as matrices. And instead of form as the specific dynamic component, he used various notions such as ferment, seed, and archeus, especially for living creatures.[10]

The archeus, source of development and activity, was related to the immaterial or spiritual realm and had special connection with metaphysical air and also with seed. In plant life the seeds were planted in the ground; for animal life the seed was the male contribution to conception. But the corporeal seed, in addition to its material husk, also had an inward spiritual essence, the archeus. Archei are multiple. In man the chief or principal archeus resides in the stomach, but other bodily functions have subordinate archei.

Van Helmont used the concept of light to tie together the various strands. Deeply immersed as he was in the Neoplatonic tradition, he had great need to establish continuity and gradual passage. And for this purpose light is excellently fitted, for it provides "luminosity" or "splendor" and these are capable of continuous gradations. To account for the specificity of living bodies, van Helmont brought together the rather vague concepts of seed, form, light, and archeus. The seed has its archeus and "in the Archeus of the seed there is contained brilliance or brightness, something like formal light." This acts as a directing force and conducts the matter to the goals appropriate to its kind. Yet we must distinguish between the light derived from God, characterized as formal light, and the splendor or brilliance which exists only in relation to nature. This latter splendor, or luminosity, comes to an end in the process of shining.[11]

Van Helmont was trying to make a distinction, but his terminology is so clouded and the words as we read them today so overlaid with the meanings of today that we have difficulty in grasping his intent. I would suggest a rough simile. Let us think of the archeus as a phosphorescent material. Then the light of van Helmont, with its divine origin, would be comparable to the incident light that acts as an exciting agent. The phosphorescent matter, after being acted on by the incident light, will under suitable conditions emit the absorbed radiation for a definite period of time, the length of which depends on various contextual factors. I suggest that in van Helmont's thought the "splendor" is comparable to the emitted light—a secondary phenomenon caused by the original incident light interacting with something else. The splendor is separable (in thought) from the incident light and will eventually get extinguished, to recede into nothingness. This splendor, still immaterial, is less substantial, that is, less independent than the incident light, which has primary status.

I would, therefore, interpret van Helmont in this sense: form and light, intimately connected, had a high ontological status. The light (of divine origin) interacted with the archeus in the seed and bestowed splendor or brilliance that have a lower ontological status, inasmuch as they are a phenomenon of nature—the realm of the transitory and the mortal. Nature receives its differentiation (*distinctiones specificas*) from the "formal light."[12]

At death the immortal soul returns to the realm of pure mind and the world of ideas and forms—the intellectual realm of Plotinus—unemcumbered by body. But so long as the mind is tied to the body, the light of the mind has limited penetration and the intellect is limited to the forms as they are embodied in nature. Thus, as long as a man is alive and his immortal *mens* is associated with the lower or sensitive soul, there is sharp restriction of intellectual powers, but a restriction dissolved at death.

In the vegetable kingdom each seed has an archeus that remains dormant until the seed is planted. Then the seed swells with moisture and acquires a ferment and ripening.[13] The process of ripening and softening, mediated by moisture, heat, and the archeus, also involves odor and taste and air, construed in their metaphysical senses. Such an intermingling of concepts had a more or less empirical basis derived from quite different phenomena, for example, the heat and gas formation that attend decaying vegetation, or the luminescence sometimes seen in rotting wood. Heat, gas, light, and odor were thus implicated in vital activity. In Helmontian terminology the air, receiving a moderate heat, gradually brings the perfection of the archeus and a disposition of forms. Air, odor, heat, moisture, gas, light were all data of direct observation. The archeus, not directly observed, was a concept that tied together all the others.

What is true of vegetables, van Helmont judged even more clearly applicable to the eggs of fish, birds, and reptiles; and especially to the "seed" of quadrupeds. Light is an intrinsic and essential part of this process. "At length a delicate, shining, and glittering light kindles the *aura* of the aforementioned Archeus, so that it may thus become vital."[14] Various factors cooperate in the generation of living creatures and light has a special role of agency.

While the reasoning process here is perhaps difficult to follow, we should realize the interaction of preexisting theory with concrete observation. Van Helmont had observed various aspects of fermentation and decay, heat formation, gas formation, along with germination of seeds. Lacking the means for critical differentiation in our modern sense, he lumped together various phenomena that we would keep sharply separate. He could not distinguish between the germination of seed and the fertilization of ova. In his attempts to clarify the obscurities he relied on his metaphysical framework in which forms, light, ferments, odors, and similar concepts had special status.

For our immediate purposes I would emphasize the role of light, affecting the archeus, which it somehow kindled into its own activity; making it "vital" instead of dormant and involving it with the forms appropriate for the particular species of life. Since the light comes directly from the Father of lights, we have a direct connection between the spiritual realm and the world of nature.

Only the light deriving directly from God has this vivifying power, which is absent in light of purely earthly origin, such as the luminescence noted sometimes in rotting wood, or in some salts, or in the sea itself. Since the "splendor" of this earthly light derives its force from nature alone, it can never result in a "vital light unless the Creator adds a specific form of light as an effective essence." This is the life of a thing, or the form, in the absence of which a fetus degenerates into a shapeless mass or a monster or else putrefies. As long as vital air and its "splendor" are present, the fetus grows. It will, however, be corrupted and soon putrefy if there is a "failure of the formal and vital light, that brings into unity the various subordinate properties." Wherefore, van Helmont continued, "only the Father of lights immediately establishes the lights of forms and the forms of lights."[15]

The archeus and the seed exert a dynamic control over the body. The human body, said van Helmont, cannot give itself a human configuration. This requires a "sculptor," enclosed in the seed, an agent, fully immaterial and yet fully real, that impresses its own image and configuration on the body. The dynamic agent is the *anima,* which, among its other functions, preserves the character of the species. All this takes place in the realm of nature. The human *mens,* although above the laws of nature in its origin, becomes subordinate to these laws "as soon as it crosses the threshold of nature" and becomes associated with the *anima.* It would be absurd, thought van Helmont, that the process of generation should take place without the cooperation of the mind. The Creator joined an immortal mind to the sensitive soul which thereby became specifically determined to a human individual, in contrast to a brute animal. The mind and soul were not united, nor was there any penetration, but only an irregular contact. In a further treatise van Helmont again described the relationships between the sensitive soul and the mind and partly summarized some of his previous views.[16]

In van Helmont's writings an important feature concerns the seat of the soul. As we have seen, the animal soul serves as the host to the immortal mind, so that the two, while metaphysically distinct, are functionally related. Van Helmont rejected the idea that the soul is located either in the heart or in the brain. Instead, on empirical evidence, he placed the site in the cardiac end of the stomach. In the treatise, "A Mad Idea," he described experiments that convinced him of this.[17] Experimenting with poison, he had ingested small amounts of aconite (*napellus,* wolf's-bane). He described the sensations. Contrary to the accustomed mode, he declared, he understood, conceived, tasted, or imagined nothing in his head, but perceived clearly and constantly that the entire functioning was taking place in the precordium and spreading around the orifice of the stomach. Even though he felt that sense and motion were extending from the head to the whole body, yet the whole faculty of speech was clearly in the precordium, to the exclusion of the head.

His experience was ineffable. To quote a bit of Chandler's translation: "That sense whereby I did perceive that I understood and imagined in the midriff [*precordiis*], and not in the head, cannot by any words be expressed."[18] Yet he insisted that he was not in a state of ecstasy, a state with which he admitted having had some experience; nor was he sleeping or dreaming or in any way ill. While the experience had its origin in a poison, he had taken only a very small amount. The whole experience, he said, passed off and although afterwards he took aconite again at different times, that particular experience never returned. Thus, for the space of two hours he perceived that nothing was acting in his head but that in an indefinable fashion the whole soul clearly was carrying on its thinking in the precordium.

This "illumination" in regard to the seat of the soul carried complete conviction for van Helmont. I would point to the similarity with the experience of Samuel Hahnemann and the illumination by which he conceived his homeopathic doctrine of *similia similibus curantur.*[19] Hahnemann, too, was experimenting with drugs, he too had a particular reaction, he too achieved his insight on the basis of one experiment.

Once convinced that the seat of the soul and the mind was in the precordium, van Helmont could find ample evidence to support this claim and to elaborate the concept. He discussed the problem in several treatises and he provided much fragmentary evidence bearing on this concept. This evidence concerned the localization of sensation around the stomach, with inferences regarding the functions of this organ. For example, he pointed out that in sudden sharp stimuli or strong emotion, the first reaction is perceived around the stomach. The unexpected noise of a gunshot or sudden bad news are first perceived nowhere except in the precordium, "that central site [*hospitio*] of the soul."[20]

If the stomach is disordered there is pallor, trembling, consumption (*siccitates*), atrophy, gripes, asthma, jaundice, paralyses, contractures, dizziness, apoplexy, and so on. The archeus, located in the stomach and controlling its functions, carries the responsibility for these various ailments. With the stomach van Helmont associated the spleen, which he thought had close vascular connections with the stomach and contributed a ferment thereto. The stomach and the spleen together constituted the *duumvirate,* the central seat of the soul.[21]

In a manner that foreshadows Broussais (1772-1838), van Helmont devoted considerable attention to the relationships between digestion and various functions of the body, especially nervous and mental disorders. He seemed especially concerned with dizziness, apoplexy, and nightmares, and their relation to disordered gastric function.

To be sure, the brain had its own special functions. It was the "executive member" for the conceptions of the soul and presided over nerves and muscles, as well as the faculties of memory, will, and imagination. Although the *anima* has its seat in the precordium, the power of memory is in the head, and the power of will in the heart. These functions represent the companions of the *anima*. This animal soul, even though it is the bond of union of the mind in the precordium, yet distributes its powers through different organs. Vision is in the eye, taste in the tongue, and touch widely distributed — these are all powers of the perishable or animal soul.[22]

Van Helmont emphasized the primary role of the stomach in various conditions that at first glance might seem to center in the head. He also stressed the importance of directing therapy to the stomach and spleen, the primary locus of disturbance, rather than to the head, which, so to speak, was only secondarily affected.

Through examples of madness and mental disorder van Helmont expounded the relations between the *mens* and the *anima,* especially as occasioned by outside causes. The bite of a rabid dog, for example, exerts its effect on the sensitive soul which "touches" the *mens*. In this process, as we have seen, light is a factor in the interaction. When a rabid animal pierces the skin with its teeth, even slightly, soon the mark (*symbolum*) of rabies is propagated in the light by which the mind and the sensitive soul are in contact.[23]

But the immortal mind is not really affected by rabies or madness or mental disturbance. These represent the affections of the corruptible and mortal *anima*. Similarly, the mind is not affected by melancholy or by changes in the phases of the moon; the mind does not get drunk nor contract madness from the bite of a rabid animal or a tarantula; rage and mental alienation are not the properties of the mind. To explain the appearances to the contrary, van Helmont declared that the mind, weary of the body, appointed the sensitive soul as its "delegate." Elsewhere he said that the *anima* takes over the activity of the mind, which consents to this process.[24]

Van Helmont glorified the immortal mind and its relation to God, but the ordinary workings of the mind, especially in disease and in physiological disturbances, are actually in the control of the lower soul, the *anima*. The *mens* recedes into an abstraction. So far as medicine is concerned, the normal functions of the *mens* do not receive any precise analysis but all the various abnormal states are attributed to causes acting through the mortal *anima*.

When we study van Helmont, we are impressed by his remarkable versatility, involving speculative philosophy, religious beliefs, and what is often called mysticism, together with natural history, physiology, and medical theory. His obscure terminology and the infelicities of the English translation have discouraged detailed study, yet his influence on the history of ideas and his place in the development of medical concepts are slowly being appreciated.

Thomas Willis

Thomas Willis (1621-1674), whom we have already met as a leading iatrochemist of the seventeenth century, was also an outstanding anatomist whose fame rests principally on his investigations of the brain and nervous system. His excellent anatomical studies he published in 1664, under the title *Cerebri Anatome*. As an active medical practitioner, with special interest in nervous and mental diseases, he also published influential works on these topics in 1667 and 1670.[25] In 1672 there appeared his important book that expounded not only comparative anatomy and physiology but also psychology and metaphysics, and in addition contributed to clinical medicine, especially in the realm of nervous and mental diseases. This work, the *De Anima Brutorum Exercitationes Duas,* provides the clearest and most significant exposition of contemporary doctrine concerning the nature of mind and its relationship to body. The English translation of Pordage, (1683), often obscure, requires reference to the original Latin.[26] The extensive secondary sources are fairly well covered in Isler.[27]

Willis, clearly influenced by atomism and the mechanical philosophy, was reacting against both the substantial form and any type of archeus doctrine. He held to "corporeity" of the soul or animating principle, but he was careful to define what he meant. He had to distinguish between the material body, the realm of physiology in the narrow sense, and what we call psychology, which concerns the immaterial. We see an interesting combination of traditional attitudes that involved neo-Galenism and religious orthodoxy, joined with the new investigative sciences, which try to separate religion and science.

One major stumbling block that the new science had to face was the concept of goal, purpose, and final cause, all implicit in the substantial form and intimately tied into the Aristotelian philosophy. The Aristotelian formulations were being totally discarded in physics. The corpuscular philosophy, so satisfactory in physics, was carrying over into biological sciences. Experimental investigations were rapidly providing new data. How to explain them? To what extent could the new be harmonized with the old? How much of the old had to be relinquished? What new formulations were necessary to "solve the phenomena"? These are some of the overall questions that Willis faced. Fortunately, his expositions and arguments, unlike those of van Helmont, follow a fairly orderly course.

At the very beginning Willis made clear his central doctrine: the soul that is common to brute animals and to man depends altogether on the body. The new discoveries regarding the structure of the animal body called for new discussions regarding the *anima* or soul. This is entirely dependent on the body, is born and dies with it, actuates its separate parts, is co-extensive with it, and seems to be totally corporeal. He did make some concession to contrary views by first surveying a variety of different opinions. Yet, while touching lightly on the differences, he was not argumentative. After the brief survey he declared that "it now remains to indicate my own opinions or rather, in an affair of such difficulty, my conjectures."[28]

Willis pointed to various sense modalities and bodily functions. There is no medium, he said, between body and soul, but the various members and parts of the body are all "organs" of the soul. Therefore, he asked, must we not believe that the soul has many distinct and extended parts to actuate the different members of the body? The soul can be divided with the body and exercises its separate functions of sense and motion even when so divided. This we see in worms, eels, and vipers, which, when cut in pieces, will still respond to stimuli. Here Willis was equating *anima* with what later was called irritability — the capacity of an organism to receive stimuli and respond to them. This responsiveness, he assumed, results from a vivifying principle called soul. Responsiveness is thus judged a function not only of the whole body but of individual parts thereof. And since this property may remain, at least for a while, in separate portions, the soul is clearly not only extended but divisible.

At this point we may refer again to the doctrine of substantial form as Sennert expounded it earlier in the seventeenth century. The substantial form was alleged to exist entire in the whole organism and also in every part. In addition, each part had its own special and characteristic form, which was also under the control of the overall form. And a similar relationship applies to the *anima*.

In the very beginning of his text, in the first paragraph of his preface, Willis made clear that the animal soul, responsible for sensation and motion, and having extension and parts, is quite distinct from the rational soul of man, and subordinate to it. Man, he said, is thus a two-souled animal. We must keep the material soul, common to man and animals, separate from the superior rational soul, immaterial and immortal.

Willis discussed at some length the properties of the soul of brutes. One great problem, of course, concerned its composition. If it is material, of what is it composed? Willis likened it to the nature of fire, extremely subtle and moveable. As with flame, the soul required a twofold food — a sulfurous substance and a nitrous substance. The animal soul, he said, has a twofold locus: in the vital fluid or blood circulating through the heart and vessels; and in the "animal liquor," or nerve fluid existing in the brain and flowing through the nerves. That aspect of the soul that inheres in the blood is comparable to a flame; the aspect within the nerves, to rays of light emanating from a flame. The soul is not constituted of blood and nerve juices but "inhabits and graces with its presence both these provinces." Regarding the soul as fire, Willis noted that in cold-blooded animals, or others "less perfect," perhaps life is not a flame, but nevertheless it is a "most thin heap of subtil particles, and as it were fiery," which agitates and actuates the members of the body.[29]

The particulate matter of the soul is not fortuitously gathered together. As soon as matter is "disposed to animation"— which takes place by a law of creation and never by mere fortuitous concourse of atoms — then the "soul, which is the *form* of the thing, and the body, which is called matter, begin to be formed under a certain species or kind, according to the model or form impressed upon them."[30] The characterization through form and matter seem inescapable. Forms, somehow, are impressed on matter. Matter is constituted of atoms. Forms, in the sense of patterns, seem to be part of eternal nature but are not subsisting entities.

Willis went on to amplify this notion, indicating that the soul, while corporeal, arises "with the body, out of matter rightly disposed," and receives its essence (or essential nature — *hypostasin sive substitentiam*) "according to the Idea or pattern foreordained to it, by the law of nature."[31] The soul, imperceptible to the senses, can be known only by its effects. When life becomes extinct the particles of the soul are dissipated, leaving no trace. Then the body quickly becomes subject to corruption. I would emphasize this formulation in reference to the doctrines of Stahl discussed later.

As soon as the soul actually exists, it performs two chief functions. First it frames the body as its domicile, and then, when that body is wholly formed, renders it suitable for whatever uses are necessary, whether for the species or the individual. And for these uses the soul is provided with various faculties and instincts.[32] These comments will take on especial significance when, in the next chapter, I discuss birth defects and the *anima* as the architect of the body.

Different souls exert different powers and faculties according to the character of the animal. Willis, noting various classes of animals, provided a splendid chapter on comparative anatomy that describes the structure of insects, annelids, crustacea, fish, birds, and mammals. All, whether bloodless, cold-blooded, or warm-blooded, possess souls.

The corporeal soul activates the blood and the nerve juices; within the blood it is kindled like a flame; it spreads through the animal juices like a light, and to perform the animal function is reflected and refracted through the brain and nerves. Willis spoke in figurative language to describe the concepts of flame and light, the former corresponding to what we would call metabolic activity, the latter to the functioning of the nervous system. But in addition there is a third aspect, an outgrowth of the "vital flame," which concerns generation. This component, growing in the blood, is chiefly light, collected especially within the genital organs, and is like a little flame, capable of kindling a further flame in a new body.

The vital flame is not destructive; instead, it "burns with a gentle and friendly heat, like a fire shut up in a *balneo Maria*."[33] This flame is subordinate to the animal soul, as to a higher form. Instead of totally destroying the blood, it acts selectively, burning some particles, letting others go. The most subtle particles — the animal spirits — are distilled into the brain and cerebellum. They then enter the cortex, to flow down the medulla and spinal marrow and then through the nerves into the entire body. The passages they traverse are wonderfully complicated.

The sensitive part of the soul, concerned with the nervous system, is extended and divisible, just as is the part having to do with the blood. The subtle particles, the "constitutive parts of the sensitive soul," are responsible for the animal functions and comprise the "hypostasis" or essence of the soul itself (*ipsiusque animae hypostasin constituere*).[34] The precise shade of meaning that we should attach to hypostasis is not clear. Pordage simply transliterates the word without attempting any translation. To me it implies an essence, not synonymous with the whole but only a core. We cannot say that the sensitive soul *is* the spirits, any more than that the corporeal soul *is* the blood. There seems to be some indefinite residue in addition to the core, but the character of that residue remains unknown.

While the animal spirits constitute the hypostasis of the animal soul, it is not easy to explain just what these spirits are, according to their own essence. As Willis phrased it, there is hardly anything in nature to which they are comparable in all respects. The chief mode of explanation was through analogy, and if a good analogy was not available, then explanation faltered and the topic remained obscure. The animal spirits are not comparable to chemical agents, such as the spirits of wine or of hartshorn, which are far less subtle. The animal spirits he compared rather to rays of light emitted from a flame, like the rays intermingled with the air and wind.[35]

Since the spirits are especially related to the brain and nerves, Willis devoted his principal attention to the structure and the functioning of the nervous system. His text is a major contribution to the anatomy and physiology of the nervous system and the relations of the nervous system to mind and its various functions. While detailed consideration of these aspects falls outside the scope of this study, I will mention a few features. Willis carefully distinguished sensory from motor function. The sensory components, consisting of images (*icones, sive, simulacra*) were carried through the nerves as through tubes, and then to the *corpora striata,* and then were represented on the corpus callosum, as on a white wall — apparently a reference to the camera obscura. From there they go to the cortex, where they constitute memory.[36] The motor aspects take place through a sequence involving imagination, memory, and appetites, that is, desire or propensity or attraction, or an "implusion toward or away from," with the animal spirits as the instruments and the nerve tubes as the pathway. And if there is a blockage or hindrance, then some function is inhibited.

In this framework it is obviously important to study the different pathways. To use Pordage's quaint translation, "Who can sufficiently admire the innumerable series of nervous fibers . . . in which the animal spirits, like soldiers sent abroad, perpetually running up and down, on this side and on that, perform the offices of sense and motion. Further, those who dwell within the head it self, the superior legion of the sensitive soul . . . lye not disorderly or loosely, but its numerous company, being limited with certain bounds and cloysters, as it were within the narrow space of one chamber, perform infinite variety of actions and passions."[37]

Willis took up in detail some properties of the corporeal soul. Regarding its origin, he declared that a "heap" of subtle atoms or of animal spirits, a "little animal soul, not yet kindled" lies hidden in the seminal humor.

When it finds a suitable hearth, a soul is kindled by the parents, just as a flame is kindled by another flame. This new soul gradually unfolds and agitates and kindles the available matter, which it forms "into an archetypal configuration ordained by the law of creation." The soul thus fashions the body according to the goals and the forms, according to the original types ordained by divine providence.[38]

The soul preserves the body from putrefaction, while in reciprocal fashion the body contributes to the soul and nourishes it. In brutes the soul has certain innate dispositions, such as the ability to select proper food, defend itself, and propagate its species. And this soul, to which corresponds the inferior soul of man, may be affected by ailments, and its flame does not always shine uniformly. However, the topics of pathology and disease we need not consider.

Man has also a rational soul, which exercises reason, judgment and will. It presides over the lower soul and regards the images and impressions made manifest to the lower soul, as in a mirror. Although brute animals do not have a rational soul, yet they do seem to have some degree of inferior reason. Willis is a little hard put to explain this. He rejected the concept that animals have an immortal soul. To explain the apparently rational behavior of animals, Willis had to fall back on divine action. God ordained that "from the soul and body mixed together, the same kind of confluence of the faculties doth result, by which it is needful for every animal, to the ends and uses destinated to it."[39]

He gave an interesting analogy. Comparing the minds of animals and of man, he offered the metaphor of a pipe organ. It is not remarkable, he said, that the wind makes a rude sound when it passes into a pipe. But we are rightly amazed when the hands of a musician, manipulating the organ, produce wonderfully harmonious and varied music. This results from the activity of a musician. Nevertheless, a mechanical contrivance, run by water power, may produce tunes sometimes equal to those performed by art. The rational soul of man, governing and directing the animal spirits, is comparable to the musician. The soul of brutes, lacking the rational soul, resembles the water-powered organ, which acts by laws and rules, according to certain prescribed and necessary ends.[40]

Animals exhibit an implanted disposition ordinarily called instinct, which dictates not only many simple actions but also many of great complexity. But in addition to their instinctive knowledge, brutes may also learn by experience, that is, through sense impressions, memory, and imagination. Brute animals can even form certain propositions from which they draw conclusions. Many actions probably resulted first from accident and then, by repeated experience, passed into habits which seem to show "very much of cunning and sagacity." Animals learn by example and by imitation. Instinct and acquired knowledge become mixed together. The most complex actions of brutes may thus be explained by reduction to "appropriate principles" of the sensitive soul.[41]

The distinction between the sensitive soul of brutes and the rational soul of man was a crucial one, involving both biology and metaphysics. In his important chapter 7 Willis compared the corporeal soul of brutes with the rational soul of man. The former is limited in its scope. It embraces the relations of material things, whereas the rational soul embraces abstractions—the immaterial—and also has the power of apprehension and discourse.

In regard to the corporeal soul, he called the "knowing faculty" the fantasy or imagination. This exists in the mid-region of the brain (*cerebri meditullio*) where it receives the sensory images. It apprehends things according to their external appearances. Since appearances can obscure or distort the true nature of things, the fantasy or imagination is often deceived. In man the intellect presides over the imagination, discerns and corrects its errors, and from particulars can derive universals and abstract concepts, distinguishing substance from accident and achieving universals like humanity, rationality, corporality, or spirituality. Going further, it can consider God and the angels, infinity and eternity, and other ideas remote from sense and imagination. This capacity to frame metaphysical concepts beyond all sensations demonstrated to Willis that the rational soul is immaterial and immortal. If it were material, he declared, it could conceive nothing incorporeal.[42]

In comparison with man animals are capable of minimal reasoning, but in man the reasoning powers are unlimited. The human reason can make deductions that transcend sense perception; can achieve axioms and the laws of logic; find causes; learn the mathematical relationships; create the arts and sciences and the "laws of political society"; make wonderful mechanical inventions and stupendous structures; and, of course, the rational mind of man can understand that God is infinite and eternal, that angels inhabit the world, that there is a heaven and a lower region, and other spiritual concepts. When compared with the functions of the human intellect, the degree to which brute animals can reason and deliberate "will hardly seem greater than the drop of a bucket to the sea."[43]

With this comparison Willis indicated the vast difference between the animal soul and the rational soul. The differences are not merely quantitative but also qualitative. The animal soul is material, the rational soul immaterial, immortal, and relates directly to God. The material, corporeal, and corruptible soul has at best only an indirect relationship to God.

The problem then arises concerning the relations between the two kinds of soul in man. Willis approvingly quoted Gassendi, who maintained that the rational soul is an incorporeal substance created by God and infused into the body as an "informing form." Willis also accepted the traditional religious view of the tripartite nature of man: he has a body; an animal life common to man and the brutes; and thirdly, "spirit, by which is signified the rational soul, at first created by God, which being also immaterial, returns to God." Man is midway between angels and brutes, communicating with both — with the latter through the corporeal soul, with the former through the "intelligent, immaterial, and immortal soul."[44]

The relationship between the two souls raises further problems. The animal soul involved the entire body, while the rational soul related particularly to the head. Willis gave various reasons why this should be so, derived partly from Gassendi, partly from his own reasonings. Among his arguments: it is not necessary for the entire corporeal soul to be occupied by the entire rational soul. The latter, purely spiritual, dwells as on a throne, within the brain, along with the imagination. Any image or sensory impression of which we are conscious is carried to the imagination. The intellect most easily exerts its rule when presiding in this "imperial throne."[45] Quoting Gassendi, Willis indicated that a king need not be all over his entire kingdom, but only in his palace. The intellect need not attend to those functions carried out entirely by the corporeal soul (that is, what we call the autonomic functions).

The rational soul plays a peculiar role in the bodily economy. For its operation it depends on the imagination (or "phantasie"). This word, of course, has numerous meanings but in the context there is a quite literal denotation, namely, the function that has to do with images. The imagination is the end point, so to speak, of the sensory chain whereby sense impressions (acting on the animal spirits) are carried to the striate bodies and then affect the imagination. All this takes place by physical means. The rational soul "will stay and preside in the court of the phantasie . . . because, whil'st in the body, it depends very much, as to its operation, on the phantasie, without the help of which, it can know or understand nothing. For it draws its first species [that is, sensory data] and fundamental ideas, by which it rears all its manner of knowledge, from the imagination."[46]

Obviously, intellects vary. One man is more capable of reasoning and understanding than is another. The essential difference lies not in the respective rational souls, but in the respective brains and imaginations. "Every disparity concerning the intellect, proceeds immediately from the phantasie, but mediately and principally from the brain": the intellect depends on the imagination and this depends on the brain. And if the brain has a bad conformation, making the spirits more dull, or if there is some other impedence, then the *phantasmata,* that is, the presentations to the imagination, are either lacking or distorted. If the intellect fails, the fault lies in the absence of *phantasmata* or else their imperfection.[47]

The concept of a rational soul enabled Willis to maintain contact with religious dogma and the prevalent metaphysics. The rational soul is immaterial and immortal, created by God, united to the body as its "informing form." It is not propagated in the ordinary fashion as is the corporeal soul, but is created by God and "poured" into the body.[48] On the other hand, the rational soul has a definite place in scientific studies, for it helps explain the observed features that eventually formed part of the science of psychology.

Unfortunately, these two distinct kinds of soul tend to run a collision course. And to avoid collision, Willis had to whittle away at the functions of the rational soul, whose properties he relegated more and more to the animal soul. This we see in the problem of inheritance, where a son resembles his father in personality, talents, and mental and emotional endowment. All these endowments Willis attributed to the animal soul. If a son resembles the father in these respects the similarity has nothing to do with the rational soul, which God created, but only with the animal soul, which is material.[49]

The rational soul has a special identity in regard to the will. Traditionally, there was always an opposition between "the will, which proceeding from the intellect, is the handmaid of the rational soul; and the sensitive appetite, which cleaving to the imagination, is the hand or procuress of the animal soul."[50] Thus did Willis express the age-old conflict between the passions and the intellect. The intellect, regarding the perceptions of the animal soul, arranges and orders them according to its will; it perceives all desires and passions in the imagination and governs them. Some it approves, others it rejects; others it will stimulate or else calm down. But the corporeal soul does not necessarily obey the rational soul and hence we have conflict and strife. Willis elaborated on this traditional conflict between the flesh and the spirit — the lower soul and the higher, the animal and the rational. But he pointed out that his discussion of the rational soul was really quite incidental to his main purpose and he eagerly returned to consideration of the corporeal soul, its actions and its passions.

The remainder of his treatise studies the anatomy and pathology of the nervous system and some of the diseases related thereto, including emotional disturbances. He had written a landmark study of the brain and its normal and abnormal functioning, but the rational soul, the immaterial component of man, really gets short shrift.

Willis, who combined a mechanistic philosophy with Aristotelian concepts, shows an intermingling of different intellectual strands. While he emphasized traditional views he veered slowly to mechanism without giving up the importance of the immaterial. When we study Willis and his precursors and successors, we see clearly the futility of pursuing any schema of paradigms. Instead, we should regard the intellectual history of science and of medicine as a sort of contrapuntal activity and we must trace the different themes, with their variations, that course through the whole.

Georg Stahl

As a scientist and philosopher, Georg Ernest Stahl (1659-1734) was all too often on the "losing side." For example, much of his contemporary reputation rested on the concept of phlogiston. When this became untenable after the discovery of oxygen and the work of Scheele, Priestley, and Lavoisier, Stahl became identified with a discredited viewpoint. Then, his medical system rested on the concept of vitalism, which came under sharp attack as biological science progressed. "Soul" as a biological force lost favor, and Stahl suffered accordingly. Yet while the main current of biological research shunted Stahl into a sort of backwater, his views have been extremely significant in the history of ideas, even if not in the mainstream of biological research.

When we try to evaluate Stahl, we realize that he was primarily a chemist and a practicing physician, and only secondarily a speculative philosopher. Yet his medical doctrines rested on his metaphysics, and only if we study his basic philosophy can we achieve any sympathetic understanding of his biological concepts.

We do not really know much about his personal life. Even the year of his birth is obscure. While most historians give the year as 1660, Gottlieb claims that the parish register in the town of his birth (Anspach, Bavaria) indicates 1659.[51] About his early life we know little. He studied medicine in Jena, received his degree in 1684, and attained considerable reputation in chemistry. For seven years he was court physician in Weimar until, at the invitation of Friedrich Hoffmann, he joined the medical faculty of the newly founded university at Halle in 1694. In 1715 he left Halle for Berlin, where, as court physician, he remained until his death in 1734.

Stahl's personality has been condemned as harsh, intolerant, and narrow, but Gottlieb emphasizes that much of the unfavorable evaluation rested on the impressions of Albert von Haller. Perhaps much of Stahl's personality emerges from what, according to Gottlieb, was his personal motto: *E rebus quantumcumque dubiis quicquid maxima sententium turba defendit, error est.*[52] For this I suggest the following: "Insofar as there is doubt, whatever the greatest mass of opinion maintains, is wrong."

While Stahl's real personality may remain uncertain, there is no doubt whatever that he was an outstandingly bad writer. Early in the nineteenth century an admirer admitted that his style was "dry, hard, perplexing; the diction is defective, very obscure, bristling with redundant particles and scholastic terminology. The reader is discouraged and is tempted to abandon the book; but just as with a difficult puzzle, if we return to it several times we finally find the answer; so too if we return often to Stahl we succeed in penetrating to his thought and, so to speak, in surprising his secret."[53]

In the present chapter I will make no effort to present the overall doctrines of Stahl nor to cover the extensive literature. In previous studies I have analyzed various aspects of his work and indicated the major primary and secondary sources.[54] Here I only want to consider some of the metaphysical concepts as they relate to topics in this chapter.

Lemoine, writing in 1864, tried to make a distinction between Stahl's vitalism and his animism, but this will not stand up under a rigorous critique.[55] Yet this attempted distinction, resting on a loose usage of terms, indicates several facets of Stahl's thought that should be made more explicit. Stahl's system depended on the concepts of soul, mind, and intelligence, complex terms overlaid with centuries of accretions. He used these concepts in what to us seems a simplistic fashion; many aspects that we would want to query he simply ignored or treated very lightly. His usage of mind, reason, or intelligence was by our standards fuzzy in the extreme, while soul combined theological and psychological components in a quite confused fashion. Yet he had certain insights that, when translated into a more modern terminology, have a significance that the older terminology might obscure.

Stahl made a sharp distinction between the living and the nonliving, and then he devoted a great deal of attention to characterizing the properties of the living. His thought centered around several key concepts: *integration* —the concern with wholes rather than with parts, with synthesis rather than with analysis; *organization*—the subordination of parts in an ordered fashion so that the parts take their significance as they relate to the whole; *control*—integration and organization, which imply an active agency; *immanence*—the active controlling agent as an indwelling force within the organism; *goal* and *purpose*—features essential for understanding vital activity; these in turn presupposed *foresight,* which in turn implied *intelligence.* If we use this vocabulary, Stahl's thought has more relevance to today's problems than might otherwise appear.[56]

Stahl's terminology emphasized the contrast between the material and the immaterial. The active agent, immanent and immaterial, possessed volition and intent, whereby foresight and goal guided deliberate choice. Such a formulation contrasted sharply with any philosophy resting on blind chance. Stahl supported his position by observation, reasoning, and concrete instances drawn from various aspects of medicine.

While Stahl's philosophical views permeate his physiology, pathology, and clinical works, there are several treatises that deal especially with philosophical problems. Three of these expository texts, the *Disquisitio,* the *Paraenesis,* and the *Demonstratio,* published originally in 1706 and 1707, were included in the *Theoria Medica Vera.*[57] Many other parts of the *Theoria Medica Vera,* especially the *Physiologia,* also reveal philosophical presuppositions. In addition, a later work of controversy, *Negotium Otiosum,* of 1720, contains relevant discussions that answer objections Leibniz had raised.[58]

Stahl tried to provide criteria that would distinguish the living from the nonliving. We can divide his arguments into two main categories, one concerned with structure and function, and the other with goal and purpose. While these all interdigitate, to some extent they may be considered separately.

The living differed from the nonliving in composition, but a more important feature centered on the concept of dissolution. The living body is always subject to a putrid corruption, which, however, does not occur during health. *The essence of life lies in this very preservation from corruption.* The bodily components exist in an ordered disposition, forming an ordered aggregate.[59] They endure for a limited time and are kept from dissolution or putrefaction by a special internal cause, totally different from anything found in nonliving compounds. The principle of conservation, preventing corruption and opposed to the corporeal and material nature of the body, permits the body to endure. This check to corruptibility is something contrary to the intrinsic nature of the body as such.[60]

This principle of life, or *anima,* is an *ens,* that is, a real existing entity. To characterize it Stahl indicated numerous features of which, for the present, we may mention the following. It is active, motive, and intelligent. It endures in time and requires instruments to effect its activity. It exists in and with the body, is concerned with the body, and cannot be separated from the body even in thought.[61]

Quite obviously, Stahl's concept of the anima has much in common with the substantial form of the neo-Galenists, as well as with the archeus of van Helmont. But Sennert and van Helmont wrote early in the seventeenth century, before the corpuscular philosophy had triumphed. Thomas Willis, coming later, created a sort of patchwork in which the primary focus rested on corpuscular doctrines, while still taking account of certain traditional aspects such as the soul. Stahl, however, held a quite different position. As an excellently trained physician he assimilated the new physiology resting on the concept of the circulation; yet he had a primary kinship with the Aristotelian and neo-Galenic viewpoints. He tried to harmonize the mechanical philosophy with concepts such as entelechy, or substantial form, or archeus, which underlay the earlier viewpoints. Stahl thus gave philosophical primacy to the old, which he modified so that it could harmonize with the new. For an overall formulation I suggest that van Helmont did not come to terms with the corpuscular philosophy; Willis embraced corpuscularianism eagerly, but without completely discarding the old; while Stahl militantly retained much of the old philosophy, which he modified to make more consistent with the mechanical philosophy.

Stahl's major problem, then, was to accommodate the mechanical philosophy into the framework of animism. This he accomplished through several separate stages, which left many loose edges, to be sure, but which brought the various doctrines together into a plausible unity. He had to define the nature of mechanism and to show how the mechanical processes related to animistic viewpoints. This he accomplished by distinguishing animism from organism and refusing to consider them in isolation.

Mechanical properties consist of configuration, size, position, and movement (either the disposition to movement or the actual motion), but mechanism lacks any goal or reason why it moves or is moved. Any necessity would be *a posteriori,* not *a priori,* and any goal or purpose would be only accidental. However, a mechanism may be an *instrument,* that is, a means for bringing about a certain end or goal.[62] Thus Stahl insisted on the distinction between the terms *facere* and *efficere* — to do and to accomplish. Only in the latter is there an agency toward an end.

An instrument involves not only motion but a direction and a regulation toward a particular end. This instrumentality forms a necessary part of organism, as opposed to mere mechanism. Essential to an organism is a "mechanical disposition," precisely adapted to achieving the goal for which it is destined. This disposition, highly specific for particular ends, distinguishes an organism. Among various examples the best is a clock, an artifact directed toward a special goal. It is mechanical, and yet an instrument (*organon*) as long as it is properly regulated. But if, through some defect, it fails to work, then it is no longer an instrument but still remains a machine.[63]

If we transpose Stahl's thought to a slightly different vocabulary, we might rephrase his views: the significant feature is neither the laws of physics or chemistry, nor the adherence of phenomena to the laws of motion. We may take for granted that natural phenomena obey these laws and that this constitutes mechanism. The truly significant question is whether the phenomena exhibit a goal or direction or end. If so, then we deal with organism, and the mechanical activities, serving as means to that end, are instruments. The mechanical configuration is then an *organon.*

Discussing this concept of end or goal, Stahl emphasized that we must not seek ultimate or cosmic ends. We must remain within what I would call proximal use. Furthermore, he concentrated his discussion on the human *anima* and hedged somewhat on the capacities and properties of the animal soul.[64] Our analysis, therefore, will remain close to the human subject.

Stahl strongly objected to any crudely mechanical explanation of vital phenomena. Mechanical principles, indispensable for understanding the physical world, certainly applied to the world of the living but by themselves were insufficient. After mechanism had said all that it could, the residue constituted the sphere of the *anima.*

Clearly, Stahl faced all the problems of dualism that Descartes had so sharply emphasized.[65] How to bring together the corporeal world and the immaterial *anima?* The answer lay through the concept of motion, which Stahl handled in a unique fashion and which played a major part in his system. Motion, obviously, formed the core of mechanical activity, yet Stahl did not deal with it in a mathematical sense nor did he formulate its laws. This was a task for the physicists who, in the seventeenth century, possessed observational techniques and mathematical sophistication adequate to define various properties of motion and, in the work of Newton, formulate its laws. Stahl did not refer to the vast quantity of relevant knowledge that had accumulated in physics.

In physiology the approach was quite different from that in physics. Zoology was "the science of living things."[66] However, there were no techniques that could apply precise measurements to the phenomena of life, and therefore Stahl, when distinguishing the nonliving from the living, dealt with motion more as an abstract concept than as a subject for precise study. He pointed to various physiological processes involving motion, such as the circulation of the blood and the activities of secretion and excretion, but there was no attempt at experimental detail. In the massive *Theoria Medica Vera* all his discussions of physiology and pathology centered around the concept of motion, but in a metaphysical rather than a concrete mode. It is wrong to say that life *consists* of motion.[67] Instead, motion is the instrumental cause, "by which the preservation of the body is achieved [and] which we call life . . . [This instrumental cause] is nothing else but a mechanical act whereby the effective preservation is carried out in a simple and directly mechanical fashion. And this is nothing else but motion, through which are removed those heterogenous substances that are not only foreign to the body but are threatening to it."[68]

This view he repeated and elaborated in the first chapters of his *Physiologia*. The body, corruptible, is preserved from corruption by motion, acting mechanically and instrumentally through "bodily machines."[69] But the motion is not blindly mechanical: it has goal and purpose and tends to conservation and maintenance of health. Mechanical necessity can characterize inanimate objects but not living creatures. Instead of necessity, we have a subordination to ends and goals.

Stahl faced the same problem as Sennert did. What metaphysical features are primary? What is derivative and secondary? What is substance and what accident? Stahl's answers were already foreshadowed in his concept of instrument. The body is subordinate to the *anima*, but the latter has no transcendental status. Instead there is absolute dependence on the body — the *anima* can do absolutely nothing without the body, can have no sensory knowledge, cannot know or think. But the reverse dependence — of the body on the *anima* — is even more stringent. The body, besides being preserved through "vital actions," provides for sensation, for local motion, and even for thought itself. It is for these purposes that the body is made. It does not exist for its own sake but necessarily exists for the sake of the *anima*.[70]

For Stahl it is motion which conserves the body and provides for the bodily needs of the *anima*. Motion is a *res*, a real existent. It differs from the essence of the body but is akin to the nature of the *anima*. Like the *anima*, motion is itself incorporeal but, again like the *anima*, it is active in the body. This motion the *anima* "regulates, directs, increases, diminishes, and bends according to its own will."[71] Motion is thus a key term in Stahl's thinking, a concept through which he brought together mind and body and "explained" the interaction and also provided a groundwork for physiological studies. For him motion could resolve all difficulties: it is a real entity, incorporeal and kin to the immaterial *anima*; yet, although totally different from the essential nature of body, it affects body.

These rather abstract assertions he elaborated in a later work, of 1720, the *Negotium Otiosum seu SKIAMACHIA*, written as an answer to certain objections Leibniz had made and to which Stahl responded only after Leibniz's death. The work is difficult, poorly organized, redundant, full of verbal quibblings, and has been little studied. Stahl himself apparently held it in low regard, as indicated by the title which we might translate as "Idle Business, or Fighting with Shadows." Rather and Frerichs have discussed certain aspects of this work and have translated a portion.[72] However, elsewhere in the *Negotium Otiosum* are passages (especially pp. 91-101) more relevant to our problem, and it is on this section that I draw particularly. Here Stahl considered and answered various objections to his concept of motion. To present-day thinking the objections as well as the responses seem to rest on verbal distinctions, but nevertheless the passages form an interesting study in medical thinking.

Stahl wanted to refute an objection: the *anima* is immaterial and motion is a property of body; therefore, the *anima* cannot move the body. In his rebuttal he distinguished between a property of body and body itself. Properties have their own existence so that body and its properties are distinct.[73] In this discussion, Stahl, even though he does not mention Descartes, was obviously referring to the latter's separation of extension and motion. For Descartes motion was separable from extension. For Stahl motion is separable from body but properties such as size and configuration remain inseparable. The simplest conception of *corpus* does not involve motion. Body must have size and configuration but need not have motion. Since motion may be either absent or present it is not essential. Motion, therefore, pertains not to essence or existence of body but only to activity. Since bodies may or may not be in motion, the two are separable.

We cannot say that motion is nothing, for if it were, and a body were then put into motion, then the activity would arise from nothing—clearly an absurdity. Hence, motion is something, even though it may not exist in this or that body.[74] Stahl made the covert assumption that what was not corporeal was incorporeal. Therefore, motion is incorporeal and does not come under the categories of dimension, extension, or configuration. Motion, since it can be absent from body without impairing the essence thereof, must have a separate existence as something incorporeal.

Motion, as incorporeal, differs from all the intrinsic or characteristic properties of body and these it does not alter. Then Stahl indicated the essential characters of motion: in its essence it is an activity whereas *corpus* is passive. Motion has degree, which has nothing in common with magnitude. Time is a condition of motion, and, said Stahl, motion regulates time rather than the reverse. Motion has proportion, limit, and progression. Furthermore, motion is not restricted to corporeal objects, for it also inheres in the incorporeal. Stahl maintained that intellectual processes or mental states consist of motion and he gave as examples reasoning, contemplation or decision, choice, love, hate, fear. He quoted Aristotle that *cogitationem esse animae deambulationem*—"thought is a progression of the mind." All action, whether mental or physical, is motion. Motion, as an incorporeal entity, presupposes a cause similarly immaterial.[75] The *anima* acts directly on the body and motion is the means of relating the immaterial and the corporeal. Motion is an intermediary that connects the *anima* and the body.

In enunciating this doctrine Stahl explicitly rejected the notion of finely material spirits. The doctrine of spirits can permit a series of transitions so imperceptibly graded that they form a continuum. We then would have a bridge to allow easy passage between seeming incompatibles like immaterial mind and corporeal matter. For this process I offer the metaphor of a gradual "thickening" of the immaterial, until it acquires the most subtle degree of materiality. This then becomes more and more coarse until it leads to the unmistakably corporeal. Typical Neoplatonism involves a graded series of celestial beings and astral bodies.[76]

This type of intermediary Stahl firmly rejected. We must not say simply, that he substituted the concept of motion for the concept of spirits. It is wrong to think of a simple verbal substitution, putting Tweedledum in place of Tweedledee. Instead there is the rejection of one metaphysics in favor of another. Stahl rejected Neoplatonism, not so much by name as by implication and inference. Instead of a philosophy of transition he adopted a schema akin to *fiat*. Motion, an entity, joins two other entities, namely, mind and matter, in a fashion analogous to some of the early immunological diagrams, whereby an antibody serves to fasten together an antigen and a cell. Appropriate receptors enable the antibody to make firm connections between disparate entities. If we assume that the separate entities are the mind and the body, then, although the analogy is rough and imperfect, it nevertheless suggests a possible model. In his own thinking Stahl himself has not avoided the "third man" fallacy, against which he inveighed.[77] He merely exemplified the biblical comment that it is much easier to perceive the mote in your brother's eye than the beam in your own. Along with Neoplatonism Stahl rejected van Helmont's concept of the archeus. Pagel has discussed this point as well as various differences between van Helmont and Stahl.[78]

The *anima* Stahl regarded as a conscious entity acting with intelligence and foresight. But since many bodily functions were carried out without any conscious intervention, Stahl had to account for this. To the *anima* he attributed two distinct functions, which he called *logos* and *logismos*, the one a simple act of intellect (that is, minimal function of the *anima*) and the other a ratiocination (that is, true reasoning involving comparison, judgment, and inference).[79] This feeble distinction is Stahl's attempt to account for the differences between unconscious and conscious (physiological) activity. He was hobbled by his own metaphysics; he had overloaded his concept of *anima*, to which he attributed too many functions, and he had difficulty in finding differential features to correlate with the data of observation.

I have already noted the interdependence of mind and body, and in this association the *anima* held primary status. The body is the *organon* of the soul, exists for the sake of the soul, and has the function of making possible the activity of the soul.[80] But why the soul in the first place? Said Stahl, the human *anima* has its own reason for being, namely, "It exists simply and absolutely for the purpose of understanding." An intelligent agent, possessing a definite goal and a volition to achieve that goal, must have organs proportionate to the purpose in view and must regulate and direct those organs in a fashion suitable to those ends.[81]

The soul, to serve its own ends, not only directs the body but also has the function of preserving and maintaining the body. As we have seen, only through the action of the soul is the body kept from corruption. This same preservative and regulatory activity of the *anima* leads to what is commonly called the healing power of nature. This aspect is substantially discussed in Neuburger's monograph.[82] Full consideration of the subject would lead us into analysis of Stahl's doctrines of pathology, a topic into which I do not want to enter here. Suffice it to repeat that the *anima* exerts its conservatory and restorative functions through motion and mechanical acts.[83] The metaphysical relations are clear, even if the concrete working out is not.

Stahl was trying to explain concrete data with what might seem inadequate conceptual tools. Today we have a powerful explanatory tool in the concept of the autonomic nervous system; we know a great deal about hormonal activity; we have considerable understanding of the controlling factors in embryological development; and so on. But the various data and theories that fill our modern texts were completely unknown to Stahl, who could rely only on the concepts available to him.

Stahl was not stampeded by the cruder aspects of the mechanical philosophy. While he kept abreast of developments in physiology, physics, and chemistry and made important contributions particularly to chemistry, he maintained a philosophic position that insisted on the reality of the immaterial. He wanted to explain total behavior rather than minute details, and for him the emphasis on fine anatomical or chemical data had little use in the practice of medicine.[84] In his day he was opposing the main current of scientific research in favor of what seemed to be an obscurantist animism. His doctrines emphasize the close ties between metaphysics and medicine. The relationship still remains, and in this area Stahl will continue to hold an important place.

SEVEN

THE POWER OF THE IMAGINATION

So quickly do we become accustomed to regularity and order that we soon take them for granted. Then what varies from the accustomed order quickly calls attention to itself to demand a particular explanation. Among such deviations from the normal the phenomena of birth defects have played an important part in the history of ideas. How do we explain the birth defects that occur over such a wide range, from monsters through many degrees of deformity to small blemishes or birthmarks? Today, we refer these phenomena to embryology and genetics. In times past we had quite different explanations, for example, that the frustrated longing of the pregnant woman could mark the baby. If, during pregnancy, the mother had a desire, say, for strawberries, and this desire was not gratified, the baby might be born with a "strawberry mark" on its skin. Other desires, as well as various emotions or imaginings of the mother might have a comparable effect on the fetus. All these different mental states of the mother were lumped together under the single term imagination.

This usage placed together many different phenomena that now are clearly separable. I might draw a comparison with the word fever, which today has quite precise definition but in times past covered a multitude of conditions, with no sharp circumscription. The history of medicine tells us how, with increasing knowledge, the meanings of fever became progressively differentiated. Similarly, the historian must study the distinct meanings that lurked within the word imagination and trace their emergence as clearly separable functions. In so doing we gain considerable insight into earlier views of the mind and the mind-body relationship.

Imagination is one function of the mind, but only one among many others, such as reason, perception, memory, emotion, will. In the seventeenth century, study of these components formed part of philosophy and only much later did there develop a self-conscious science in its own right called psychology. Philosophers—and the leading physicians were philosophers as well as healers—had to consider all these various components of mind, their relationships to each other, to the body, to the rest of nature, to God, and to the supernatural.

Within the realm of mind the different components overlapped. Perception had a direct relationship to the real world, to something that existed outside the mind and that stimulated the sense organs. Memory involved the recollections of what had once been perceived, while imagination involved some internal stimulus, not corresponding to anything "out there," but drawn from within, that is, a mental state having no direct correspondence to reality. Hoffmann phrased the distinction that in memory "the mind attends to the traces of a past impression, and causes absent bodies to appear present"; while in imagination the "traces of things impressed on the senses are gathered up and similar thoughts are then excited in the mind."[1]

So long as we deal only with normal functions there is no great confusion, but difficulties appear when we deal with the abnormal. Then the line between memory and imagination becomes blurred; so too with the relationship between imagination and reason. Under normal conditions the reasoning process might seem to be independent of imagination. But where reason seems disturbed—as in hallucinations or delirium, or misinterpretations, which today we call a delusional system—these states were interpreted as disturbed imagination. In terms of a naive realism, to say that something is imaginary is to say that it is falling away from reality. When the reason is not in "proper" relationship to what is "really" out there, then imagination has taken over.

Mind thus has many interrelated aspects, and metaphysical views, whether explicit or only implicit, determine the way the mind fits into the whole scheme of things—how it relates, for example, to body, life, soul, nature, God. The neo-Galenists held views quite different from the corpuscularians or the chemists. We cannot talk blandly of the influence the mother's imagination might have had on the unborn fetus unless we consider the metaphysical bias of the authors in question. Does this involve the concepts of form and matter? or an archeus? or merely particles in motion? Must we consider the devil as one of the influences acting on the imagination or perhaps other aspects of the supernatural? Different philosophical systems gave different answers.

We cannot study imagination in the seventeenth and eighteenth centuries without placing it in a proper context and yet the area is so enormous that only a small portion can be analyzed here. In my discussion I will not take up the problems in biology that engendered so much dispute, such as the conflicts between the preformationists and the epigenicists, or between the animalculists and the ovists. These important topics are discussed in a variety of recent texts and monographs.[2] For a good overview of the relation between the imagination, literature, and medicine, the papers of Rousseau are extremely helpful.[3]

Sennert

Daniel Sennert (1572-1637) wrote before the great upsurge in embryological research triggered by Harvey's *De Generatione Animalium* (1651).[4] Sennert had built his medical system chiefly on the Aristotelian principles of form and matter and on the Galenic faculties, spirits, and humors. Although to explain certain facets of the corporeal world he introduced some atomistic and chemical concepts, these did not diminish his overall reliance on neo-Galenic thought. This we see clearly when he dealt with mind and its functions. The possible influence of the mother's imagination on the fetus posed a serious problem, which Sennert attacked by analyzing first the powers of the imagination in general and then attending to the imagination of the mother as a special case, wherein the mind could affect the fetus. By using this approach he revealed his philosophical bias and provided a clear idea of his position.

Many remarkable phenomena, such as producing and curing disease, were attributed to the imagination. Yet Sennert emphasized at the very beginning that these effects do not derive directly from either the imagination or the mind. An idea or notion (*phantasia*) is a phenomenon of consciousness (*cognitio*) and does not itself produce any local motion, and any activity involving local motion is quite distinct from an idea. Mental phenomena do not directly affect the body. Thus, if a man has sexual thoughts and imagery, the "humors and spirits" will move toward the genital organs, and by this motion of the humors and spirits certain obvious physical changes take place. But the physical changes in the sex organs do not result directly from the image as such. Instead, the imagination affects the natural faculties, for example, the faculties of attraction, retention, or expulsion, whose function it is to move the humors and spirits.[5] There is a sequence: the imagination acts on the faculties, which act on the humors, and this latter activity produces the physical changes in the body.

We must not think of this as any sort of Cartesian dualism, with its sharp separation between mind and body and a limited scope for interaction. On the contrary, we have a rather vague unity, involving mind and *anima*, forms and faculties, with emphasis on function. Form and matter, mind and body go together, but there are distinct sequences, which the scientist can study, sequences that involve orderly progressions and functional separations. To explain the interrelations Sennert relied in large part on the concept of consent or sympathy. Any of the natural faculties may be affected by consent and thus be excited to act.[6] Thus, to take a different example, the image or idea of a purgative medicine may induce evacuation of the bowels. Through the imagination the natural motor faculty is "drawn into consent," agitates the humors, and these, when agitated, stimulate the expulsive faculty with the resulting excretion. Sennert gave many examples, all indicating that the imagination acts only *mediately*, not *immediately*. The imagination sets off a chain reaction whereby the humors and spirits are the proximal (or direct) cause and the imagination the remote cause.[7]

Critics who regard this as pure verbalism must remember that Sennert was subjecting experience to analysis, separating off individual sequences involving both mind and body, and indicating the connections between them. The term sympathy points to some definite connection, whose details were admittedly unknown. When, after much careful research, some of the intermediate details were eventually discovered, the idea of sympathy became enshrined in the more precise term sympathetic nervous system.

The imagination by itself cannot produce disease, for if it did the result then could only be an imaginary disease. In conditions such as melancholia or in delusional states the actual causal factors are the emotions, the *affectus animi*—grief, fear, terror. Sennert also discussed the belief that some persons fall victim to the plague through their imagination.[8] But in such instances the imagination acts only where there is already a predisposition and where the germs of plague lie latent in the body. The malignant humors are set into motion by the emotions of fear or terror and then these movements induce the plague—the fear and terror mobilize the malignant humors that were latent.

He gave other instances that would come under the category of delusions, for example, a man believed that his body was too big to pass through a door. The physician, to cure this delusion, ordered the man to be forcefully carried through the door, whereupon the patient bewailed loudly that in this process he was completely broken up inside. Shortly afterwards he died. Sennert attributed this case report to Marcello Donato (died about 1600). Rather noted the same case in his study of Thomas Fienus (1567-1631).[9] Said Sennert, such a patient actually had a disease and died from the disease, not from his imagination. If the imagination had anything to do with the disease it was only *per accidens*, that is, in connection with sadness or fear or similar "passions of the mind." In the instances that Sennert gave there were no autopsies, and to the modern temper this absence impairs the force of his argument. Yet we must grant force to his contention that the imagination acts on the emotions and the emotions, through their effect on the humors and spirits, can intensify any physical state already existing.

The mind can affect diseases. It is very well known, he said, that anger or joy can have an altering effect on the humors and in this way a long continued or intense imagination can cause many diseases. Thus, through the imagination, spirits and "vapors" may be attracted to the head and then the actions of the other parts of the body are not properly carried out.

Imagination can cure as well as cause disease, but only in this same indirect sense, *per accidens* and not *per se*. A cure of disease takes place not through any single action but rather through a number of different coordinated actions—alteration, coction, excretion, changes in the disposition of the parts that provide or receive the humors. The imagination can take part in this process, for it induces changes in the mind whereby the spirits are moved to overcome the disease. Confidence, acting on the mind (*animus*) gives rise to joy or pleasure. This stimulates the native heat and the spirits, whereby the food is better digested, harmful humors are overcome, and the disease eliminated. What is pleasing to the mind results in better digestion. On the other hand, foods which are, so to speak, "restrained" by the emotions of care, fear, or grief, are not properly digested. Such foods then become corrupted, crudities and harmful humors accumulate, and diseases arise or increase.[10]

Significant here is the emphasis on interaction among a variety of functions. Some of these Sennert identified as faculties; others as affections of the mind; others as notions or imaginings; still others as movements of the bodily components — the humors and spirits; still others as foods, subject to various changes, some beneficial, others harmful. The emphasis rests not on any distinction between body and mind, but rather on interaction and process, on total activity. Here the imagination can have a mediating effect, as part of the total process.

Imagination cannot act at a distance, unless through an appropriate chain of intermediaries. Sennert gave an interesting example. "Beyond all doubt" a menstruating woman can taint a mirror into which she looks. This is not at all a matter of witchcraft but happens by way of spirits, vapors, and effluences, which serve as intermediates. In some fashion the imagination can direct these spirits and humors. Through strong emotions such as hate, anger, or envy, they are directed to the eyes and flow out more abundantly. Sennert's term *copiosius* implies that normally there is some degree of outflow, increased during emotion. The effluences bearing a malignant quality can affect and injure external objects to which they extend. And since the eyes ordinarily abound in very subtle humors, it is not remarkable that a menstruating woman can affect an object more through her eyes than through other parts.

From our standpoint the important feature is Sennert's willingness to concede that the imagination can in some indirect fashion induce action at a distance but only at a modest distance where intermediaries can be traced. It is utterly absurd, he declared, to believe that this action can occur over long distances, such as many miles. We must not attribute to the imagination any effects greater than its own powers. He utterly rejected such claims that imagination could cause someone at a distance to fall off a horse.[11]

Sennert provides a striking combination of uncritical acceptance and critical awareness. He had a deep concern for facts, the basis of all theory and all explanation. But by our standards he was not at all rigorous in examining his facts. He accepted various assertions as *extra dubium* — not to be questioned by any reasonable person — and on the basis of these he constructed his theory. Then he used his theory in a critical fashion as a touchstone by which other allegations of fact might be judged. His theories allowed a limited chain reaction between various mental and physical states. This harmonized with the claim that a menstruating woman could affect a mirror into which she looked. But action at a great distance conflicted with his theory and therefore was rejected.

In this connection — action at a distance — we may compare the views of Sennert to those of his somewhat later contemporary, Sir Kenelm Digby. The later also dealt with action at a distance, namely, the healing of wounds through the "Powder of Sympathy." This I have discussed elsewhere. [12]

After this preliminary survey we can examine the specific problem: what effect can the imagination of the mother exert on the fetus? Some persons, Sennert admitted, denied any effect whatever but, he went on, so many observations prove that the fetus is altered through the imagination of the mother that doubt indicates either ignorance or obstinacy. [13] He referred to individual instances, some taken from the reports of others, some from his own experience.

Among other cases he mentioned the incident related in Genesis, Chapter 30, verses 31-43, wherein Jacob made an agreement with Laban to receive as his wages all the cattle (the sheep and goats) that were speckled or spotted. Laban agreed, but first he removed from the flocks all the animals that were spotted and handed the remainder over to Jacob. Then Jacob, noted for his sharp dealing, took rods (branches) of poplar, hazel, and chestnut that were streaked and set them up near the watering troughs so that the animals might conceive while looking at the rods; or, if pregnant, that they might see the mottled rods during gestation. And then, reports Scripture, the females that conceived under the influence of the streaked and spotted rods brought forth young that were streaked or spotted. These animals now belonged to Jacob, who became very rich.

This narrative from the Bible provided support for the doctrine that the environment, acting on the sensorium of the mother, could alter the fetus. We may query whether the mental process of the sheep, as they gazed on the parti-colored rods, involved what may properly be called imagination. But as I have indicated above, this word was by no means univocal in its denotation. In studying maternal influence on the fetus we are on more secure ground if we think of mental content of the mother rather than imagination in the strict sense.

Sennert related incidents from his own experience: for example, when a pregnant woman passed under a mulberry tree, several berries fell on her. She gave birth to a daughter who had papillomatous growths like mulberries, on those very parts of the body corresponding to the places where the berries had fallen on the mother. In a further case, a pregnant woman who saw a butcher cleave with an ax the head of a swine then gave birth to an infant whose upper jaw and lip were split up to the nostril (cleft palate).[14]

These and other examples Sennert offered as instances of disturbed imagination in the mother, but how the imagination affected the fetus he admitted was obscure. The action certainly did not occur immediately and simply, for in an infant the proximal cause of the bodily configuration and growth was the creative faculty (*facultas conformatrix*). Growth of the fetus cannot be directly altered by any sort of image but only by motion of the humors and spirits acting on this creative faculty. Affections of the mind can, through the humors, influence the creative faculty.[15]

The changes that might overtake a fetus Sennert divided into two categories, which he called respectively the common and the determinate. More consonant with present-day idiom might be the terms nonspecific and specific. The former changes, affecting the fetus in a rather gross fashion, involved the size and number of component parts (for example, absence of limbs or gross monstrosities) or even abortion or death. The specific changes, however, had a precision about them, a definite similarity to some external object, for example, a mulberry or cherry, or animal, that had affected the imagination of the mother and produced the so-called marks on the infant.

The imagination could bring about the nonspecific changes by means of the passions or emotions and the movements of the humors and spirits. Such movements served as the instruments of the formative faculty as it shaped the fetus; when these movements were in turmoil, the formative faculty was correspondingly disturbed and might generate parts that were larger or smaller than normal, greater or less in number or that lacked the proper configuration. Such bad results occurred by chance and did not follow any particular pattern.

But the specific changes — the imprinting on the fetus of some "determinate" image — could not be explained in this fashion. The marks on the fetus — the verruca like a cherry that the mother had desired, or the skin blemish resembling the mouse that frightened the mother — were also properly referable to the imagination, but in these instances, to connect the imagination with the formative faculty was, Sennert admitted, very difficult. He recognized many different opinions. It is safest, he thought, to hold that the imagination directed the faculty by means of examples or models.[16]

Anyone who wonders that the formative faculty can recognize a model and respond to it should remember that all the faculties in man derive from the single *anima*. Thus they have some communication among themselves even though, he added apologetically, we have no clear idea how this takes place. We do not know how the image, received in the brain, is carried to the formative faculty in the uterus. Sennert felt sure of his facts, that the imagination *was* involved, but he was offering only conjectures in regard to the mechanism.

Sennert doubted that the spirits and humors carried any image to the uterus. He invoked instead the unity of the anima, which nevertheless had separate faculties appropriate for each organ. Excitement in one part can induce a change in some other part, and yet the *anima*, the overall directing force, remains the same. He was thus invoking the concept of sympathy. It is not remarkable, he declared, that what moves the powers of the mind in the mother can also excite the faculties in the seed and involve the fetus.[17]

Central to Sennert's juggling was his firm belief that the imagination did, somehow, produce the mark on the child. He fully realized that his own explanations were not entirely convincing. The concept of sympathy was at best vague, but this was not important, for *theoretical difficulties should not negate facts*. Although Sennert did not express himself in these precise terms, his discussion pointed in this direction. And as we shall see, Bablot's treatise on the same subject a hundred and fifty years later embodied the identical reasoning.

Despite his vague theories, Sennert did not neglect the collection of data. The formative faculty, he noted, seemed to operate on a sort of timetable and the changes induced by the imagination could occur only at specific times. Some changes, he believed, could take place at the moment of conception (wherefore, he said, some believe that the imagination of the father might be effective). However, in the later months of pregnancy the imagination cannot induce changes in the total configuration. When nature has once formed the fetus, the imagination cannot then change the number or configuration of the parts. And hence, he declared firmly, many of the reports that had been handed down were mere fables.[18] Nor, he continued, can the imagination imprint *any* sort of mark on the fetus but only those for which the material of the body was appropriate. Thus, the force of the imagination cannot produce on the fetus any feathers, scales, or horns. The materials for forming these are not available to the formative faculty.

The discussions in which Sennert indulged tend to be rather long-winded. For the purposes at hand, I would stress the following points. Sennert was a neo-Galenist whose theories derived from primacy of the substantial forms, as discussed in Chapter 3. His explanations depended on forms and faculties, but these terms, so easy to deride, did indicate the importance of the time span, of specific sequences, interrelationships, and essential unity. These all derived from empirical observations, even though cloaked in what seems to us harsh and redundant nomenclature. Furthermore, Sennert brought into clear relief the interrelation between theory and fact. Facts determine the contents of our theories, but in reciprocal fashion the theories help determine what we will accept as facts (and what we discard as fables).

Neo-Galenists, as we have seen in previous chapters, went into apparent eclipse before the splendors of the mechanical philosophy. And yet the problems remained: does the mother's imagination affect the fetus and, if so, how? These problems interpenetrated the entire intellectual fabric of the eighteenth century.

Descartes

Descartes (1596-1650), rebelling against the scholastic philosophy and neo-Galenism, substituted his clear-cut dualism based on a corpuscular philosophy. Nevertheless, in regard to maternal influences on the fetus, he accepted the same data as did Sennert, even though he dealt with the topic in a rather casual fashion.

In *De l'homme*, not published until 1662 but written apparently in the early 1630s, Descartes indicated that the traces of ideas pass by the arteries toward the heart and spread through the blood.[19] And then he declared, casually as a sort of aside, that they might be determined by certain actions of the mother, to be imprinted on the limbs of the infant being formed in the uterus. But he did not indicate any pathway or mechanism by which this took place.

Descarte's usage of the word idea is complex and not entirely consistent. In the present context, ideas, as Hall points out, have a corporeal status, as an impression on the animal spirits as they leave the pineal gland.[20] In his treatise *On Vision*, Descartes similarly hinted that he could show how sometimes the images could pass from the brain, through the arteries of the pregnant woman, to reach the limbs of the infant, "and there produce those marks of desire that cause so much wonder among the learned."[21]

In his *Passions of the Soul*, written in 1646, he again contented himself with indicating the data, without showing any stepwise explanation. He referred to the various idiosyncrasies that we today attribute to allergy, that some persons cannot endure the scent of roses or the presence of a cat.

He either attributed the phenomena to early unpleasant experiences or else claimed that the affected persons have "shared in the feelings of their mother, who has so suffered before they were born. For it is certain that there is a relation between all the movements of the mother and those of the child in her womb, inasmuch as what is harmful to the one is hurtful to the other."[22] But Descartes did not try to provide any stepwise explanation of the way this might come about.

Malebranche

The Cartesian disciple Malebranche (1638-1715) examined the topic in somewhat greater detail. Malebranche was a Catholic priest and theologian who first became acquainted with Descartes's *De l'homme* in 1664 and thereafter became an ardent Cartesian. He devoted many years to close study and in 1674 published his major work, *De la récherche de la verité*,[23] which went through many editions in his lifetime. In the course of this text he discussed the problems of maternal influence on the fetus and in so doing he gave us an insight into the current knowledge of embryology as well as the degree of credulity and of critical acumen that informed the writings of a leading intellectual of that era.

Malebranche did not hesitate to make sweeping statements; if he did not know any information to the contrary, he considered his assertions completely valid and on their basis he would proceed to build theoretical elaborations. Thus, he declared that the fetus was united to the mother "in the strictest possible" fashion.[24] Hence, although the fetus had a separate soul, the body was not separate from the mother. The infant sees what the mother sees, hears the same sounds, receives the same impressions, and is moved by the same passions. The body of the infant is the same as that of the mother — "the blood and the spirits are common to both" — and so the movements of the fluids in the mother are necessarily communicated to the infant. Hence the passions and feelings and all thoughts are common to the mother and the infant.

These all appeared indisputable to Malebranche. He buttressed his assertions by particular and familiar examples. For instance, a pregnant woman frightened by a cat will give birth to a child that will have strong emotions at the sight of a cat, and strange effects may ensue. We can only speculate whether Malebranche had in mind what we now call allergy or was referring merely to fright.

In his presentation, Malebranche made two methodological statements of extreme significance. First, he said what he offered was only a hypothesis (*une supposition*) that he believed would be sufficiently demonstrated later, that is, by further examples. Then, he declared, "every hypothesis that can satisfactorily resolve all the objections one can raise, must be accepted as an indisputable principle" (*un principe incontestable*).[25]

With this theoretical background he pointed to the process of "sympathy," whereby emotions and their physical counterparts are communicated among adults. Moreover, infants still *in utero* have a delicacy of fibers infinitely greater than that of mature persons. Hence, he inferred, the movement of the spirits must produce greater changes in the fetus than in the adult.[26] Then he gave examples to clarify and prove these points.

Malebranche described a case of considerable importance, subsequently much discussed.[27] A young man of some 20 years of age was born feeble-minded (*fou*) and with bones that had been broken at the same places as in a criminal whose body was "broken on the wheel." Malebranche indicated the cause: the mother, while pregnant, had witnessed this ferocious torture inflicted on the criminal. Every blow had forcibly affected the imagination of the mother and "by a sort of *contre-coup*" also affected the delicate brain of the infant. The fibers of the mother were firm enough to resist the violent movement of the spirits, but the cerebral fibers of the infant were dissolved. That is why the infant was born feeble-minded. In the mother the animal spirits went forcibly from the brain to the parts of the body corresponding to those where the criminal was struck, but the bones of the mother, being quite firm, could resist the violent motions of the spirits and were not injured. Not so, however, with the tender bones of the infant, which could not resist the forceful influx of spirits. Malebranche went on, that if the mother had "determined" the violent spirits to other parts of her body, the infant would not have had broken bones. Instead, the fetal injuries would have corresponded to those parts of the mother where the spirits had gone.

For the more common birthmarks, consequent on the desires of the mother, Malebranche had a comparable explanation. If the mother, for example, strongly "imagined and desired" pears, then the fetus would imagine and desire the same thing. And if the fetus were not yet *animé,* that is, not sufficiently matured to have its own mind, then the spirits, stimulated by the image of the desired fruit, would nevertheless spread through the body which was sufficiently tender to undergo alteration. "The poor infants come to resemble those objects that they desire with excessive intensity."[28] The body of the mother, however, lacks the delicacy whereby it might take on the configuration of the desired object.

The differences between Sennert and Malebranche are striking and illustrate the distinction between a physician-scientist, however misguided, and a speculative theologian who did not have much concrete experience in the study of nature. As a Cartesian, Malebranche had dismissed the whole concept of faculties and he thereby gave up features that characterized the best of the neo-Galenists: concern with observation, critical discrimination, isolation of observable sequences. Sennert, writing more than a half century before Malebranche, nevertheless had a sharper insight into natural phenomena than did the latter and a keener sense of what might be "according to nature." And he had a greater humility regarding the difficulties in finding a satisfactory explanation.

Sennert wrote before the tremendous upsurge in embryological studies that took place in the second half of the seventeenth century, but Malebranche was exposed to the many new currents and had taken substantial interest therein. Yet even by 1712, the date of the best edition, Malebranche's views on the imagination of the mother seem much less critical than those of Sennert, despite the more modern metaphysics and much of the newer embryology.[29]

Boerhaave

Since Boerhaave (1668-1738) was the outstanding physician of the first part of the eighteenth century, his views on the imagination would hold considerable significance for understanding the thought of the era. But it is difficult to track down the temporal relationships of his ideas. His two most important works, the *Institutiones Medicae* and the *Aphorismi de Cognoscendis et Curandis Morbis*, were first published in 1708 and 1709 respectively.[30] The first dealt with the equivalent of our present-day basic sciences, the latter with clinical problems. The texts were relatively brief aphoristic statements, more or less in the Hippocratic tradition, contrasting with the massive treatises of many seventeenth century authors. Hoffmann's *Fundamenta Medicinae* of 1696 was an earlier example of this revival in the aphoristic style.

Boerhaave's thought, published so tersely, was expanded in his lectures. The printed text served as a skeleton, so to speak, and the spoken word provided the flesh. Much of what Boerhaave said in lectures had been preserved in student lecture notes. After Boerhaave's death, Haller (1708-1777) collected this material and published extensive notes to explicate various key terms in the compressed original text. This fleshed-out version is a major source for understanding Boerhaave's ideas. Haller also provided further notes of his own, giving additional personal comments and abundant references. The original text had gone through many editions and translations in Boerhaave's lifetime. Haller's version, under the title *Praelectiones Academicae*, first appeared in 1739-1744, with numerous translations and other editions.[31]

We thus get the thoughts of Boerhaave principally through the minds of his auditors, particularly Haller. We must assume that the commentaries reflect the master, and certainly for the most part this assumption seems reasonable. We must realize, however, that Boerhaave first gave his lectures in 1701, first published his abbreviated text in 1708, while the text *in extenso* appeared some forty years later. We have little indication of the way Boerhaave may have changed his ideas in light of new advances during this period. In the extended notes we have occasional references to work published after 1708 but not often.

Boerhaave's views on clinical medicine offer the same problem. The extended commentaries of van Swieten (1700-1772) provide the best and most detailed exposition. In van Swieten's massive work the first volume of the first edition appeared in 1741, and subsequent volumes appeared over a period of years. There were many editions and translations.[32] Some of the text presents van Swieten's own thoughts and observations but most of it is Boerhaave's. There is sometimes difficulty in distinguishing between the master and the pupil.

Because of these posthumous publications we are necessarily studying "Boerhaavian thought" rather than the exact words of Boerhaave. For general purposes of intellectual history this raises no difficulty, except where, for comparison with other physicians, precise chronology might be important.

To the subject of generation Boerhaave devoted a substantial discussion, covering many aspects of physiology and embryology and indicating many of the current problems. He included the question, does the imagination of a mother affect the fetus? Can the mother, in any way, govern the form of the fetus? Boerhaave expressed the opinion that the mother does not have any voluntary power of changing the fetus, nor does the strongest imagination as such have any effect.[33] Yet the imagination can produce an effect when there is a sudden irrational *horror*. The translation of the Latin here causes difficulties, since this word, in the Latin, has two distinct senses: a physical reaction, with shaking and shivering, such as we have in the first stages of a fever, and an emotion of terror or dread. Boerhaave used both these senses but the standard English translation does not adequately distinguish them.

Boerhaave said that we have a horror at miserable sights and our blood and humors act in an unaccustomed fashion. By this "horrifying imagination" the fetus suffers the same changes as occur in the body of the mother.

Boerhaave, juggling with the word horror, makes his point in an oblique fashion. A marked physical reaction, such as occurs in a fever, might affect the fetus in a direct physical fashion. *Horror* in this sense involves physical mechanism, although the step-by-step relations are not clear. Sennert had already set the stage for this modality. But by also equating *horror* with acts of the imagination, that is, mental states, Boerhaave offered a pathway whereby the imagination, without "shivering," could similarly affect the fetus. Thus, he reported a case that he saw with his own eyes. A pregnant woman walked under a mulberry tree[34] and a berry fell on the tip of her nose. The berry became depicted on the tip of the infant's nose, with the same configuration, color, acinar structure, roughness, and a few hairs. The mark became exacerbated whenever mulberries ripened on the tree. The possible objections, that this might be coincidence and that the infant might have had the mark even if the mother had not walked under the tree, Boerhaave dismissed as improbable and unworthy of a philosopher. Instead of meeting the arguments on their merits, he contented himself with the statement that ignorance regarding the cause of a phenomenon offers no grounds for conclusions.[35] He accepted similar cases, that infants were born with hare lip or six digits, because the mother had seen similar persons. And he drew the conclusion that the mother can add or take away or change something in the fetus, although not by simple will or knowledge.

Boerhaave accepted an empirical correlation, between the experience of the mother and the marks on the infant. He excluded any mechanism of deliberate volition but otherwise he left the mechanism unexplained. These various cases do not, he admitted, conform to the laws of nature as we know them, yet the facts cannot be denied except by someone who has perfect knowledge of all the laws of nature.[36] In other words, while we cannot offer an explanation at present, only a complete knowledge of all the laws of nature (which obviously we do not have) could permit us to deny the data of experience. He accepted "facts" and was willing to wait for the future to provide the explanation.

In his *Aphorismi* Boerhaave and van Swieten returned to the possible effects of the imagination. In discussions of epilepsy and its various and quite diverse causes, one of the alleged mechanisms is that the mother, when pregnant, might have been shocked by seeing a person in an epileptic fit.[37] Van Swieten expanded on the subject at considerable length. In the causation of epilepsy he recognized a hereditary aspect, a "hereditary morbid taint." Quite different from this was the effect of antenatal influence — what we might call environmental effect. If the mother had been frightened by seeing an epileptic fit, the imagination of the frightened mother communicates with the fetus and then the infant from birth is immediately subject to epilepsy. The disease is thus congenital. To be sure, infants may have convulsions at birth from other causes, such as an "acid acrimony irritating the intestine," but in such instances, if the acid acrimony is corrected, the convulsions cease.[38] In the particular case he was describing, however, the paroxysms were not relieved and the infant patient died in convulsions.

Van Swieten appreciated the possible criticisms that could be leveled against his viewpoint and the possible charges of credulity. Maternal influence was denied by some who "cannot conceive how a change of thought in the mother can so affect the fetus." Van Swieten admitted not understanding the connection between a cause acting on the mother and the effect appearing in the infant. He could not understand why the mother should not have been rendered epileptic rather than the fetus. But he fell back on the familiar argument that, even if we do not know the cause, we must not therefore deny that such a thing really happened.[39]

He adduced many other cases of the alleged effect of the imagination on the fetus. Van Swieten depended on a combination of empirical observation on the one hand and an admitted lack of knowledge on the other. He defended himself against charges of credulity by pointing to some other phenomena for which no cause could be offered: for example, why the menses cease during pregnancy, or why the breasts enlarge after delivery, or how the placenta is produced, or how the fetus is connected to the umbilical cord, and many others. Even the most subtle philosopher, he said, would have difficulty in offering a cause for these effects. But we do not therefore deny the facts. "Wherefore the effect of the mother's imagination upon the foetus cannot be more justly denied for this reason, because the manner is not understood by which this change of the foetus has been produced."[40]

These various instances indicate his attitude toward experience and the relations between experience and reason, topics in the logic of science that I will discuss further in Chapter 10.

Blondel

An important study in this era was a book by James Blondel (died 1734) that climaxed an exchange between the author and another physician, Daniel Turner (1667-1741). The latter, firmly believing in the power of the mother's imagination, expressed his views in a book he wrote on skin diseases.[41] In 1727, Blondel attacked this idea in a smaller work, whereupon Turner counterattacked. Blondel, in turn, returned to the battle with a book whose full title summarizes the dispute: *The Power of the Mother's Imagination over the Foetus Examin'd. In Answer to Dr. Daniel Turner's book, intitled A Defense of the XIIth Chapter of the First Part of a Treatise, De Morbis Cutaniis.*[42]

Since Turner originally wrote on skin disease, he paid special attention to the naevi, the congenital skin blemishes supposedly resulting from the maternal imagination, and he mentioned other familiar cases of the types already discussed. How to explain congenital abnormalities of various types, from monstrosities, through all stages of deformity, to small skin blemishes or birthmarks?

Much of seventeenth and eighteenth century medicine took the form of polemics, whose chief goal seemed to be to destroy an opponent rather than to attain truth. Yet out of this polemical attitude there gradually developed the scientific method as we now recognize it. The touchstone lay in the twin categories of reason and experience. To these all opponents made equal appeal yet differed regarding the meanings that they attached to the terms. What constituted experience? In modern terminology we might rephrase the question, what do we mean by a fact? We have the further question: what constitutes sound reasoning? When are our inferences correct and reliable? Both these questions are age-old. The medieval philosophers honed reason to a very fine edge indeed, but however effective this tool was in dissecting abstractions, it did not seem to cut deeply into the sensible world, the world of experience. The relations between reason and experience have been troubled.

Commonly we think of the Renaissance as the era when sensory experience began to take a more important part in the total scheme of things. Be this as it may, by the seventeenth century a combination of experience and reason replaced any earlier tendency to some sort of disjunction. By the end of the seventeenth century the conjunction was firmly established. Yet even when joined to experience, reason without qualification was not enough. It had to be sound reason. And the concept of soundness progressed from a vague indefinite status, through stages of increasing precision, to attain the monumental status it enjoys today. The ways in which reasoning became more and more sound correspond to what I call growth of critical judgment. We appreciate this growth in retrospect, and the writings of Blondel illustrate the process admirably. They are worth detailed examination.

The search for clarity was one of his virtues. In the preface he stated his position clearly: he was attacking the "vulgar error . . . the common opinion that marks and deformities which children are born with, are the sad effects of the mother's irregular fancy and imagination."[43] And this error, he said, is contrary to experience and sound reason, as well as anatomy. He dismissed the usual defense: that "long experience of many ages . . . attested by so many creditable witnesses" is adequate proof of the fact. We cannot rely on generally accepted hypotheses. There are too many examples of fallacious but widely accepted beliefs, and *post hoc* does not mean *propter hoc*.

He carefully defined imagination. In his context it meant "a modification of the mother's thoughts upon certain outward objects,"[44] for example, the longing for a particular thing; a sudden surprise; the abhorrence

of an ugly object or, conversely, the pleasure from contemplating something delightful; fear or apprehension; an excess of anger or grief or, conversely, of joy. In his definition we thus have a combination of imagery,
perception, and emotions, all bundled into one concept.

That the mother *could* affect the fetus was indisputable, for "the pros-
perity of the fetus does depend on the welfare of the mother," and whatever harms her may be indirectly prejudicial to the fetus. Thus, distempers, falls, blows, poor diet, excessive exercise and bodily agitation may
affect the infant. Similarly, the fetus "may also suffer by the affection of the
mother's mind." Disappointment, for example, may impair a woman's
sleep or appetite and indirectly affect the child. Various emotions and agitations of the mind are accompanied by agitations of the body, with concrete physical changes. "Vehemence" in the blood "may separate the placenta and cause an abortion."[45] Violent actions of the diaphragm are
physical forces that press upon the uterus and can cause damage. In all this
we recognize the first category that Sennert had distinguished.

Then, without reference to his predecessor, Blondel turned to the further distinction regarding determinate or specific impressions on the child,
such as the image of a cherry. And this effect Blondel strongly denied. In
his argument he gave criteria for evaluating experience. There must be a
sufficient number of observations which should relate to different aspects;
experience must rest on evidence of the senses, and not on "occult qualities,
suppositions, conjectures, hear-says, and casualties [chance]." There must
be uniformity and not contradiction. Furthermore, there must be a sufficient number of cases to counterbalance "counter observations." We cannot, for example, consider a drug effective if it cures only one case in a
thousand. Then he indicated factors relevant to the testimony of others:
hearsay evidence must be received with great caution; credibility diminishes proportionally to distance in time or space; witnesses must be impartial and "without any interest to cheat"; they must not be "credulous, nor
prepossest, nor too hasty"; and those who have been proved wrong in the
past are not to be trusted.[46]

Then Blondel examined the data supporting the belief in the power of
the imagination, noting the lack of agreement in regard to persons, time,
and extent. Some persons deemed the imagination of the father an effective cause; others thought the imagination effective at a distance, comparable to a magnet; some considered the imagination operative at any time
during the nine months of gestation, from the moment of conception to the
moment of delivery but others restricted the time factors. And then there
was a wide range in the particular changes attributed to the imagination.

In contrast, the ancients accounted for monsters by "more rational
causes," such as defects in the seed, deformities of the parents, bad con-

formation of the uterus, violent accidents, even the anger of God.[47] But more recently all defects have been blamed on the imagination. Blondel concluded that the imaginationists cannot rely on the antiquity of evidence as a point in their favor.

After discussing the evidence in general, Blondel took up specific points that John Stuart Mill later elaborated in his canons of induction. Thus, we may have acts of the imagination without any subsequent marks or deformity; we may have marks or deformities "without any precedent imagination"; and there are marks considered as subsequent to the imagination and yet deemed to be the effect thereof.[48] Blondel took up each of these problems in turn and presented particular cases to support his own claims. In retrospect, of course, his evidence lacked cogency, for he selected instances that fitted into his own views and did not show us that they derived from specially reliable witnesses. He did, however, introduce enough evidence contrary to the "vulgar opinions" to cast doubt on the latter and to induce a verdict of "not proven."

Then he made a quantitative estimate on the basis of probabilities. From the bills of mortality he calculated that in 20 years about 500,000 children were born, and he conjectured on the number of birth defects. Monsters were exceedingly rare. Deformities such as hare lip or defective limbs, not quite so rare, he estimated at one for every 1,000 to 2,000 births. Of skin marks or moles he suggested an incidence of one to 100 to 500. Thus, per 100,000 births he estimated only 300 instances of abnormalities — deformities and spots, together. Then he estimated that out of 100,000 births at least 25,000 mothers would have been "exposed to the danger and fury of imagination," while only 300 infants would have had marks on their bodies. He thus calculated the odds against imagination as 24,700/300.[49] But this concedes too much, for perhaps half of the latter children had their deformities or spots "without any preceding imagination." Hence he revised his odds to 24,850 to 150 against imagination having been a factor. Still further revision of the figures was necessary, to take account of "credulity of witnesses," as well as cheats, misrepresentations, "false and ridiculous stories," accidents, and various other factors. To support this claim he gave several instances of impostures and of utter absurdities. He particularly criticized Malebranche for lack of critical sense, gullibility, failure to consider other explanations, and ignoring other cases that were relevant but did not support his claims.

Then he turned to his more immediate opponent, Dr. Turner, and considered in detail some of the cases the latter had taken from the literature as proving the power of the imagination over the fetus. These sources ranged from Hippocrates and Hesiod to various seventeenth century authors. Blondel's critique indicated in some cases that Turner had misinterpreted his authorities; other cases rested on remote hearsay and lacked credibility; in others there was fraud and deliberate misrepresentation; others provided no adequate evidence of alleged imagination; and so on. In his discussion of one case of congenital lameness, Blondel remarked that "the reality of the lameness is not in question, 'tis the cause which is in dispute."[50]

He summarized his long analysis by the following points: the "imaginationists" changed their hypotheses from time to time "according to their humour and fancy"; imagination often has no sequellae; marks and deformities appear without previous imagination; various testimonies are doubtful, false, or irrelevant; mathematical odds are against imagination as a factor; and positive cases can be explained as due to chance.[51] So much for experience. Then he attended to "reason and anatomy." The appeal to reason dealt principally with inconsistencies and seems largely quibbling, adding little. The appeal to anatomy, however, is far more significant.

Certain of his points were quite general. There is no communication of nerves between mother and child. The child has its own soul and mind, with no direct connection with the mother, so that the mother cannot communicate her thoughts to the mind of the fetus, as Malebranche had claimed. Blondel elaborated on the absurdity of this view. He recounted briefly and with some confusion the contributions of Harvey, de Graef, and Leeuwenhoek. He himself inclined to the view that the animalculae (the sperm) contain the preexisting organs and that the ovum is the *nidus* in which the animalcula lodges and is nourished. The parts of the fetus thus preexist before conception.[52] Hence the imagination of the mother cannot act on the fetus in any stage of its development. Turner had claimed a common circulation from the mother to child and back, but Blondel indicated the absence of circulation in common between mother and child, and into this topic he went in great detail.

How, then, to explain the actual birthmarks and deformities? He offered possible causes in five categories: "1. the variety of particles, and of their combinations. 2. the distempers of children in utero. 3. the interruption of the increase of some parts in the child. 4. force and violence upon the body of the foetus. 5. misfortunes from inheritance, and the transmigration [passage] of the ova."[53] For each of these he gave explications and examples, which we do not need to consider specifically.

Blondel was motivated largely by the spirit of controversy. He criticized the evidence offered by others and the theories founded thereon, but he did not himself provide new data. His contribution to science was critical rather than substantive, but nonetheless important, for the question what can be accepted as evidence underlies all scientific endeavor. And Blondel helped create standards for evaluating assertions before they serve as a basis for theories.

Critical judgment depends on underlying philosophical concepts. If we compare Sennert with Blondel, we realize that Sennert was a neo-Galenist who, even though he adopted some of the corpuscular notions, remained firmly committed to the concepts of form and matter. His explanations had to accommodate themselves to this underlying requirement. The data accepted as facts were filtered through the concept of form.

Blondel was a corpuscularian. His own views he considered "clear and intelligible, and easily deduced from the laws of motion, which God has established among bodies."[54] And he insisted that explanation should be free from occult qualities and other doctrines of the neo-Galenists. It was easy for Blondel to be highly critical of assertions to which his basic metaphysics was opposed. He was less critical of assertions that seemed to favor his own basic views.

We must recognize this fundamental point in scientific methdology: theory depends on facts but also helps determine what we accept as facts. We thus have a circular process and we must accept the circularity.

Maupertuis

As we approach the mid-eighteenth century we perceive a great change in medicine and the biological sciences. The older physicians, hitherto dominant, had had their training in the late seventeenth century and reflected the thought modes and struggles of that era. A new generation, coming to the fore, had been spared the tumult of conflicting systems, for by now the mainstream of science centered firmly around the mechanical philosophy that had vanquished the neo-Galenists and absorbed the chemists. To be sure, the rather crude mechanical doctrines were undergoing transformation around the middle of the eighteenth century, as Robert Schofield has so well discussed.[55] Physicists appreciated that the forces affecting the particles of matter were more subtle than had originally been thought. Attraction was a force to be reckoned with and the cruder mechanism, such as that of Baglivi and Pitcairn, no longer had the appeal it had exerted in the first two decades of the eighteenth century. This whole transformation of scientific thought in mid-century involves many different strands. I want to restrict the discussion to the specific area of the maternal imagination.

In this problem an important figure was Pierre Louis Moreau de Maupertuis (1698-1759), physicist, mathematician, astronomer, geographer, one of the most brilliant minds of the century but a rather stormy personality who engaged in extensive controversy. Voltaire took part in the quarrels, and his literary skill and malice darkened Maupertuis's contemporary reputation. Bentley Glass provides an excellent brief summary of these episodes which have figured most prominently in the history of the physical sciences.[56]

Maupertuis made important contributions to biology, particularly in the broad fields of reproduction, embryology, heredity, and evolutionary theory. There are sound expositions in Glass, and in histories of embryology.[57] Maupertuis's most famous single work in these fields was his *Venus physique,* published first in 1745.[58] He rejected the *emboîtement* theory, hitherto dominant in embryology, in favor of epigenesis. The conflict between the two rival doctrines is a major feature in eighteenth century biology but rather oblique to our purposes. Maupertuis also made important studies on the inheritance of birth defects, particularly of supernumerary digits. Glass has provided a splendid discussion of these contributions.

In his book *Venus physique* Maupertuis, expounding many doctrines in regard to heredity and generation, devoted a brief chapter to the maternal imagination and its possible effect on the fetus.[59] He emphasized the point to which Sennert had already drawn attention, that we must distinguish two types of phenomena, the one having to do with severe malformations, the other with the marks on the skin. Maupertuis found no difficulty in accepting the concept that violent emotions could affect the whole process of fetal development. Between the fetus and the mother there is certainly a connection sufficiently intimate that a violent commotion in the spirits or blood of the mother could be transmitted to the fetus and deform its delicate tissues.

As a support for this doctrine, Maupertuis accepted the phenomena of "sympathy." He saw nothing surprising in the case of Malebranche, of the infant whose limbs were broken in the same places as the criminal's whose execution the mother had witnessed. But he objected to the claim that the mother could impress on the fetus the configuration of an object that had startled her or that she had desired to eat. The fear a woman might experience at the sight of a tiger could cause the infant to perish entirely or to have major deformities but not cause the child to be born brindled or with claws (unless, he added, this was purely the result of chance, having nothing to do with the fright from the tiger). The child with the broken bones would be much less remarkable than one with the cherry-like imprint induced by the mother's desire.

Birthmarks that supposedly resembled animals were very common and he had seen many, but he took little stock in the asserted resemblance. To him the marks seemed merely black hairy spots, although to some observers an animal shape appeared clearly outlined. And then he made the telling point that mothers do not recall various desires or fears until after they have given birth to a marked infant. And it would be most strange if in a nine-month period a woman had never been frightened by an animal or wished to eat some fruit. In modern terminology Maupertuis was criticizing reports for being retrospective rather than prospective. The latter would be convincing, the former not.

Maupertuis shed no new light on the imagination but his account is significant in several respects. As one of the most eminent scientists of his era, he had a highly critical mind. He also had unusual expertise in the problems of generation, an expertise derived not merely from the literature but from direct investiagation. Although he did not make the distinction explicitly, he did tend to differentiate between the emotions, which could affect the fetus, and the "imagination" in a stricter sense, which had no effect on the fetus. The emotions, through their effect on the blood and humors, could induce alterations in the fetus in a gross fashion, although Maupertuis was not critical about any possible mechanism by which the phenomena might take place. That the superficial marks might be due to the mother's imagination he completely rejected, denying the fact and not even bothering to criticize any of the alleged mechanisms. We can regard Maupertuis's views as representing the attitude of an outstanding mid-century scientist.

Buffon

Georges-Louis Leclerc, Count de Buffon (1707-1788), mathematician and naturalist, was one of the luminaries of the French Enlightenment. As a leading biologist he was intensely interested in the problems of generation, which he studied intensively to arrive at his own theoretical formulations.[60] His views rested on a sort of dualistic atomism with two kinds of primitive bodies, the organic molecules, the basis of life, and those that were inert. Both kinds entered the body when food was ingested. There was separation and purification during digestion, and the molecules entered the blood to supply nutrition and bring about growth. From the blood each organ was able to select what was appropriate, through a mechanism he called the internal mold (*moule intérieur*), which we can regard as a sort of template, distinct for each organ, whereby what is suitable gets accepted and all else rejected. What is thus selectively removed from the blood enters into the proper tissue.

When growth is complete, at the time of puberty, there is a superabundance of organic molecules. These then get carried from all parts of the body to the organs of generation, which provide a locus for combination. The organic molecules, coming from all different parts of the body, can combine into an organization *in parvo* similar to the body as a whole.[61]

These minute organized bodies appear in the generative fluid of each sex (that is, in the fluid of the Graafian follicles as well as in the seminal fluid of the male) but cannot develop until the male and female components mingle in sexual congress. Then a new individual is formed. There is thus emphasis on organization and development, with the organic molecules serving as the ultimate elements whose qualities and distribution determine the characteristics of the fetus.

Buffon elaborated his views in considerable detail so that they could explain various observed phenomena, including certain data of heredity. Without going into details, we can appreciate his emphasis that mechanical laws are totally inadequate to explain the facts of generation. He rejected the simplistic mechanical views so popular earlier in the century.

In one long chapter dealing with the development and growth of the fetus, Buffon discussed the problem whether the imagination of the mother might affect the fetus.[62] His arguments, although resting on the newest embryological data, are not significantly different from those of Blondel. Buffon did, however, offer other metaphors and examples. Pointing out that there is no direct vascular connection between the bloodstream of the mother and that of the fetus, he claimed that the fetus *in utero* is in essence independent of the mother, just as the egg is independent of the brooding hen. As for the naevi at birth, he pointed out that the marks necessarily have some sort of configuration, which may resemble one or another object, but any resemblance depends on the imagination of the viewer rather than of the mother.

He denied that imagination can produce in the infant any "real" representation of objects that excited emotions in the mother. In regard to the famous case of Malebranche, of the infant born with broken limbs, he made this trenchant comparison: we might just as well expect a brooding hen that sees a rooster having its neck wrung, to hatch out a chick with a twisted neck.

Buffon declared, however, that emotion can induce severe bodily changes in the mother, which can shake, compress, agitate, and otherwise affect the uterus. If this commotion is sufficiently violent, the fetus might perhaps receive a trauma that would kill or wound it or deform the parts struck with particular violence. But the commotion could not produce in the fetus anything similar to the thoughts of the mother.

But how to explain the fact that the infant *was* born with these deformities? Said Buffon, by sheer chance. The rare and the unusual happen with the same necessity as the common and the ordinary, but less frequently. Even the most extraordinary arrangement of matter must occur eventually. One can wager that in a million or a billion births, sooner or later an infant will be born with two heads or four legs or with the bones broken, or with whatever deformity one might indicate. It might even happen that such a monstrosity may be accompanied by a particular state of mind in the mother. It is more likely that such a phenomenon will happen by chance, than that the mother's imagination should have played a causative role.

Buffon also pointed out that despite the relative independence of the fetus certain diseases can pass from mother to infant. He specified syphilis, which affects the bones. He thought that the case of Malebranche might have suffered from this disease; or perhaps rickets, which, he pointed out, produced "callus" in the long bones.

Only credulity, said Buffon, rendered this case marvelous, yet many persons will accept it as true, despite our reason and our philosophy. Prejudice based on the marvelous will always triumph over reason, he said, and this should not astonish a philosopher. He had no hopes of persuading women that the marks on their children were unrelated to their unsatisfied desires. Yet he pointed out that before delivery we could ask a woman what unsatisfied desires she might have had and what marks the child should therefore bear. He himself, he said, had asked these questions but all he did was to vex the women without convincing them. Thus, in modern terms, he sought in vain for prospective and predictive evidence.

Haller

Albrecht von Haller (1708-1777) was the leading physiologist of the eighteenth century. In his massive text, *Elementa Physiologiae* (1757-1766), he devoted a considerable part to generation, and in his discussion he commented on the problem whether the imagination could affect the fetus.[63] His concern here was rather indirect, for he approached the topic not as a controversialist, like Blondel, but as an investigator who had an underlying interest in the mechanisms of embryology. He wanted to eliminate the idea of any immaterial force, any *anima* that controlled the development of the fetus and he explicitly condemned the doctrine of an intelligent spiritual force, an *animae vis fabricatrix*, directing the formation of the fetus. Haller also condemned the doctrine that assumed some sort of spiritual force that would differentiate the unformed matter of an animal. He also rejected any "seminal idea," "plastic idea," or other similar doctrine.[64]

Those who adhered to the idea of some type of soul were laying particular stress on the occurrence of birthmarks. Certainly, the imagination, as a mental function, was immaterial. And if the mind of the mother could affect the development of the fetus, such an action would bring back into embryology a kind of animistic causation, which Haller was striving to eliminate. Although he did not phrase his argument in these words, this formulation seems entirely consistent with his views.[65]

Haller discussed the topic of malformations and the possible role of imagination. Extremely erudite, with a profound knowledge of the literature, he provided extensive references to various predecessors and their claims. Indeed, the main threads of his argument get obscured by the very mass of detail.

He recounted the various cases that had been adduced as evidence, of the kind we already have met, and he reviewed the familiar claims alleged as mechanisms, for example, that ideas of the mother reached the fetus by way of the blood or the nerves. No one, he said, "seriously believes that he understands how the mind of the mother would change the fetus."[66] Yet those who claimed that the imagination would affect the fetus, while admitting that they could not explain how, declared that the effect was *true* and that there were many other effects that demanded credence, even though no one could provide a mechanical explanation. For this view he named Boerhaave as the chief proponent. Without accepting this argument, Haller seemed willing to allow some sort of indirect influence on the fetus from severe maternal emotional disturbance.

As for various birthmarks, he regarded these as a form of skin disease, and he gave some conjectures regarding the pathology, for example, the retention of blood in veins whose membranes were rendered more translucent. (He could not know, of course, the fine details of hemangiomas.) Other lesions he considered a kind of verruca, or an "enlarged sebaceous gland" — brown, swollen, more or less rounded, showing some firm hairs. When these lesions are larger, they may be likened to the skin of a deer, or a bear, or a hare. Many of the tumors, allegedly signs that resemble this or that object, are of similar character. He considered the various cases to be disease, "especially congestions of the gelatinous material in the subcutaneous spaces."[67]

Various other deformities were harder to explain but some, at least, he was ready to attribute to uterine pressure. Others, such as superfluous digits, he did not try to explain but referred to a familial incidence without any question of maternal fright. That various other deformities were due to maternal terror, he considered incredible. And the famous case of Malebranche he ascribed to a physical cause, the separation of the epiphyses.

Severe congenital deformities are common in animals as well as in man — for example, infants with one arm or no feet. These he believed resulted from some unknown type of arterial compression. Similarly, a lack of nourishment could impair development of various parts such as the parietes covering the viscera. Or there might be too much blood. "Weakness" of the cellular tissue he judged the cause of hare lip.[68] The different examples of congenital deformities he attributed to physical causes, although these were conjectural rather than demonstrated.

Haller also repeated the now familiar arguments: that many pregnant women had various emotional disturbances without any disturbance in the fetus; and on the contrary, many deformities occurred without evidence of prior terror. Furthermore, there are disturbances in the development of plants without any question of mental upset. He believed that in the seeds of vegetables and in the ova of animals there lay hidden the cause of the future development, eternal for each species, but other factors can supervene, such as abundance or lack of nutrition, excessively strong or weak "pressure," or other less known causes. These can induce changes in structure, which nevertheless remains within its own limits. A tulip bulb never produces an iris, nor a woman a cat. And regarding the powers of the imagination, Haller wanted to wait until he had more convincing examples of markings that had been forecast ahead. Like Maupertuis, he wanted a prospective investigation.[69]

Bablot

As a sort of anticlimax we may examine briefly a book published in 1788, *Dissertation sur le pouvoir de l'imagination des femmes enceintes*, which supported the earlier views on the power of the imagination.[70] The author, Benjamin Bablot (dates of birth and death not known), who described himself as Conseiller-médecin-ordinaire du Roi, à Châlons-sur Marne, strongly defended the concept that the imagination of the mother could act on the fetus.

The first part of the book he devoted to evidence supporting his own viewpoint. He began with the scriptural account of Jacob and Laban, and then, with a considerable amount of skipping around, continued almost to his own time. He included Hippocrates, Aristotle, Pliny, Galen, and many others. In addition, he inserted a long discussion of animal magnetism and drew on the report of the commission that the king had recently appointed to investigate the claims of Mesmer. From this fascinating document Bablot drew much consolation, and he emphasized the surprising effects that the mind could exert over the body — the phenomena we now call hypnotism. This, to Bablot, indicated the power of the imagination of one person over the imagination of another.[71] He did not, however, show the relevance of these mesmeric phenomena to the problem of marking the infant. He was eagerly embracing any evidence that indicated a relationship of imagination to physical changes, and simply assumed its relevance.

He covered a vast amount of sixteenth and seventeenth century literature, picking out excerpts that supported his contentions. Yet he was completely uncritical of his sources and lumped together many different kinds of phenomena such as the general influence of mind over body, the concept of sympathy, and some factors of inheritance. By slippery textual analysis he even drew support from the adverse comments of Maupertuis.

This first portion of Bablot's work provides a slanted review of the literature. More significant for the history of ideas is the second part, wherein he tried to refute specific objections to the views he was advocating. To answer the objection that there was no direct communication between the blood and humors of the mother and those of the infant, Bablot pointed to transmissions across the placenta of various maternal states and affections, such as syphilis or smallpox.[72] But more important, he simply denied the anatomical claims and quoted "authorities" who had asserted a common blood circulation between mother and fetus.

A second objection concerned the analogy, that the fetus in the uterus was as independent of the mother as the chicken in the egg was independent of the brooding hen.[73] Bablot replied that the analogy was quite faulty, the comparison specious. He admitted that we cannot explain how the imagination produces its effect, but he continued to assert that the effect did take place.

In his discussion he pointed to various accounts wherein persons with delusions — considered to be disturbed imagination — returned to normal solely through mental therapy. We have here the germ of the later "moral treatment" wherein mental disturbance was treated by psychological means only. But with Bablot the single term imagination was used indiscriminately to cover all the various phenomena, and then the different results were freely transferred from one category to another. Psychological cure of mental disease involved the imagination; so too did the phenomena of animal magnetism; and so, allegedly, did various birth defects. The data in any one category were thought to support the claims in the others.

A third objection concerned the nervous system and the lack of direct communication between spirits in the brain of the mother and those in the brain of the infant.[74] This Bablot dismissed rather cursorily, for he pointed out that there are many phenomena for which we cannot offer any explanation, but we cannot therefore deny the fact. And facts always stand above the best possible reasoning. He made no effort to provide any criteria for establishing facts, nor did he try to evaluate his authorities or distinguish degrees of credibility. He accepted authority as the touchstone. Yet on the other hand Bablot was skeptical about the validity of any given hypothesis. He preferred even a wobbly "fact" to a closely reasoned theory.

The fourth objection seems forceful: our sensations do not resemble the objects that cause them, and hence it is impossible for internal emotions to produce a "real" representation of a particular object.[75] In other words, the perceptions of an object cannot produce a material object. To answer this, Bablot indulged in some conjecture drawn from Fienus, on the way that the imagination of the mother might produce "real" representation of an object. He compared the mother to a painter and the fetus to a canvas. The intervention of spirits (that is, nerve fluid) plays the role of the painter's brush. As the imagination of the painter produces a picture on the canvas, so the imagination of the mother can sketch on the fetus the features of different external objects that she had thought about.

Another important objection concerns the disturbances and monstrosities that occur in plants and are comparable to the alterations in animals.[76] Bablot, however, indicated that the imagination is not responsible for all abnormalities. It would be absurd, he said, to hold the mother's imagination responsible for such monstrosities as a fetus with two heads or three arms or only one leg. In the vegetable kingdom monstrosities could be attributed to faulty circulation of the nourishing sap.

These instances provide an adequate sampling of Bablot's reasoning. But perhaps his viewpoint is best summarized in his conclusions, where he discusses the assertion of Buffon, who tried to induce pregnant women to announce their unsatisfied desires before delivery and then examined the newborn infants for birthmarks. Bablot, instead of answering this objection on its merits, argued *ad hominem*. He took his stand with the great men who, from ancient time to the present, believed in the power of the maternal imagination. Among others he mentioned Empedecles, Hippocrates, Soranus, Galen, Plato, Plutarch, Avicenna, Cicero, Pliny, St. Jerome, St. Augustine, and St. Thomas Aquinas. In modern times he included Fernel, Aldrovandus, Thomas More, Montaigne, Paré, Fienus, Descartes, Riverius, Riolan, Digby, Lemery, Malebranche, Maupertuis, Boerhaave, van Swieten. In view of these authorities, said Bablot, no one should lightly dismiss the power of the maternal imagination over the fetus. It is the height of impertinance or madness to regard as visionaries, ignoramuses, or imposters all the great men who have declared themselves in favor of an opinion that rests on the experience of more than 3,000 years.[77]

Bablot contrasted the process of reasoning with the simple assertion of van Swieten, "I have seen, I have examined." Can any amount of reasoning, he asked, outweigh the existence of a single fact?[78] Clearly, the concept of fact and the relation of fact to authority are the critical features of this dispute. There is a great temptation to smile at Bablot's naiveté and his lack of scientific attitude. But there are some important features that deserve explicit comment here.

Impasse

Approximately 150 years intervened between Sennert and Bablot. In this interval there were enormous changes — in basic metaphysical viewpoint, in sheer quantity of information, in cultural patterns and attitudes,

in degrees of critical acumen. Yet in regard to the imaginationist controversy many of the ideas persisted with little change. The assertion that the
imagination of the mother was a causal agent retained its force throughout
the whole period.

We can see certain reasons for this persistence. There was failure to clarify just what was meant by imagination. The term, covering a multitude of
functions, lacked precision. The imaginationists and the anti-imagina-
tionists might be referring to different aspects of the broad category that
imagination embraced, so that there was no real meeting of minds.

Then, the disputants failed to specify in compelling fashion any stepwise
mechanism by which the imagination might exert its effect. To be sure,
there was one school of thought that invoked a spiritual force, an archeus,
between the activity of the mind and the physical manifestations. But, as
the mechanical philosophy displaced neo-Galenism, the concept of
archeus, or a similar entity, came under severe attack. Any such immaterial force was rejected, yet, as we saw in Haller, the imaginationist view
seemed to suggest a persistence of this archeus-like entity, and confusion
resulted.

We must appreciate the enormous increase in volume of biological
knowledge. There were vast advances in microscopy. The discovery of the
sperm and of the Graafian follicle were quite epoch making. (Of course,
the discovery of the ovum came only much later.) These led to the disputes
of preformationism versus a true development of bodily parts from an un-
differentiated substance. Important studies clarified the stages of the developing vertebrate embryo; there were major discoveries in parthenoge-
netic reproduction of certain insects; in metamorphosis; in regenerative
capacity inherent in certain low animals like the polyp; there was increasing knowledge of placentation and of the anatomical relations between
fetus and mother; there were early investigations of inheritance of abnormalities — these were a few of the ways in which knowledge increased
between the mid-seventeenth and the mid-eighteenth centuries. Yet despite the overwhelming wealth of data, the interpretation and explanation
— the theory — remained confused.

We see this in the *Encyclopedia Britannica,* the first edition of which appeared in 1771. In the article, "Generation," the author briefly expounded
current views, with special reference to Buffon and Maupertuis, and closed
the brief essay with the statement, "Whoever reads this short sketch of the
different theories of generation that have hitherto been invented, will
probably require no other argument to convince him that we are still as
ignorant of the nature of this mysterious operation as they were in the days
of Noah."[79]

Literally, of course, this is nonsense, yet the author was referring not to bits of information which had massively accumulated but to the lack of any cogent explanation, of any theory that compelled assent either among scholars or among the rude and unlearned. This, clearly true regarding overall theories of generation, was equally true in the specific area that dealt with malformations. Malformations ranged from gross defects like meningocele or hare lip to minor abnormalities like birthmarks. But the explanations were in dispute.

Since explanatory theories rest on facts, the choice between theories will depend on what we accept as facts. The word itself is ambiguous. On the one hand it has a connotation of immutability. It *is*. It represents reality, indisputable. In a second sense it is only an assertion, an allegation that some will accept, others not. As such it is subject to dispute. We could unify these two senses by using the term alleged fact in all contexts. This, while accurate, is clumsy and not generally used, yet if it were, much dispute would be avoided.

The whole point of the imaginationist controversy rests on the acceptance or rejection of allegations. And this, in turn, involves the distinction between fact and theory. Bablot epitomizes one viewpoint clearly: the influence of the mother's imagination on the infant is a fact. To be sure, he could not explain it but, since fact is irrefutable, this lack of suitable explanation did not worry him. This viewpoint represents one of the continuous threads that extend throughout the entire dispute.

The opposite point of view declares that the deformity or abnormality is a fact but the causative role of the imagination is only an allegation, not a fact at all. As merely an alleged theory, it is subject to criticisms and doubt and must conform to tests of validity. This view, of course, was not explicitly stated in these particular terms but is implicit, for example, in Blondel's comments.

A severely critical attitude was becoming more and more prominent in the early eighteenth century, in a wide variety of intellectual activities. Blondel's writings provide an excellent example of such critical acumen in the field of medicine. Yet the only cogent way of refuting an alleged explanation is by offering an alternative explanation whose links and details are overwhelmingly clear and convincing and which account for the data in an inescapable fashion. The imaginationist controversy in the seventeenth and eighteenth centuries indicates the way men groped for explanations but lacked key terms that would make any explanation convincing. The controversy is, indeed, an important landmark in the history of ideas.

EIGHT

THE PROCESS OF EXPLANATION

The physicians of times past, like those of today, tried to bring order into experience. They did so by creating explanatory theories. Quite naturally, any given period regards its own theories as sound, those of its predecessors as outmoded, inadequate, perhaps naive, illogical, or even absurd, and in any case "wrong." Yet for the historian these wrong explanations are further data. With their truth or falsity he has no real concern. He must, however, study their origins, their growth and acceptance, and their decline, and thereby place them in perspective.

The medical historian finds an enormous range of theories. Broad philosophic concepts merge with those specifically medical. Cudworth, for example, combined Greek philosophy, especially Neoplatonism, with Christian theology to provide an overall explanation of the world; Gassendi combined classical atomism with Christian theology to provide a quite different explanation. Both were influential in medical theory. We can contrast Cudworth and van Helmont, Sennert and Boyle, Pitcairn and Stahl, all differing markedly from each other. We can pass from grand philosophies to more restricted theories, from those that explain the whole universe to those that deal with a minute aspect of experience; we can study the explanations that involve the devil and witchcraft and others that involve genes and nucleic acids. In all these examples, from the most sublime to the must mundane, someone is offering an explanation. What do these different pronouncements have in common? What characterizes them as explanations?

Philosophers may distinguish different kinds of explanation — scientific from historical, psychological from logical, causal from descriptive — and offer criteria to separate the valid from the invalid. The historian, however, must have a definition that will cover the wrong as well as the right, the outmoded as well as the current, the general as well as the specific.

Rather than offer an initial definition we might better note some concrete examples of the explanatory process. First, however, let me offer my definition of two technical terms. I call the *explicandum* that which is to be explained, while the *explicans* is the statement offered in explanation, that is, the answer to the question why or perhaps how.[1]

The word explanation comes from the Latin *planus*, meaning smooth. Literally, explanation is that which makes smooth (referring, of course, to a state of mind, not a physical object). The explanation resolves some intellectual problem or difficulty. It smooths over a rough spot in the under-standing, clears up a puzzlement, permits a sense of satisfaction or rest to succeed some particular mental unease.

This we can call the psychological aspect of explanation, as distinct from the logical. The psychological aspect we see to best advantage in the small child of three or four. He is sufficiently adept with language to frame questions and at the same time is distinctly aware of particular events that, since they do not fit in with his previous limited experience, provoke a sense of unease. This attitude the child expresses in questions. Why is the grass green? Why does a dog bark? Why is the sun hot? Ordinarily it is the bright child who asks questions, for he is actively examining experience and dis-tinguishing the familiar from the unfamiliar, comparing *this* with *that*. The comparison turns up discrepancies, and the child, aware that the new does not harmonize with the old, seeks explanation.

All of us, children and adults alike, view experience in certain patterns that vary in complexity according to the maturity of the individual and the environment in which he moves. Carl Becker, examining "climates of opinion," mentioned the satisfaction we get when we regard things in a pattern. He went on, "and mental satisfaction is always worthwhile, for the simple reason that when the mind is satisfied with the pattern of things it sees, it has what it calls an 'explanation' of the things — it has found the 'cause' of them."[2]

In a different context Basil Willey expressed what I consider to be a comparable idea. Said Willey, "The clarity of an explanation seems to de-pend upon the degree of satisfaction that it affords. An explanation 'ex-plains' best when it meets some need of our nature, some deepseated demand for assurance. 'Explanation' may perhaps be roughly defined as a restatement of something — event, theory, doctrine, etc. — in terms of cur-rent interests and assumptions."[3] This presentation, I maintain, is equally applicable to the four year old pestering his mother, to the physician trying to explain an illness to a patient, or to the biologist trying to account for his experimental data. In all these there is a pattern that needs to be enlarged and an initial sense of puzzlement. Explanation expands the pattern in such a way as to provide an inner satisfaction. When the child is satis-fied, he stops asking questions. Indeed, if the mother allays his curiosity, the child ordinarily says Oh — a sign that a satisfactory resolution has been achieved.

Is the explanation "true" or "correct"? Can the mother, for example, give a sound, logical, and correct account of why the grass is green, or the sun hot? This is a quite different problem. The correctness or truth of an answer need not affect the sense of satisfaction that the answer conveys. Explanations will vary in the degree of satisfaction they offer, that is, the degree to which the answer resolves preexisting intellectual patterns into a state of satisfaction. The truth of the explanation refers to quite different criteria.

This degree of satisfaction involves what I call the psychological aspects of explanation, crucial for any generalized account of the explanatory process. An extreme example of this psychological component we find in the story of two Scottish farmers early in the last century. The recently invented telegraph was transmitting messages from Glasgow to Edinburgh. One farmer, seeking an explanation, asked how it worked. The other replied, "Well, if they stretched a dog from Glasgow to Edinburgh, and stepped on his tail in Glasgow, he would bark in Edinburgh. But since it is not convenient to stretch a dog that far, they stretch a wire instead." The first farmer presumably replied with the classical Oh—his curiosity was satisfied, his pattern of universe now embraced the new phenomenon. He had received and accepted an explanation.

A critic might point out that the supposed explanation was only a faulty analogy but even though this analogy does not conform to sound logical criteria, it does conform to one major facet of explanation, it made smooth the puzzlement of the inquirer.

Apart from the psychological aspect a second component of explanation we may designate as logical, having special relevance to science. For an example I will note a common experience. In certain cases of injury the sensation of pain comes perceptibly later than the sense of touch or pressure. Thus, if we receive a blow, we are aware of the tactile sensation a small but identifiable interval before we feel the pain. In comparable fashion, if we accidentally touch a hot stove, we jerk our hand back before we are aware of the pain. Why does this happen? How can we explain it?

At this point we must introduce the further term "universe of discourse." I define it as any set of experiences that can form a class, that has some sort of unity and provides a fairly distinct context separable from other contexts. Stamp collectors, gourmet cooks, turf enthusiasts, mathematicians, all represent separate classes, each with its special vocabulary, special procedures, special concepts, not shared by others, and each comprising a universe or realm of discourse. In simplest terms this merely represents a class sufficiently well defined to be talked about. We deal with many different realms of experience. When we saunter down the street at noon, enjoying the sunshine and the crowds, we are in one realm; when we read a work of fiction, in another; and when we study biochemistry or pharmacology, still another.

Logical explanation, I suggest, involves the passage from one universe of discourse to another. Thus, if while we are walking down the street, we are caught in a sudden shower, we explain the onset of rain not by our perceptions while walking but by specialized information within the realm of meteorology. This is a universe of discourse quite distinct from the street on which we are walking. To explain the phenomenon that we feel touch before pain, we refer not to the stone on which we stubbed or perhaps broke our toe, but to the realm of physiology, more specifically neurophysiology. This has its own distinctive terms and concepts.

Let us examine part of the universe of discourse we call neurophysiology. If we look at a peripheral nerve under a microscope, we note a vast number of fibers that differ greatly in diameter. Careful experimental study has shown that the nerve impulse travels faster in the thicker fibers than it does in the finer ones. Further experiments proved that the stimuli resulting from touch pass in the larger fibers, while stimuli from pain travel in the finer fibers. We can put these data together into a pattern that will clarify the original phenomenon—the nerve impulses corresponding to the touch travel relatively quickly; those arising in pain receptors travel relatively slowly. Therefore, the impulses corresponding to touch or contact should reach the centers of consciousness more quickly than the impulses arising from the pain receptors.

We started with observations in one level of discourse—the ordinary naive experience of stubbing our toe. To explain the puzzlement about touch and pain, we selected data from another universe of discourse that we call neurophysiology. We choose enough data to make a coherent pattern of information. With this pattern, drawn from a specialized subject, we try to resolve the puzzlement in the original universe of discourse. In the original puzzle—the *explicandum*—there is now proffered an *explicans* from a different universe of discourse. *The explanation consists in achieving a smooth passage from the one to the other*—the joining together of the two realms of discourse. The conjunction permits a stepwise progression that is psychologically satisfying.

In the present instance the *explicans* is the data regarding the transmission of the nerve impulse. However, reliance on these data alone is not sufficiently rigorous. An *explicans* may be acceptable to one person but another might consider it inadequate and not satisfactory and hence might reject it. In our particular example, the pattern of information regarding the speed of the nerve impulse may satisfy a layman, but anyone with a substantial knowledge of neurophysiology might not find it adequate. There are too many unresolved points, and the expert sees difficulties not apparent to his less sophisticated brother. Thus, there is more than one kind of pain and of touch, and the *explicans* must take into account more than the speed of transmission in the peripheral nerves. There are connections in the central nervous system involving chains of neurons. What are the various pathways? How many relays are there? How was the nerve impulse transmitted across the synapse? What about the intrinsic physiologic capacities of the different neurons? The structure and conditions within the central nervous system, in vast detail, are relevant to the *explicandum*, and to satisfy the expert we must go considerably beyond the data for the peripheral nerves. Is it possible that some findings in the central nervous system may modify or even invalidate the simple correlation found in the peripheral nervous system? The initial relationships between two universes of discourse are merely a first approximation, which deeper study in neurophysiology can elaborate. Further study may confirm the relationship, to convince even the skeptic; or it might invalidate the initial correlation, in which case the explanation is incomplete or untenable.

In science there are many universes of discourse at progressively "deeper" levels, and each level may be "explained" by reference to an *explicans* on a more abstract level. This involves the problem of reductionism. Suffice it to point out here that as we get into deeper and more basic levels, the explanation — the relationship of *explicandum* to *explicans* — appears smooth to fewer and fewer persons. Many persons will admit that they no longer understand the asserted relationships. This means that the passage from one universe of discourse to the other is not smooth. The puzzled person, perhaps, may not know the content of the *explicans* — for example, he may not be sufficiently knowledgeable in mathematics or in organic chemistry. As an alternative, the inquirer may know the terms but simply may not "see" the asserted relevance, so that the puzzlement is not resolved. He does not get what the psychologists call an Ah-ha reaction — the illumination that characterizes acceptance. This state of affairs is often resolved by a more detailed stepwise demonstration or a more skillful exposition. Or, perhaps, the skeptic may see the asserted relationship but he has other information that makes the assertion unacceptable — not necessarily false but not acceptable. In such cases, again, the smoothness necessary for an acceptable explanation is not present.

As a generalized statement I suggest three components to the explanatory process. First, a puzzling experience — a datum or fact or concept — in some universe of discourse. This is the *explicandum*. Second, a pattern of data and of concepts in some other universe of discourse — the *explicans*. And third, a relationship, a bridge, whereby the questioner can pass readily from one area to another. Explanation is a passage between the two universes of discourse whereby the original intellectual roughness is made smooth. With this formulation we can better analyze the bewildering succession of theories and explanations that the historian encounters.

We face the major question, why does an explanation, acceptable for a long time, finally get rejected? I will offer four separate examples that illustrate different facets of this complex process.

Why Does Opium Put You to Sleep?

Underlying the acceptance or rejection of a given explanation is the total world view, that is, the basic metaphysical outlook that a person might hold. Sometimes, philosophers make this world view highly explicit and carefully articulated. More often the world view is part of the general intellectual environment, accepted without question. Francis Bacon had a great deal to say about this when he described his famous four "idols" that affect man's thought. The "idols of the tribe" represent the basic limitations of the human mind. The "idols of the cave" refer to the "predominance of a favorite subject, or . . . partiality to particular ages"; the "idols of the marketplace" concern the confusion of words with things — the "names of things which do not exist" or "names which result from fantastic suppositions and to which nothing in reality corresponds"; the "idols of the theater" concern "the various dogmas of philosophy." These idols, obviously, influence the acceptance or rejection of any given explanation.[4]

The historian must note the different ways in which the idols manifest themselves. For example, concern may shift from the hereafter to the here and now; from the abstract to the concrete; from speculation to demonstration; curiosity may veer to new directions and address its questions to different groups of persons, to scientists rather than priests, or experimentalists rather than logicians. If such changes occur, the idols might seem to be wearing different robes yet have not changed their role in affecting the acceptance or rejection of any given explanation.

Bacon's formulation is especially relevant in understanding the implications of the *virtus dormativa*. In earlier chapters I have discussed at some length the neo-Galenic philosophy and the reasoning that underlay the concept of occult qualities and substantial forms. We have seen that Molière, in the third quarter of the seventeenth century, satirized this doctrine as it applied to medicine. The *virtus dormativa*, as an occult quality, became a symbol of empty verbalism that contrasted with the modern approach of the new science. It also contrasted with the new critical philosophy that rebelled against the scholastic subtleties.

David Hume combined these currents when he scornfully remarked that nature has consoled philosophers for their disappointments. "This consolation principally consists in their invention of the words *faculty* and *occult quality* . . . they need only say, that any phaenomenon, which puzzles them, arises from a faculty or an occult quality, and there is an end of all dispute and enquiry upon the matter."[5] Since an occult quality is only a facet of the substantial form, this latter concept must bear the brunt of all criticism.

Why did the substantial form, acceptable as an explanation at one time, become a source of merriment or scorn for a later era? The answer, I believe, lies in a changed attitude toward reality and, as a necessary corollary, a changed attitude toward the *explicans*.

In our present example, the *explicandum* is "opium puts you to sleep."
For the earlier physicians the *explicans* was the occult quality, the *virtus*
that derived from the substantial form. For Sennert and like-minded physicians, the substantial form was real. For Bacon, Molière, and Hume, it
was not real but merely an empty sound.

Clearly, for any explanation only something real can serve as *explicans*.
If we try to explain some event by means of a good fairy, or an Easter
bunny, or Santa Claus, or a gremlin, we cannot satisfactorily resolve a
puzzlement.

The attack on substantial forms and occult powers had its philosophical
support from the school of thought known as nominalism. For this school
the universals so dear to the scholastic thinkers were deemed not real but
only a name, only a *flatus vocis*. Francis Bacon clearly had this in mind
when he described his version of the idols of the cave and condemned the
reliance on mere names to which, he thought, no reality corresponded.

According to the nominalist position, if we explain the soporific action
of opium by invoking the *virtus dormativa*, then we are saying that opium
puts you to sleep because it has a putting-to-sleep power. For the nominalist this statement adds nothing. It is purely analytic or tautological and
simply restates the original *explicandum* in different words. In essence, to
the query "Why does opium put you to sleep?" we receive the answer "Because it does." Such an answer is not an explanation at all, for it does not
take us from one universe of discourse to another. The original area of
puzzlement, the *explicandum* is brought into relation with nothing new.
Thus, in the nominalist position the alleged *explicans* is not real and the
alleged explanation is only a delusion.

However, suppose we reject the nominalist position and maintain that
the substantial form and its derivative occult qualities do represent something real. Then we would have a universe of discourse quite distinct from
the *explicandum* and we would meet the formal requirements of a proper
explanation. The substantial form, as *explicans,* involves a realm quite
distinct from that of everyday experience. It is a realm of immaterial
entities, which exert force and direction, which control activity through
qualities.

The criticisms of Hume appear forceful but we must remember that he
was directing his shafts of wit against a degenerated doctrine and not
against that doctrine in its full flower. By the eighteenth century the occult
qualities or virtues had decayed into a purely *ad hoc* term, aimed at a
single phenomenon and not related to any other activity. In a more modern setting the *virtus* would be comparable to a gremlin, which accounts
only for the single event for which it is invoked.

But for Sennert a *virtus* was a truly viable concept, and the occult quality
that induced sleep was only one aspect of the more general entity, the sub-

stantial form of the poppy. And for Sennert the substantial form was certainly real. As we have seen, an occult quality is one that can be detected not by direct sensory perception but only by its results. Its existence was inferred, not directly observed. We might compare it, say, to a subatomic particle whose existence is inferred from the track that it makes in a cloud chamber. We do not see the particle directly; we see only the traces it leaves behind. Similarly, we do not perceive the occult quality; we see only its effects. The occult quality, known by its effects, participates in a complex immaterial world of respectable philosophical lineage.

For the neo-Galenists the occult qualities are real; we might rephrase the neo-Galenic position as a series of propositions: heat exerts activity; heat is a perceptible quality; qualities exert activity; whatever exerts activity is a quality; some qualities that exert activity are not perceptible and are properly called occult; qualities are instruments of form (substantial form); forms are real. In this chain of reasoning there may be faults; the reasoning may be wrong, but it certainly is not absurd or ridiculous.

The occult quality can serve as a genuine explanation, provided we accept the reality of the total *explicans*. However, scientists of the late seventeenth century rejected the occult quality as an explanation because they adopted a different metaphysics. The new science, based on the mechanical philosophy, rejected the entire universe of discourse from which the neo-Galenists derived their *explicantia*. The new science, therefore, left the *explicandum* standing isolated, with nothing to relate to. Eventually the new scientists had to furnish a totally different universe of discourse from which to derive a new *explicans* and build a different bridge to the *explicandum*. When a different conception of reality became dominant, the explanation resting on the old metaphysics collapsed, for its *explicans*, reduced to tautology, no longer represented a real universe of discourse. Without two universes of discourse brought into relation, we cease to have an explanation.

Incidentally, as an exercise in logic, I recommend that my readers try to find out why opium does put you to sleep, according to modern views of pharmacology and neurophysiology. The search will not be easy, nor necessarily satisfactory.

Humoralism and Solidism

Textbooks of medical history describe a long succession of theories, each of which tries to explain the phenomena of pain and disability, that is, disease. These various theories we can, if we want, categorize in different ways and give them different names: animistic or naturalistic; humoral or solidist; mechanical or chemical; cellular, ultracellular, or molecular; or any other classification we may choose. But for our present purposes we can well regard these theories as illustrating the dynamics of the explanatory process, and in so doing we may perhaps gain a clearer insight into the theories and their interrelations.

The expression "explain a disease" has a certain ambiguity. We can try to tell how the disease came about — in technical terms, indicate its pathogenesis. This we usually do in terms of causation. Thus, in an animistic philosophy, we can explain a patient's disease by saying, "The gods are angry with him." Or, in a naturalistic philosophy, we can account for a child's illness by saying, "He went out in the rain without his rubbers." These statements would point to an early link in a chain of causes. On the other hand, instead of explaining how the disease came about, we can try to tell what it *is*, according to the concepts of the era. For the Greeks a given disease might be deemed a disproportion of the humors, and today a streptococcal infection. Explanations of this character, that tell what a disease *is*, avoid the problems of pathogenesis. Since I discuss causation in the next chapter I will here concern myself with what I call the existential aspects of explanation.

In our schema, explanation consists of drawing a suitable relationship between the *explicandum* — in this instance a disease — and another universe of discourse — the *explicans*. The latter, in the present context, is a composite of structural detail, functional properties, and conceptual elaboration, all combining in a theory.

Let us begin our analysis with the so-called humoral theory of disease, which goes back at least to Hippocrates and has maintained a measure of viability ever since.[6] We can profitably note the various ways in which this theory expanded and changed, while still preserving its explanatory function.

The concept of the humors had its basis in experience. The bodily fluids are readily and directly observable; they show considerable variation in health and disease. Perhaps because the Greeks saw special significance in the number four, the primary humors were thought to be four in number — blood, phlegm, yellow bile, and black bile, present in varying proportions. There were obvious variations in the appearance of the various humors. Thus, cerebrospinal fluid, saliva, nasal mucus, and the gastric juice were all considered to be phlegm. The Greeks, lacking analytical tools, saw a unity in this diversity. Behind all the different appearances there was, they thought, an essential unity of the particular humor.

Within certain limits predominance of one or another humor accounted for (or explained) the different temperaments; a disproportion beyond normal limits explained disease. In any given disease an individual humor might become disproportionate in amount, assume different appearances that vary in color and consistency but maintain an identity despite considerable change. Thus, in the course of a common cold, the nasal mucus undergoes a series of changes in amount, color, and consistency and yet remains phlegm. Restoration of health occurred when the disproportion or alterations were eliminated.

This theory, suitably elaborated, comprised a coherent body of doctrine that served as *explicans*. In many instances its relationship to the disease — the *explicandum* — was clear: a coryza, a dropsy, a diarrhea — clearly identifiable patterns — fitted beautifully into this schema. For other diseases the relationship was less clear, but the physicians could still find a reasonably smooth passage between the two universes of discourse.

The concept of humoral composition, with suitable proportions in health, disproportion in disease, served as a satisfactory *explicans*. It was well grounded in concrete experience and involved only moderate abstraction. To be sure, it rested on a limited base — it paid little attention to the solids — and it might require hypothetical elaboration to fill in some rough spots. At times the relationships between specific diseases and the humoral explanation might seem tenuous, yet there was no serious inconsistency with the available body of knowledge.

We can readily understand why the original humoral theory paid little attention to the alterations found in the solid organs. In ancient medicine the internal organs could not be examined during life and autopsies were rare. There was too little information about the solid organs to correlate with disease states. Gradually, however, the significance of the solid components became apparent. Among the ancients there developed an increased interest in anatomy, especially in the Alexandrian school. New medical speculation, such as the Methodist doctrine of *strictum* or *laxum* and the materialistic views of the atomists, undoubtedly were relevant factors. There was a slowly increasing number of autopsies that could reveal changes in the viscera.[7] Gradually there developed a substantial knowledge of the solid components of the body. Furthermore, the increasing knowledge indicated that the fluid components far exceeded in number the original four humors described by the Greeks.

In the previous example we studied the occult qualities as *explicans*. That theory was quite rigid and could not readily adapt itself to new data. The humoral theory, however, could easily make such an accommodation and could embrace new components without difficulty. As the theory grew, it had to share its explanatory functions with other theories derived from additional fields of knowledge. But this humoral theory, even while serving as only a partial explanation applicable in a limited area, harmonized with the new concepts in a way that the substantial forms, for example, could never do.

We readily perceive these factors if we examine some of the medical literature published in the early eighteenth century. By that time the list of humors had expanded far beyond the original four. Lister offered the following classification.[8] Common to both sexes were: chyle; blood (serum, lymph, globules); urine; bile; sweat and tears; insensible perspiration; saliva, phlegm. Unique to the male was semen; unique to the female were the menstrual flow and milk; peculiar to the embryo was amniotic fluid. Boerhaave had a comparable list of humors: sweat, perspiration, tears, ear wax, sebaceous matter, mucus, saliva, sputum, "mucilage," lymph, serum, bile, semen, oil, milk, fat, and so forth.[9] This multiplicity indicates sharper empirical discrimination and allows better correlations with individual diseases than did the original four humors.

The humors, however, could no longer serve as principal explanation for all diseases. Boerhaave clearly distinguished diseases due to disturbances in the fluids from those correlating with disturbances of the solids. He recognized the appropriate specificity of each category. Furthermore, the growing science of chemistry could also enter into the same expanded universe of discourse. Boerhaave, avoiding narrow partisanship, adapted chemical concepts to explain certain diseases involving the humors. The acid acrimony and the alkaline acrimony of the humors became important concepts. By the eighteenth century we can regard the humoral theory as the handmaiden of chemistry, on which it depended for further development. The humoral theory of the ancients had become transformed into a rudimentary biochemistry. The role of the bodily fluids in health and disease remained significant but in an altered context.

In this survey we began with a universe of discourse that included ancient humoral theory as the major component. This theory expanded in both scope and depth so that by the eighteenth century there was an enormous range of data that could be subdivided into subordinate classes enjoying a reasonable (even if not absolute) harmony. Fluids and solids, chemistry and mechanics could at least meet on common ground and furnish *explicantia* for disease. I suggest that this process reveals the normal growth of science, wherein theories expand and change, eliminating some features as they embrace others. Such a universe of discourse is not static but it has dynamic properties comparable to a living organism. The eclecticism of Boerhaave lets us perceive the overall unity of that universe of discourse.

However, two important features call for comment: first, the subdivision within the total universe of discourse and a resulting type of reductionism; and second, an opposition between the abstract and the concrete. It will be simpler to begin with the latter problem.

Early Greek humoralism had one great advantage: it was quite close to direct experience. Anyone could readily see the phlegm or the blood, and only slightly less readily the yellow or black bile. These humors were concrete, not abstract, and despite some hypothetical properties remained close to immediate observation. Subsequent developments of science, however, involved progressively greater degrees of abstraction and postulation of additional hypothetical entities.

Progressive discrimination played an important role. A fever, for example, might be attributed to a disorder in the blood. Observation might show that what seemed to be a single febrile disease could be separated into two types. Could we make a comparable separation in the *explicans?* Observation .and inference might, perhaps, lead us to distinguish different states of the blood — for example, acid acrimony and alkaline acrimony — to correspond with the distinction between the two kinds of fever.[10] A discrimination in the *explicandum* thus could lead to a comparable discrimination in the *explicans,* but the latter distinction was more hypothetical, further removed from direct experience.

As science progressed explanatory concepts became further removed from experience. When we read Boerhaave we are impressed by the various hypothetical entitites that he invoked as *explicantia:* the "least fibers," the invisible particles in the blood, the invisible vascular channels, the chemical substances, and, of course, the ultimate atoms of which everything was composed.[11] All these entities rested on evidence elaborated by reason, but they were progressively more general, more abstract, and correspondingly further removed from direct experience.

Francis Bacon, early in the seventeenth century, had warned us against this process. The mind, he said, "longs to spring up to positions of higher generality, that it may find rest there." But this is fraught with danger, lest our abstract notions be "confused and overhastily abstracted from the fact."[12] Bacon, of course, favored a slow and cautious induction and a gradual ascent from particulars to generalizations.

At this point I must emphasize the difference between concrete and abstract terms in our explanations. In the early eighteenth century the process of abstraction, characteristic of so-called rationalism, was dominant, and the explanatory process relied more and more on hypothetical entities or abstract terms as the *explicantia.* But the directly opposite trend became increasingly important as the century progressed. This we can readily trace to the growing importance of the autopsy. Pathology had always been a part of medical science, with the principal function of explaining disease. It contrasted with physiology, which dealt with normal phenomena. As more and more autopsies were performed, there accumulated a great mass of anatomical detail to correlate with clinical appearances. These anatomical details were particular and concrete, and the physicians began to depend on them as the *explicantia.* Curiosity sought its answers in empirical demonstration of specific gross lesions. The autopsy provided such demonstration and the concrete data of the autopsy became more significant than the shadowy general concepts that lacked demonstration.

Only after the death of Boerhaave (1738) did autopsy pathology begin to realize its full potential as an explanatory force. Morgagni's *Seats and Causes of Disease*, first published in 1761, was a great landmark, both in the history of pathology and in the theory of explanation.[13] Previously there had been abundant published autopsy reports, of which the *Sepulchretum* of Bonetus was the most important.[14] This compilation had recorded autopsy data quite uncritically and offered little correlation between clinical and anatomical findings. Morgagni, on the other hand, connected the two in remarkable fashion. He arranged his cases in series, according to the region of the body affected; and then, with little generalization or theory, described the anatomical findings, which he correlated with the clinical course. By making the correlations he built a bridge between these two realms and explained the clinical findings in a manner completely acceptable to his readers.

Let us examine a more or less random example. A 59 year old woman was "seized with an apoplexy." The "right limbs had neither feeling nor motion . . . the eyelids of the right eye were paralytic, and almost closed . . . [but] she had no difficulty in swallowing fluid." At the autopsy there was considerable interest among the students, "because, if the injury in the brain was organical, they hoped they should certainly see it on the left side, according to the observations of Valsalva." (He was referring to recent empirical observations suggesting contralateral localization in the brain.) In the brain he found "on the external side of the left thalamus" an area that "was very soft, and liquified, and was found to be mixt with a certain bloody fluid . . . so that nothing but a disagreeable smell was wanting to make us pronounce it absolutely rotten." He considered this an "apostem," that is, an abscess. Today we have no hesitation in pronouncing it a bland infarct. In interpretation Morgagni declared, "You see this doctrine confirmed, that the injury of the brain is found in the hemisphere which is opposite to the paralytic side of the body."[15]

The autopsy "explained" the clinical diagnosis of apoplexy in the following fashion. The disease represented an organic lesion (in contrast to a functional or, as we might say, hysterical disorder); the lesion, he thought, was an abscess; and it had a definite localization in a specific part of the brain. He had correlated data in one universe of discourse (clinical observation) with those in another (anatomical description), and the connection he made satisfied the curiosity of his audience. He did not offer a schema of pathogenesis; he did not indicate the progressive steps that led up to the disease. He made what I call an existential rather than a causal explanation.

Today, of course, our students would not be satisfied. They would want to know a great deal more about, say, arteriosclerosis, the process of thrombosis, the microscopic changes, the specific nerve tracts involved, and so on, in perpetually widening circles, whose expansion we call scientific progress. But the universe of discourse embraced in these subjects did not exist in Morgagni's time.

It was Morgagni who really introduced the great era of clinico-pathological correlation that culminated in the early nineteenth century, with the magnificent achievements of Laennec, Bayle, Bretonneau, and others of the Paris School.[16] These physicians, who so greatly advanced our knowledge of specific diseases, depended on autopsy dissection and gross examination of organs. They used the same techniques that had been available for hundreds of years, but they observed more carefully and in greater detail and correlated more precisely. As a result they made vast progress in the explanation of diseases.

New techniques created new universes of discourse and new levels of explanation. At the end of the eighteenth century Bichat had made a start in developing the science of histology, that is, the study of individual tissues rather than of entire organs. He distinguished the different components of the bodily organs, for example, connective tissue, serous membrane, mucous membrane, muscle, bone, and the like, and described many of their properties. The notion of constituent tissues allowed more precise correlations. Diseases could be referred not to disorders of entire organs but to specific components of those organs. Histology thus provided a "deeper" level for explaining disease.

Bichat did his work without the advantage of microscopy. Later in the nineteenth century the microscope became a truly useful tool. It led directly to the so-called cell theory, propounded by Schleiden and Schwann, which truly revolutionized biology, including the study of disease. The cell theory carried one step further the chain of explanation that began with organ pathology and continued with tissue pathology. Students of disease could find an *explicans,* first with gross organs, then with individual tissues, and then with cells, that is, with progressively finer components. Each stage, however, remained firmly anchored in observation and seemed to be carrying out the recommendations of Francis Bacon.

Morphology, with its present culmination in electron microscopy, was only one line of progress in explanation of disease. Biochemistry underwent enormous development. Whereas even half a century ago the pathologist — the "morbid anatomist" — had the principal role in explaining disease, today the chemist has the preeminent position. Instruments of exquisite precision make possible minute discriminations, which play a role in explanatory processes. The humoral pathology of the ancients has become modern biochemistry. But whereas ancient humoralists attended to the bodily fluids and neglected the solids, the moderns have achieved an integration. The distinction between fluids and solids is blurred. We study chemical substances; their reactions and their loci, whether in cells or interstitial fluids or the circulating blood; the excretions; or the intercellular substances. Solids and fluids may still provide convenience for discourse, but they now form a unified system whose components are constantly interacting. But the process of explanation, the "satisfactory" relation of a given phenomenon to some other universe of discourse, remains the same.

The study of disease involves many different sciences, each of which can be regarded as a separate universe of discourse. Yet the separation is only approximate. While gross pathology can serve as *explicans* for a particular disease, the gross appearance of the organs can itself be explained by the data of histology. The *explicans* in one context becomes the *explicandum* in another. The phenomena of histology, in turn, find an explanation in physiology and biochemistry and genetics, and these in turn may find their *explicantia* in physical chemistry and molecular physics. The ancient atomists tried to reduce all explanation to the dance of atoms. The modern biological scientist is, perhaps, a kindred spirit who differs from his ancient predecessor more in methodology and critical acumen than in goal.

When we try to explain disease we must keep in mind the different levels of explanation. How far down the line do we want to go toward the ultimate reduction? This, of course, will depend on the questioner, on the degree of curiosity that he has, and on what might be necessary to satisfy his curiosity. The layman, the medical student, the general practitioner, the specialist, the "basic scientist" will each want a different answer. Each of them will be drawing on different universes of discourse, but for each the *process* of explanation, the relating of an *explicandum* to an *explicans*, remains the same.

The Reliance on System

In the previous section we noted some broad aspects of the explanatory process, relative to diseases, generally. Now, in contrast, I will turn to a quite specific feature in medicine, namely, the different kinds of secretion that we find in the body. How does it happen that we have so many different types? How can we explain the phenomenon?

One answer, of course, would be to consider each secretion, each "humor," as primary, independent, and coordinate one with the other. The original four humors of the Greeks followed this pattern. No one derived from any of the others. However, this view became rapidly untenable as knowledge of physiology developed and the concept of the circulation was firmly established. The blood, clearly, was a mother fluid that circulated all through the body. The blood passed through different glands, and from each gland there was secreted (or excreted) a different kind of fluid. Particular secretions were closely correlated with particular organs or locations. The nose produced mucus, the mouth saliva, the stomach its own juice; the pancreas, the liver, the testes, the breasts, each yielded a specific fluid distinct from any other. There was also the lymph, associated with the small bodies commonly (even if erroneously) called lymph glands. The circulating blood was the common factor prior to all the others. How did it happen that from this single substance, blood, there was derived milk in one area, semen in another, perspiration in another, and lymph in still another?

The modern student who faces this question immediately falls back on the common knowledge of today—the cell theory—and explains the specificity of secretion by sepcificity of cells. And this, in turn, he correlates with specific structural and functional aspects. But such a view depends on information not available in the eighteenth century. It is a little difficult for a modern student to try to live again in the frame of reference prevalent 250 years ago. We have trouble imagining what life was like without planes, automobiles, television, radio, or electric lights: it is even more difficult to enter into an intellectual environment different from our own.

However, the process is easier if we think of a common thread, namely, the search for an explanation. In 1700 the data to be explained—the secretions—were much as they are today; but the universe of discourse that served as *explicans* was very different. Boerhaave is a spendid example for study, for he provided an explicit set of concepts as *explicantia*. As a medical systematist he furnished a beautifully articulated collection of terms that, in the aggregate, could "explain" almost anything in physiology or pathology. His system makes us aware of two distinct aspects of the explanatory process, namely, the logical and the veridical. These correspond to the questions "Is it formally valid?" and "Is it true?" If we study Boerhaave's explanations we find formal validity, even if the relationships he drew are not true.

Secretion, the elaboration of special fluids in special loci—is a subdivision of the more general problem of the way transformation of blood components takes place. How, for example, does the food we ingest become transformed into blood and then into specific components of the fluids and solids? Food undergoes a series of changes in the stomach and intestines; the altered material enters the lacteals and thoracic duct, and then the subclavian vein and the right heart; from the right ventricle the blood, relatively crude, passes into the lungs. Here, he thought, occurs the finer transformation and attenuation whereby the coarser particles are broken down, "polished and rounded." They receive an "intestine motion" and agitation. "It is necessary for a large number of globules to be prepared of different sizes, that every series of vessels may be supplied with those that fit their diameters."[17] All this attenuation, he thought, took place in the vessels of the lungs.

For Boerhaave, as I have suggested previously, the vessels were the equivalent of our modern cells, having vast differences in size and function.[18] For us the various metabolic transformations take place through cellular action. For Boerhaave these specific changes took place through the "action" of the blood vessels, particularly those of the lung. Thus, for Boerhaave, vessels were functional units that existed in many orders of magnitude, corresponding to the different magnitudes of the blood components.

In the late seventeenth century Ruysch, with his new injection techniques, had provided a powerful tool for extending anatomical knowledge. He perfected methods of injecting blood vessels with a waxy mass, permitting subsequent maceration of the tissues in water. In this way he produced splendid preparations of the vascular system, filled with the injection mass. Such preparations—some of them still existing in Holland—show an unexpectedly rich vasculature and various patterns characteristic for different organs. Although structural details did not of themselves provide knowledge of function, accurate structural data could permit inferences and could give us reliable new knowledge, just as satisfactory as direct observation itself.[19]

Why does the blood, serving all of the glands indiscriminately, yield bile in one locus, mucus in another? Before presenting Boerhaave's formulations we can note the manner in which he disposed of alternate theories and showed that they could not serve as satisfactory explanations.[20] Two other theories had been popular, one mechanical, depending on pores that acted as sieves; and the other chemical, relying on specific ferments. The Cartesian philosophy had recently revived the old doctrine of invisible pores, which, through their configuration, could permit some particles to pass while others did not. Boerhaave pointed out that secretory ducts are exceedingly small and delicate, and the shape of any pores would readily change. This would obviously impair the specificity. But even if the pores were "immutable," there still could not be any real specificity, for "whatever be the figure of a pore it will admit all sorts of particles whose largest diameters are less than its own," an argument that Pitcairn had already advanced. The pore theory, in brief, will not stand up to rigorous examination.

The theory of ferments fared no better. A ferment, Boerhaave said, was a substance that, when mixed with another, "changes the latter into a different nature from what it had of itself without the ferment." But if the glands are composed of vessels through which blood flows, then simple reasoning shows that fermental action is impossible. There is no locus for them to act, for the blood is in flux. Hence, since it is "logically" impossible for ferments to act in vessels and since glands, he thought, were composed of vessels, he concluded that "ferments have no existence in the body, and that they are incapable of mixing with the blood, and promoting its secretions."

What, then, is the right answer to explain the specificity of the secretions? To answer this question Boerhaave had to draw a relationship between the *explicandum* and some other universe of discourse as *explicans*. This latter he found in a fusion of anatomical data with the laws of mechanics, especially of hydrodynamics. He indicated a number of features that might serve as differential explanation. To appreciate their significance we must keep in mind that for him glands represented congeries of vessels in which hydrodynamic principles were operative.

For convenience I will enumerate several points of discrimination and the significance he attributed to them.[21] The various alleged factors are not mutually exclusive.

1. The "distance" of the afferent artery of the gland from the heart. This feature, he thought, affected the velocity of the bloodstream, for "the blood which is nearest the heart will be different in the motion and combination of its particles from that which is more remote, since the last will go on very slowly and retain but little of force which the heart impress on it."

2. The "situation" of the artery leading to the gland, relative to its parent stem. This refers to the angle that the branch artery made with its parent stem. For Boerhaave this seemed important. As concrete evidence he pointed to the angle that the mammary artery made with the subclavian artery and noted that this differs from the angle that the carotid artery made. Correlatively, "the secretions derived from both are equally different." The angle, he thought, would affect the degree to which particles of different mass would leave the main bloodstream and pass into the branches.

3. Different "complications" of vascular branches, that is, their different patterns of distribution. For evidence he relied on Ruysch, who had demonstrated the various patterns distinct for each individual gland — the small vessels might be straight, or brush-like, or serpentine, or show networks of different kinds. This variability, thought Boerhaave, would affect the velocity of the blood particles and the degree of friction. As the motion

of particles is affected, "attraction between the parts will then take place, and they will combine variously."

4. The "velocity" of the blood. For Boerhaave this had extreme importance and in one or another fashion entered into most of the differential points. In the present instance Boerhaave seems to have had in mind the relation between velocity and viscosity. "The blood's fluidity is in proportion to its velocity; for by rest or a slow motion it becomes thick, but by a swift circulation it dissolves, and becomes more fluid."

5. The "proportion" of the branch to its parent trunk, that is, the diameter of the branch relative to its parent. This feature, again, he related to the fluidity, for, he said, the smaller the branch relative to the trunk, "the more fluid will the liquor be which flows into it."

6. The "force both external and internal" that may act on the "discharge" of the humors. Boerhaave had in mind the relationships that we today connect with pressure, rate of flow, and volume. Knowing nothing about blood pressure or vasoconstriction, he nevertheless pointed to the variations in urine secretion according to the amount and quality of ingested fluid. Among other examples he also referred to the variations in secretion induced by emotional stress.

7. The effect of "stasis" on the secretion. A secretion like nasal mucus that stands in its "receptacle" will become inspissated. The mucus is fluid when first secreted but becomes thicker if it accumulates and dries.

8. The degree of "absorption or exhalation" of the fluid part of the secretion. This is obviously akin to the preceding, although he gave different examples.

All of these, as representative factors, varied in different glands, so that no two organs had the same combination. And, he went on, even if we neglect all the conditions of which we are ignorant, ten different factors will permit 362,880 different possible combinations. No wonder that the character of one secretion would differ from that of another. Each gland, he implied, had a combination of factors specific for itself and distinct from every other. By joining the evidence of our senses with inferences from the laws of mechanics and the knowledge we have concerning the nature of the humors, we can "understand the vast number and variety of the secretions and excretions throughout the body."[22]

Boerhaave's formulation shows some interesting features. His explanation takes this form: different glands have specific secretions (a fact of observation); different glands have more or less characteristic vascular patterns (another fact of observation); these distinct patterns, when combined with the principles of hydrodynamics, serve as the *explicans* for the specificity.

Why did he consider the asserted relationship cogent? Supposing he had said different glands have different secretions; different glands have different colors; the difference in color explains the specificity of the secretions. No one would consider this persuasive, Boerhaave least of all. If we compare this with the assertions he actually made, we find a marked contrast. The vascular pattern is a datum that forms part of the complex system, woven together of laws and principles, of observations and abstractions. The whole system (of which we note only a very small part here) brings together anatomy, physiology, pathology, clinical medicine, physics, and chemistry into a well organized whole, a triumph of what we call rationalism. In this system the vascular pattern plays an important part; the color of the glands plays no part at all. The force of Boerhaave's explanation depends, therefore, on his system as a whole, which provides meaning and cogency to all the individual correlates. He had explained the individual secretions and their specificity by relating them to a "system-as-a-whole."

When we actually study his concepts in detail we find a circularity involved. Boerhaave said in effect, "My system explains secretion in this way," but the process of secretion as he envisaged it forms a prominent support for his system. Furthermore, we may note the lack of any step-wise demonstration to validate his asserted correlations. He made bland general statements without any specific correlations. Just *how* do the factors account for the observed differences in secretion? What is the connection between the specific vascular pattern and a specific quality of a secretion? Does *this* vasculature correlate with, say, a high fat content, and *that* vasculature with a high salt content? Even a few such intermediate correlations would have greatly strengthened both the system as a whole and the specific derivative explanations. In the early eighteenth century, however, sufficient data and adequate techniques were not available for any such discrimination. From the technical standpoint Boerhaave did not have the means, and from the intellectual or critical standpoint he did not see the need.

Boerhaave had said, in effect, *this* had something to do with *that* — the *explicandum* and the *explicans* are connected. He asserted a "togetherness." He had, so to speak, placed them both in an "envelope" and declared that in essence these two sets have an inner relevance. The relevance, however, depended on a systematic formulation, which, in turn, relied on hypothetical entities, far removed from experience. The system provided a formally valid explanation, applicable, on an *a priori* basis, to a wide range of phenomena. But it provided no means of translating the asserted relationships back into observational data. We can see the marked distinction between the approach of Boerhaave and that of Morgagni. Yet the differences in approach must not blot out the similarities in the dynamics of explanation.

The Confusion of Witchcraft

An earlier example referred to Morgagni and the way in which certain anatomical findings explained particular clinical aspects of disease. The phenomena to be explained were straightforward and so, too, were the terms of the explication. Everything was on a relatively simple factual level. In contrast, the example of the *virtus dormativa,* given previously, was quite complex. The difficulty was not with the problem itself — Why does opium put you to sleep? — but rather with the terms in which the explication was couched. Did the explanation involve a real entity or only a *flatus vocis?* The answer entailed a choice between the neo-Galenic philosophy and some competing philosophy. Thus the questioner faced alternative explanations.

For my present example I choose a problem wherein there are not only alternative *explicantia* but where, in addition, a confusion attends the *explicandum*. There is difficulty in making clear just what we are trying to explain, and just what its relationships are. These difficulties occur when we study certain aspects of witchcraft.

Any examination of witchcraft revolves around the twin concepts of natural and supernatural. These I have discussed in general terms in earlier chapters. Here I would merely point to nature as the realm of the impersonal, regular, and predictable, while the supernatural, which involves God and other spiritual beings, has its essence in personality and volition, combined with power. We may think of these two aspects as the foci of science and of theology, respectively. Each has its own theoretical superstructure, its own terms and relationships, and each can serve as *explicans* for particular phenomena.

The history of thought shows a gradual demarcation between these alternative modes of explanation. In the world of experience more and more phenomena were becoming recognized as natural, that is, as coming under the rubric of "natural law," not affected by any divine will. Correspondingly, the phenomena receiving a supernatural explanation diminished in number. At one extreme God, the "first cause," established the world and the laws of nature. Then, having created the world, God stepped aside and did not again interfere. Nature became autonomous. At the opposite limit God did not step aside after the creation but remained constantly in touch. He had established the laws of nature but he was not in any way constrained thereby. He could lay them aside or modify these laws whenever he wished. Any such modification or suspension we call a miracle.

We must distinguish between the phenomena alleged as witchcraft and those considered as miracles. The miracles not only transcended the ordinary course of nature but also had the quality of beneficence — they brought about some favorable or desirable goal. However, other events might also seem to lie outside the range of natural law and yet bring only harm and suffering. For example, misfortune might befall the righteous and torments afflict the godly. The believers in witchcraft would hold that these did not follow merely from the laws of nature but resulted from volition of a supernatural being. These harmful events could be attributed not to God, who wrought only good, but to the devil and to his agents. Malevolence was the motive force.

Let us imagine some concrete instances. A farmer had a quarrel with his neighbor; the next week the farmer's cow, previously quite healthy, died suddenly. A woman scolded her indentured servant and that very night had an attack of severe abdominal cramps. A church deacon refused to shelter some gypsies, and the next day the deacon's horse stumbled and broke a leg.

How did these events come about? How do we explain them? On the phenomenological level certain data are clear — a quarrel and a death of a cow, a scolding and an attack of cramps, a conflict with the gypsies and a stumbling of a horse with resulting broken leg. Did the death, the cramps, and the broken leg occur independently of the prior quarrels? Or did the antecedent quarrels play a role, so that without them the misfortunes would not have taken place? The latter alternative entails certain presuppositions: the misfortunes did not occur through ordinary impersonal cause-and-effect relationship, but malevolence played a part in the causal sequence. This malevolence was translated into harmful results through supernatural forces mediated by the devil or his agents — witches and warlocks — who could exert special powers known as demonic magic, or similar designation.

Important here is the interpretation of fact. What is it that we are trying to explain? What is the *explicandum*? What are the facts and what is their degree of circumscription? For the believer in witchcraft the fact consisted not in the death of the cow, but in the sequence "death of the cow brought about by the magical incantation of the witch." The *conjunction* of the events is the fact, and to explain it we must identify the factors through which the whole conjunction came into being. However, for the skeptic the sequence represented only a series of disconnected events and not a conjunction. Disputes regarding witchcraft centered largely on the questions: What *are* the facts? Do they lie in the realm of nature or of the supernatural? The answer will determine the choice of *explicantia*.

In a dissertation of 1703, Friedrich Hoffmann addressed himself to these problems, even though he used a different terminology and a different frame of analysis.[23] Hoffmann did not concern himself so much with witches (who, after all, were only intermediaries) as with the devil himself and the powers he might have over man. Concerning the existence of the devil and of demonic powers there was no doubt. Like most intellectual leaders of his generation, Hoffmann believed that God was beneficent and omnipotent, and the devil malevolent but limited in power and subordinate to God. The devil cannot negate the works of God, cannot overturn the laws of nature. God had established the laws of nature and only God could abrogate them. Hence it follows that the devil cannot perform miracles. For example, he cannot bring the dead to life, he cannot create living creatures out of inanimate objects, he cannot transport persons through the air. These would all be contrary to the laws of nature.

Hoffmann's denial that the devil could transport witches through the air struck at the heart of demonology, for in popular belief the devil enabled witches to fly long distances to attend the witches' Sabbath. Such an alleged action, since it ran counter to natural law, must be unequivocally rejected. An alleged witch might assert that she had flown through the air to attend a witches' Sabbath but her assertions are untrue and must find an explanation other than the power of the devil. Hoffmann recounted a story of a poor woman who obstinately maintained that she attended such a witches' Sabbath. Secret observers noted that before she "departed" on such a flight she annointed herself with an ointment and then fell into a deep sleep that lasted until the next day. When she awoke she stubbornly maintained that she had attended a witches' congregation and she could not be convinced otherwise.[24] Here, clearly, her assertion would find an explanation not through demonic activity but in natural phenomena in the area of drug action. Demonic influence did not form a proper part of the *explicans*.

Because Hoffmann was a scientist, he dismissed as mere fables many assertions of alleged demonic action that contravened natural law. He showed what the devil could *not* do: he could not transgress the laws that God has established. Any report that alleged such a transgression was either a fable or a fraud, or else a product of a diseased imagination. And as we will see, disorders of the imagination could be explained by natural causes. But having shown through logic what the devil could not do, Hoffmann faced the real problem, to determine what the devil could do, that is, to determine the facts and then to explain them.

The devil was pure immaterial spirit, having no extension, no material property. How, then, could what is purely immaterial act on body? One answer involved the concept of intermediaries, which I have called the Neoplatonic maneuver. As a model we can think of the mind-body relationship. The mind also is immaterial but nevertheless obviously acts on the body. The action occurs through very subtle fluids — the finely material spirits—that pass through the nerves. By means of the nerve fluid the mind, which is of spiritual origin, brings about movement. Mind acts on body "through the intervention of another agent." Similarly, the devil, as spirit, can exert his will on natural objects through intermediaries. As an immaterial spirit the devil cannot act directly on solid bodies but he acts through his influence on subtle fluids that serve as intermediaries.[25]

We can draw an analogy to the human will, which can choose, say, to move the body to the right or to the left. The decision, once made, is implemented through the exceedingly fine animal spirits, and once the decision is made, the activity takes place according to the laws of physics and mechanics. But the initial directing force comes from the immaterial mind. The spirits represent the intermediary that entrain a course of physical phenomena.

The activities of the devil are entirely similar. The devil, exerting his will on finely material fluid (or spirits), can induce results that accord with the natural law. The devil does not in any way overturn the laws of nature but uses the properties of nature to impress his evil will on the world. He does not break the laws of nature but merely bends them to his will. Through volition he brings into being events that would not otherwise happen. But when they do happen the events are entirely "natural"; the devil only provides a malevolent direction. After the movement is initiated natural law takes over. While the devil is part of the supernatural realm his powers are limited by "natural" sequences. His supernatural activities consist in imposing a special direction on events.

Here we must distinguish between the world at large (the macrocosm) and man (the microcosm). In the macrocosm the subtle fluid is the air and ether that surround the earth. Because the devil can affect these subtle fluids, he can bring about various atmospheric disturbances, such as rain, hail, and lightning, and thus wreak harm on man. Hoffmann also thought that certain manifestations of insect life, such as hordes of locusts, spiders, and caterpillars, resulted from changes in the weather and thus could harm man by damaging crops. Hoffmann did not directly say that the devil caused these plagues, but he phrased his belief in the words that everyone who blames the devil for these things will not be speaking nonsense.[26]

There is a close parallel between man and the great world around him. Analogous to the air and ether there is in man an extremely delicate fluid, a spirituous matter that is a most subtle air mixed with delicate sulfurous particles of the blood. And this finely material substance Hoffmann equated with the animal spirits that mediate both bodily and mental activity, including the imagination.[27]

According to the contemporary views the imagination depended partly on the mind and partly on the body. Said Hoffmann, "Imagination is nothing else than the impression on the fibrils and the pores of the brain, of those ideas which external objects communicate to the senses." Ordinarily the sense organs receive external impressions which get transmitted to the sensorium by means of the animal spirits and leave traces that play a part in memory and imagination. But the ideas impressed on the brain may have an "involuntary internal cause." Hoffmann was thinking of delirium or "perverted reason" but the statement is equally applicable to demonic influence on the animal spirits. Since the devil can act on these animal spirits he can influence the sensorium and thus affect the imagination. The devil can make imaginary things seem real and make witches believe in the external reality of impressions that are purely internal. The devil can thus induce various types of illusion.[28]

Having established that the devil acts only on the animal spirits, Hoffmann concerned himself with the physiological mechanisms or physiological data that would correlate with the phenomena. For example, if the devil may distort the imagination, why does this happen only in some persons and not in others? There must be some difference in receptivity to the devil's influence, and these differences Hoffmann related to the circulation. Those persons, he said, who have abundant thick blood that circulates rather slowly through the cerebral vessels are more susceptible to the activities of the devil than are those whose blood is thin, motile, and florid. Other factors such as temperament, sex, age, diet, and climate may also render individuals susceptible to demonic influence. In France and Italy, where people drink wine and engage in intellectual disputes, we hear little about witchcraft. But in northern and colder climates, such as Lapland, Finland, and Sweden, or in Westphalia and Pomerania, where people drink thin beer and eat a harsh diet of beans, heavy bread, and pork, we have many examples of witches, incantations, specters, and "other demonic illusions."[29]

The illusions and delusions caused by the devil have physical bases: they are grounded in nature and represent the actions of natural law, but the activity is initiated not by human will or by poisonous substances but by demonic intervention. Yet the devil cannot operate as he pleases, but only if there is some prior disposition, especially in the blood.

Disturbances in the animal spirits can result not only in disordered imagination but also in various somatic ailments, especially those involving motor activities such as convulsions, spasms, and "epilepsy." In his textbook Hoffmann had defined convulsions and spasms as "violent and disordered movements of the spirits into the nerves and muscles which do not obey the directions [*determinationi*] of the common sensory, as they should."[30] Convulsive disorders can thus become a ready field for demonic activity, since the devil need only redirect the spirits to produce the disturbances. Furthermore, the devil can also induce those disorders that result from diminished force of the spirits, such as melancholia, or impotence, and states where the "tonus" of the fibers might be relaxed.

But here we meet a great difficulty, for many conditions wherein the devil might have some dominion can also occur from exclusively natural causes, without demonic intervention. There is a great affinity, said Hoffmann, between "natural diseases" and "supernatural diseases."[31] Disordered animal spirits are at work in both instances, but in the one the disorder resulted solely from natural causes while in the other the disturbance of the spirits was initiated by a demonic malevolence.

Here we have a deep diagnostic problem. Some instances of a disease may result from purely natural causes but in other cases the devil may play the initiating role. How can we discriminate and tell one category from the other? What criteria can we use? To help the differential diagnosis Hoffmann offered seven criteria that could suggest a demonic influence. These are: a sudden attack in a previously healthy man, such that suspicion of poison might arise; the use of blasphemy and obscenities; knowledge of the future and of secret events, especially in unlearned persons; the knowledge of foreign languages that the affected person had never heard; vast physical strength that greatly surpasses the normal; the excretion (or expulsion) of various monstrous and heterogeneous objects such as nails, hair, wood, thorns, flint, bones, and teeth; and finally, the failure of the established remedies to cure the disease.[32]

We may intercalate here a brief comment on the movie *The Exorcist,* which had such a vogue a few years ago. This movie, about a case of supposed demonic possession in present-day life, used several of these criteria as evidence that the illness had resulted from the action of the devil. The movie clearly reflected advanced medical thinking, but medical thinking of the year 1703.

The explanatory process, I have emphasized, demands the reference of some phenomenon, the *explicandum,* to some other universe of discourse. When Hoffmann tried to explain an event attributed to witchcraft, he faced alternative *explicantia,* not entirely harmonious with each other: natural philosophy (or science) involving natural law; and theology, involving the devil as a real but immaterial being of malevolent will. Hoffmann tried to provide some sort of unification. He felt that witchcraft could indeed be studied in a scientific fashion. By analyzing the workings of the mind under various conditions (some of which would be deemed natural and others supernatural), he tried, in a vague groping fashion, to set up a science of the mind.

The empirical study of mental phenomena was in its early stages. John

Locke had contributed greatly to its progress and so too had the physicians who noted the psychosomatic correlations that received much attention in the seventeenth century. Yet the mind was intimately related to the theological concepts of soul, immortality, freedom of the will, and the like, which dovetailed with further theological entities such as the devil, his attributes, and his powers. The whole concept of mind hovered between the material and the immaterial, between the empirically based concepts of science and the revelation-based concepts of theology. The imagination, as we have seen in this and the preceding chapters, was a connecting link between the body and the mind, and mind was a connecting link between science and theology.

Hoffmann attempted to circumscribe the different components and yet include them in a single explanatory formula. We see this in the criteria by which he tried to distinguish, in cases of supposed demonic possession, the demonic factors from those purely natural. He attributed to natural law those aspects that harmonized with the knowledge of his day, and the features he could not explain by natural processes he attributed to the supernatural. The realm of the supernatural contained the pheonmena that the science of his day could not clearly and satisfactorily explain.

Hoffmann might have said, "At the present moment our scientific concepts cannot satisfactorily explain all the components of alleged witchcraft, but the gradual increase in future knowledge will certainly enable us to explain these aspects in terms of 'nature.' " With hindsight we realize that such faith would have been completely justified, for all the features that Hoffmann attributed to the devil we can today readily explain in psycho-physical terms without invoking a devil. Hoffmann lacked faith that in time we could bring these facets under the rubric of science. He chose to retain his faith in the supernatural and to bring the two separate realms together to serve as a conjoint *explicans*.

He ignored the incompatibility or, in different phraseology, he did not perceive that there was any incompatibility. He saw only harmony, and hence the relationships that he drew between the *explicanda* and the *explicantia* were to him smooth and satisfactory. To us, today, these relationships are not acceptable. Perhaps what we call progress consists in finding the rough spots in a relationship that had previously seemed smooth and harmonious.

NINE

THE CAUSE OF DISEASE

Every time we use the word cause or phrases such as "due to . . ." or "resulting from . . ." we are indicating a special connection between events that we call a causal relationship. What is the nature of this relationship? For 2500 years or more philosophers have disputed its meaning, with profound subtlety but without agreement. Today, as in times past, we tell our medical students that the proper way to cure disease is to remove the cause. *Tolle causam,* as an exhortation that goes back to antiquity, represents admirable advice. But unfortunately, it is easier to exhort than to specify. What *is* the cause of any given disease? Physicians, in answer, have readily named this or that feature as cause, but the assertions of one group would find bitter contradiction from some other group; and even if there were agreement, it would not last very long.

By treating patients and noting successes and failures, a physician gains some insight into the causes of disease. However, this practical activity, although vastly important, is only one aspect of the problem. There are more abstract considerations—for example, what is the essential nature of the causal relationship?—that concern philosophers rather than physicians. In any such philosophical analysis Hume and Kant stand out as giants of the eighteenth century, but their concepts had little direct influence on eighteenth century medicine. For the physicians of that era, notions on the basic nature of causality derived from traditional medicine, especially the Galenic strands that in turn go back largely to Aristotle. When seventeenth and eighteenth century physicians dealt with causality, they used terms that sound quite harsh today. To make this terminology meaningful we might use an approach quite different from the usual historical method. Instead of starting with the earlier stage and coming forward in time, we can attack the problem more effectively if we reverse this procedure, start with modern usage, and then work backward to the seventeenth century. The present-day medical usage of "cause" has at least a ring of familiarity, and if we work backward from the present, we can use this familiarity to clarify the earlier meanings.

Let us look at a contemporary textbook and examine a well studied disease, typhoid fever. Our text, beginning with a definition, says unequivocally, "Typhoid fever is an acute, often severe illness caused by *Salmonella typhi* and characterized by . . ." a list of symptoms. Noteworthy here is a simple and direct statement, the cause *is* the bacillus, or conversely, the bacillus *is* the cause. Similarly with malaria, in which there are four major clinical types. The textbook declares flatly, "It is caused by four species of the genus Plasmodium."[1]

These two examples are infections in which specific microorganisms have been isolated — in the one case a bacterium, in the other a protozoon. The infectious agent is called *the* cause. In both diseases a physician can suspect the diagnosis on the basis of the symptoms alone, that is, on clinical grounds. But any diagnosis reached in this fashion remains tentative. Assurance — certainty — comes only when the offending organism has been identified. Clinical suspicion is the first step. Precision comes when we have found the organism and then we say that the laboratory has confirmed the diagnosis. Without this additional step we cannot be sure that the patient *really* has typhoid fever (or malaria). The organism, so glibly called *the* cause, is thus the necessary criterion by which we determine with assurance that the disease is present.

Let us now go back to the end of the nineteenth century and consult William Osler. I choose the third edition of his textbook, written in 1898. In his discussion of malarial fever Osler also began with a definition, but the word cause did not appear. Instead he defined the disease only on its clinical features, that is, as characterized by certain symptoms. However, Osler did go on to say, "With the disease are invariably associated haematozoa described by Laveran."[2] This term haematozoa, of course, referred to what is now called the plasmodium.

When Osler wrote, relatively little was known about the plasmodium but he fully appreciated the association between the organism and the disease. This constant association, he realized, might serve as a tool whereby the doctor could identify the malaria and distinguish it from other kinds of fevers. Although typical malaria had a distinctive clinical course, many cases were obscure, and in such instances a diagnosis was at best a matter of guesswork. Any sort of "constant association" could furnish a reliable criterion and take the guesswork out of diagnosis. As Osler stated, "To be able, everywhere and under all circumstances, to differentiate between malaria and other forms of fever is one of the most important advances which has been made of late years in practical medicine."[3]

But he noted many gaps in our knowledge. He did not know, he declared, how the parasite existed outside the human body, nor the manner in which the infection came about. The available evidence, he thought, suggested the respiratory tract, although he admitted that proof was lacking. While he mentioned casually that the mosquito had been suggested as an intermediate host, he paid no special attention to this suggestion. To understand his views, we need only realize that he wrote his text just before the scientific breakthrough that identified the anopheles mosquito as the intermediate host transmitting the disease.[4]

Although Osler did not call the parasite the cause of malaria, he did discuss many relevant factors, gathered together under the heading of etiology. Here he talked about topics such as geographical distribution, the association of the disease with marshland, the beneficial effects of drainage, the special seasonal incidence, the relationship of heat, moisture, wind, and elevation. The term etiology seemed to gather together all the miscellaneous factors that might have some sort of relevance to the disease. But what sort of relevance? There was no way to tie together a seasonal incidence, a swampy terrain, and a specific parasite. These all seemed somehow relevant but did not fall into a unified pattern.

In common usage the term etiology refers to the aggregate of factors that have some sort of bearing on a disease. The dictionary defines this word as the study of causes, and the crucial feature here is the plural usage—causes are recognized not as one but as many. There is an enormous difference between the causes of disease—multiple or plural—and the cause of disease.

Particularly among medical students the question arises: what is the difference between cause and etiology? When we study the history of diseases we find a clue. Etiology applies to the entire mass of factors that relate, somehow, to the disease in question. The singular term cause seems to refer to a specific factor that defines the disease in a unique fashion. When that factor is present, the disease may be diagnosed with assurance. When that factor is not identified, the diagnosis remains in doubt, regardless of all other factors.

This distinction becomes clearer if we go back to the mid-nineteenth century. I choose a text of Thomas Watson, of 1847, long before the plasmodium was discovered or the role of the mosquito even suspected.[5] In his presentation Watson analyzed the various clinical types such as quotidian, tertian, and quartan, and the intermediate or obscure forms. He could provide no sharp criteria, no unequivocal definition, and the distinctions rested on clinical features alone.

In his discussion Watson did use the word cause but not in the sense of a sharp criterion. Instead he fragmented the term, so to speak, and gave each fragment a more or less distinct meaning. The cause was broken up into subgroups, into different kinds of cause. The various circumstances that seemed to favor the disease tended to fall into clusters. For example, all individuals are not equally susceptible, but some persons seem to be especially predisposed. The responsible factors, whatever they might be, he lumped together as the predisposing cause of the disease. However, there must supervene something else that he called the "exciting cause," that is, the factor "without which ague would never occur at all." This factor he considered to be "certain invisible effluvia or emanations from the earth," constituting a specific poison.[6] The effluvia "are probably gaseous or aeriform . . . they are imperceptible by any of our senses. Of their physical or chemical qualities we really know nothing. We are made aware of their existence only by their noxious effect." Watson was seeking some unknown factor that acted as the inciting agent, at whose properties he could only guess.

If the exciting cause of ague is a specific poison in the air, Watson understandably showed concern with the conditions under which this poison might develop. He realized that a certain degree of warmth and moisture was required. There was a seasonal incidence. Marshland seemed to favor the disease but marsh water, when examined under the microscope, gave no clue to the pestilential agent. The poison seemed more active at night, yet the miasma might lose its harmful properties by passing over water. Watson mentioned examples of ships that had anchored near malarious coasts. Sailors who went ashore contracted ague, sailors who remained on the ship sayed healthy. One authority had suggested 6,000 feet of water as a critical distance.[7]

Yet there was no single coherent pattern into which all the data might fall. Today, our knowledge of the plasmodium and the mosquito clarifies the data that so puzzled Watson. Lacking precise knowledge, he nevertheless recorded the facts he considered relevant and categorized these into various kinds of cause. The distinctions were a means of imposing some sort of order on the great number of individual facts that were somehow related but whose interconnections were obscure. To avoid a chaotic mass of discrete data, Watson, following the custom, fragmented the notion of cause into subordinate types. In this way he could introduce order into the confused mass of data and could handle them more readily. Etiology was a catch-all; subdividing the term cause offered a better means of understanding.

A key to the better understanding of causality lies with the implications that attend the usage of *the* cause as contrasted with *a* cause. With malaria (and other infectious diseases) the usage of *the* cause — without qualification — became prevalent only when the specific plasmodium was identified and its role in the pathogenesis clearly explicated. All other factors — seasonal incidence, swampy terrain, the mosquito, the life cycle of the parasite, and so on, in great detail, are all relevant in producing the disease, but they stand in a different relation to the disease than does the parasite itself. A logician calls the parasite the necessary cause of the disease, the *sine qua non,* without which no person can have malaria.

In common usage, as a manner of speech, we can call the plasmodium the cause, thus granting it special recognition. But we do not mean that the specific protozoon, acting solely by itself and *independently of all other conditions,* can induce the disease. There are various accessory requirements—the organism must enter into the bloodstream and find there an environment suitable to permit multiplication. We call this susceptibility, which implies, among other things, the absence of inhibitory factors such as anti-malarial drugs or antibodies.

Susceptibility, in any infection, usually involves complex genetic and immunological features. The older physicians as well as the logicians called it the predisposing cause but were not able to specify the details. In present-day textbooks, once the necessary cause has been identified, all other factors are usually placed in a scrapbag called etiology, and some of them are woven into a section called pathogenesis.

However, if the necessary cause is not known, then we do not ordinarily speak of the cause. Instead, we today speak loosely of etiological factors. The older authors, who considered multiple factors as causal, subdivided them into definite subcategories (such as predisposing or remote causes), attempting thereby to achieve precision. Watson did this, and in so doing he was using a much earlier terminology.

Many infectious diseases, then, have a demonstrable agent that we now call the necessary cause or, in a loose sense, the cause; but the situation is quite different in many noninfectious disorders. A good example is gout, which Hippocrates recognized and which physicians ever since have studied. Particularly in the last 50 years an enormous mass of relevant information has accumulated, but no one speaks of the cause of gout.

In modern textbooks gout is considered to be a group of diseases involving the metabolism of the chemical substances known as purines, and the end product, uric acid.[8] The diseases we call gout are ordinarily identifiable by an increased level of uric acid in the blood—hyperuricemia. But of all those who have hyperurecemia only about one in six has clinical symptoms, of which arthritis, subcutaneous deposits known as tophi, and stones in the kidneys are the most common. All these manifestations result from local deposits of uric acid salts—sodium urate.

There are thus two major problems: why should there be a high uric acid level in the blood; and what brings about the clinical manifestations?

In regard to the first problem we find several possible variables, any or all of which may play a part. Since uric acid is an end product of purine metabolism, there may be an excessive intake of purines or their precursors (exogenous origin); excessive synthesis may take place in the body (endogenous origin); the metabolism of purines may be disordered (faulty chemical transformation); or the excretion of uric acid may be diminished. These variables may or may not act in concert and may show varying

degrees of interconnection. All gout thus represents a chemical derange-
ment that we know has a genetic origin and a familial trend. The term
coined by Garrod, an inborn error of metabolism, is both popular and
accurate. For simplicity, we will not consider the nonhereditary forms of
gout.

In regard to the second problem we must realize that a patient does not
go to the physician and say, "Doctor, I have a high uric acid level in my
blood." Instead, he goes complaining, say, of intolerable pain and swelling
in his big toe; that is, he complains of the actual clinical signs of disease.
These do indeed result from the excessive uric acid level in the blood. We
know from impeccable evidence that gouty arthritis arises when microcrystals of sodium urate are precipitated from the blood into a joint and induce there an intense inflammatory reaction. Yet of all patients with
hyperuricemia less than 20 percent will have clinical gout. Why does an
attack occur in one patient rather than in another or at one time rather
than another? Our textbooks tell us that an acute attack may come on
suddenly and may follow trauma, illness, operation, dietary indiscretion
or, on the other hand, may have no discernible stimulus. But how these
various stresses get translated into the acute inflammatory reaction is not
known.

Modern research has given us an enormous mass of information regarding purine metabolism and the factors at work in the production and excretion of uric acid, and the ways in which these may be distorted in
patients with gout. But despite our vast knowledge regarding the congeries
of diseases we call gout, we know no single factor we can call *the* cause. In
gout we cannot point to anything comparable to the plasmodium of
malaria.

Let us now go back to 1900 when we did not have nearly as much knowledge and when biochemical studies were rudimentary. Yet, despite the
lack of details, the broad correlations were clearly appreciated. Gout, we
read, was the expression of "a peculiar diathesis, or constitutional bias,"
either inherited or acquired. Characterizing this diathesis is the "tendency
to a) the accumulation of urates in the blood, and b) to the deposition of
urates in the tissues." The deposition of sodium biurate crystals "is the
actual excitant of the arthritic attack in gout."[9]

After this background statement, the author discussed the various conditions which "engender, or tend to engender, the gouty state."[10] Some he
called intrinsic causes, inherent in the individual, such as age, sex, heredity, "bodily conformation and individual peculiarities." Other factors,
extrinsic causes, include excesses in diet, such as in eating meat and in
drinking alcoholic beverages. As exciting causes specific incidents such as
exposure to cold or a fit of anger sometimes might precipitate an attack,
but any such factors cannot act without a constitutional predisposition.

The nomenclature is that of the older authors and seems splendidly appropriate. And clearly, the main relationships of the disease were well appreciated.

If we go still further back into the era when uric acid and its salts had not been identified, the analysis of causal factors followed the older general pattern. In 1826, John Mason Good said that gout depended on "a peculiar diathesis or state of the constituion." In some instances this was hereditary, in others not. The diathesis "may remain quiescent and not discover itself for years til it meets with some occasional cause of excitement." (Occasional cause is the same as the exciting cause.) Then the particular manifestation will depend on the temperament, constitution, and personal peculiarities of the individual. The incident that might trigger an acute attack — intoxication, excessive eating, strong emotion, exposure to cold — could produce a "general disturbance" in the body.[11]

Good recognized the general clinical correlation but he could not trace any specific interactions nor offer any connecting links. He knew that "some morbid material" was separated from the "system" and "thrown off" during the paroxysm, but he could not define the nature of the morbid material nor tell how it acted. Good merely noted various relevant factors and called them causes with one or another of the qualifications that hold so much significance.

Let us now go back to the older authors of the seventeenth century and see how they regarded the notion of cause. Compared with nineteenth century physicians the older writers seem vague indeed, yet their concepts formed the mother lode from which were refined the modern ideas. For the analysis I draw on Sennert and his younger contemporary Riverius. They fairly represent the numerous physicians of the sixteenth or seventeenth centuries who dealt with causation as part of their study of medicine.

We must realize that the early physicians worked within a framework quite different from our own. They had but a scanty array of facts (although of this, of course, they were not aware), and they valued not so much the discovery of new facts as the logical disposition of the facts they did have. They worried especially about the different categories of cause. We might regard their efforts as verbal quibbling, but such an attitude would be merely parochial and presentistic.

Riverius

Riverius dealt explicitly with causality in relation to disease. He offered this definition as the most completely general statement: "All those things are given the name of causes which contribute anything to the production of disease in any way whatsoever, whether *per se* or by accident, mediately or immediately [directly or indirectly] or maintain or exacerbate the disease, or have some effect in any other way at all."[12] So broad is this definition that it excludes virtually nothing. Almost any factor might have some degree of relevance, even if quite remote. To have practical value the concept of cause must be subdivided.

The physicians in the first half of the seventeenth century were still writing in the shadow of Galen and followed a tradition transmitted by medieval and Renaissance authors. Part of this tradition was the Aristotelian doctrine of the four causes, which had served as the framework for logical analysis. According to Aristotle, to understand the process of change we can ask four types of questions. The answers correspond to the four causes (*aitia*) — the formal, material, efficient, and final. These categorize the answers to the four questions: what is it? (the formal cause); of what is it made? (the material cause); by what agent? (efficient cause); and for what end? (final cause).[13] As Randall states, these are the necessary conditions for understanding a process and rendering it intelligible.

How do the various specific causes of disease harmonize with the canonical four causes of Aristotle? Renaissance physicians disputed the answers. Both Sennert and Riverius agreed that the causes of disease were all to be subsumed under efficient cause. Some contrary views, such as those of Argenterius, need not detain us.[14]

After discussing the cause of disease in general Riverius proceeded to differentiate the kinds of cause, offering, so to speak, various categories that might apply to some factors, although not necessarily to others.[15] The arrangement is not systematic. He did not imply that the divisions were either complete or exhaustive. Rather, he merely enumerated types of causal relations, usually in contrasting pairs, that we can find when we examine disease. All the different groups show much overlap.

Cause *per se* produces its effect by its own internal force with nothing else intervening. This contrasts with cause *per accidens,* which excites some other factor by whose intervention the disease is produced. Thus, cold water *per se* has a cooling effect, but if the cold renders the skin more compact, there can result a heating effect. A purgative *per se* is "hot," but by evacuating the bile and the hot humors, it has a cooling effect and cures a fever. The principal cause is that which, by itself, provides the initial stimulus to the effect or may be capable of doing so. The adjuvant cause cannot produce the effect by itself but may aid the principal cause. The cause *sine qua non* is that without which an action cannot occur. By itself, however, it produces no effect.

To illustrate all this Riverius gave the example of the gout. His terminology sounds strange when compared to the modern views. The principal cause, he said, was the cold constitution of the air and the abundance of the humors to be excreted. The adjuvant cause is the delicacy of the humors, and the cause *sine qua non* is the "weakness of the joints and the laxity of the pores." Into this archaic terminology we might place the modern concepts: as principal cause, hyperuricemia; as adjuvant cause, the microcrystals of the deposited sodium urate; as the cause *sine qua non,* the hereditary disposition (or weakness).

For the next division Riverius gave the remote as opposed to the proximal. A cause is remote when between it and the disease there intervenes something else. The proximal cause is that which immediately gives rise to the disease. The extreme importance of the proximal cause will emerge later in this chapter, but we should note that Riverius paid it little heed. Only later, when logical analysis was sharpened and more data became available, did this category take on the special significance that we will discuss later.

Riverius was more concerned with the distinction between external and internal causes, a distinction that at first glance seems straightforward. The internal causes of disease are those which lie hidden in the body and are known not by the senses but by a process of inference. He included humors, spirits, material to be excreted, breath, vapors, the component particles of the parts and whatever is related thereto.

The term external causes he applied especially to that group of factors known as the "six non-naturals."[16] These he enumerated as air, food and drink, motion and rest, the excreta and retenta, sleep and wakefulness, and passions of the mind. And he admitted that it might seem odd to consider some of these as external. But since physicians generally accepted them, he went along also.

Necessary causes he defined as those that affect us necessarily — we cannot avoid them. The nonnaturals came into this category, for we necessarily relate to air, food, rest, excretion, sleep, and emotions. But although they unavoidably affect us, they need not cause disease. They do so only under conditions of abuse, as we shall see later. The opposite of necessary is contingent — what may or may not happen, for example, the bite of a wild animal. There is a necessity to breathing or eating, but not to the bite of a dog.

Riverius further contrasted the antecedent cause, that which is prior and brings about the disease mediately, from the conjoint cause, which produces the disease immediately. To illustrate this rather murky distinction he gave the example of a "continued fever": the material capable of becoming putrid is the antecedent cause, but that which actually becomes putrid he called the conjoint cause. A conjoint cause can also be external.

All causes, said Riverius, might be divided into procatarctic (or occasional), antecedent, and conjoint. He distinguished the conjoint cause *simpliciter* from the continuing cause. The distinction is highly significant. When the conjoint cause *simpliciter* is present, the disease occurs, but when this cause is taken away, the disease is not removed. An example is the wound caused by a sword thrust. Remove the sword, yet the wound remains. In contrast we have the continued cause. When this is present, the disease is present, when it is taken away, the disease is removed. He gave the example of a calculus or other substance that gave rise to an obstruction. When the calculus is removed, the obstruction is also eliminated.

This terminology sounds strange to modern ears, yet Riverius, following a long tradition, was trying to analyze the connections between a disease and various relevant factors, and to find some element of necessity. He sought a factor such that, when we have it, we necessarily have the disease, and when we take it away, the disease is necessarily removed. The classical statement, widely found with one or another variation, would be *qua posita, ponitur morbus; qua sublata, tollitur morbus.* Many factors, obviously, do not have this relation to a disease. But physicians tried to find what did bear such a relation.

The seventeenth century usage of the terms necessary and sufficient diverges somewhat from the nineteenth and twentieth century usage, yet deals with the same problem. More recent logicians have expanded the implication of the older rendition to give greater generality—they speak of the reciprocating cause, by which they mean "that not only does the phenomenon occur when the cause is present, but that the cause must be present whenever the phenomenon occurs; so that we may safely argue from either to the other."[17] If we have such an intimate and reciprocating relationship, then when we remove the cause we necessarily remove the effect. I want to keep this concept in mind as we analyze further the seventeenth and eighteenth century notions of causation as it relates to disease.

When we study what Riverius wrote on the causes of disease we become familiar with a series of traditional terms that he expounded in a terse and dogmatic fashion. He enumerated and explained briefly many different kinds of cause, but he did not provide any systematic overview of the nature of causation nor did he come to grips with problems that today seem important. We must realize, however, that sixteenth and seventeenth century physicians, trying to understand disease and its causes, had rather different interests from what we have today. The older physicians fully realized the importance of establishing causal connections and whenever possible wanted to show that *this* had some sort of relation to *that*. Hippocrates, for example, had pointed to various environmental or bodily factors that he could relate to disease. This is in the best tradition of medicine.

Thoughtful physicians, in the present as well as in the times past, always search for relationships between a disease and prior events or factors.

Today, with elegant technical means at our disposal, we emphasize the empirical data, the facts, which we try to make as precise as possible. In the sixteenth and seventeenth centuries physicians were content with broad indefinite correlations. Not having technical means for precise discrimination, they were satisfied with vague data. The physicians devoted intellectual energy not to making the data more precise but rather to making the relationship precise. They were not troubled if a given datum was indefinite and of doubtful validity, but they devoted great effort to analyzing the kind of relationship that the datum bore to the disease. They elaborated a complex arrangement of causal categories. Interest lay, above all, in assigning a given factor to the "proper" category of causes. Whether a given factor was a principal or an adjuvant cause seemed quite important.

Sennert

When we go from Riverius to Sennert, we note the same basic concern with the kinds of cause, but we have a more detailed presentation in which Sennert, incidentally, paid rather argumentative attention to other authors and made frequent reference to Greek, Arabian, and Renaissance writers. Virtually all the terms that Riverius mentioned Sennert also discussed but in different order, with different emphasis and a much sharper focus.[18]

One major feature involved the problem, whether anything intervened between the cause and the effect. If nothing intervened then we have the proximal or immediate cause. If, however, some additional factor does intervene, then we have the mediate or remote cause. The question of immediate versus mediate, underlying as it does all the earlier analyses of causation, involves the topic of necessity. The proximal or immediate cause is always necessary. We see this clearly if we transpose the question into somewhat more modern terms and ask, what is the proximal cause of death? Until very recently we might have answered, the cessation of the heart beat. Between this cessation of the heart beat and death there is no intervening factor. (For simplicity we will not consider "brain death" or enzyme systems or other concepts unknown in the seventeenth century.) The cessation of the heart beat is certainly necessary for death to occur. When we have thus given the proximal or immediate cause of death, we have also given a definition, namely, that death is the state in which the heart has (permanently) stopped beating. As we shall see in the next section, Boerhaave gave special attention to the relationship between proximal cause and a definition.

Quite different are the remote or mediate causes of disease. The patient might have had pneumonia or cancer or meningitis or any number of other conditions. Any of these is mediate, since between it and death there intervened other events, including the cessation of the heart beat. And obviously, none of these diseases is a necessary cause of death, since many patients with these diseases recover.

The remote causes can be classified in many different ways. The two most significant categories are the procatarctic, corresponding roughly to a trigger agency; and the proegumenical, the predisposition on which that trigger (or exciting cause) acts. Various authors had disputed the finer shades of meaning of these terms, but into these disputes I do not want to go. I will try merely to give Sennert's own interpretations.

The procatarctic causes, according to Sennert, are those that "excite and set into motion the causes latent in the body so that they affect our body in a way that is manifest and evident to the senses." The procatarctic cause thus requires some preceding morbific disposition on which to act. It can never by itself induce a disease. Nor can it ever be a proximal cause since, to become operative, it always requires some other factor, namely, the predisposition. But not every cause of disease needs a predisposition. A sword thrust, for example, is the proximal cause of a wound, but it is not procatarctic since it does not excite any latent cause.

The proegumenical causes are predispositions latent in the body and must precede the disease. As examples of such predispositions Sennert mentioned a diathesis or a cachochymia. These, whose usage goes back to Galen, would be antecedent causes of disease. To the modern ear they represent only ignorance, that is, some vague state of unknown type, present in some patients but not in others, that preceded the development of a given disease. But for seventeenth century writers these terms were meaningful.

To render these distinctions more concrete, let us consider cerebral hemorrhage as a disease. Then, as antecedent cause we could say hypertension, and antecedent to this we might say chronic glomerulonephritis, and antecedent to this we might say scarlet fever. All of these would be proegumenical causes of apoplexy. Another example of interrelations between categories would be a fracture due to a fall. In a normal person, a minor trauma would have no effect on the bones, while a severe fall could result in a fracture. In the latter case the trauma (in the normal person) would be the immediate cause of the fracture, but, since there is no additional factor involved, not a procatarctic cause. However, if we had a patient with carcinoma of the lung and metastases in the femur, then a relatively minor trauma would result in a fracture, although a normal person would have been unaffected. In this instance the trauma would be a procatarctic cause (but not a proximal cause). The metastasis, of course, would be an antecedent or proegumenical cause; and antecedent to that would be the original cancer.

Sennert knew nothing of scarlet fever, glomerulonephritis, hypertension, or carcinoma metastases; but following a long tradition he did recognize the complexities of the causal relations and the different ways of interpreting them. Modern medicine has brought greater precision to what was then but dimly perceived.

The antecedent causes we may regard as potential determinants of disease. They do not necessarily produce the disease but they are capable of doing so, that is, of becoming actual, as other factors supervene. They are remote causes as well as potential, and cannot be included in any definition of a disease. If we remove the predisposition we may prevent the disease. To use a modern example, if we relieve hypertension we may prevent the development of cerebral hemorrhage.

Sennert and his contemporaries, as well as his predecessors, were quite concerned with the question whether accessory causes were internal or external, whether part of the bodily economy or of the environment. We must try to enter into the values of these older physicians. As we have already noted, the physicians attended more to classification than to discovery. They saw great importance in finding the "proper" classification and subsumption, the correct logical connection. But all the various subtle distinctions diminished in importance as medical knowledge increased.

The conjoint cause had as its synonym the continued cause. The definition would be some factor in the body, proximally connected with the disease, such that when the factor is present the disease is present, when the factor is removed, the disease is eliminated. The example, already familiar, is the obstruction resulting from calculus or inflammation. The obstruction is the disease, the continued cause is the obstructing calculus. In such an example, the disease persists only when maintained by the continuing cause and is eliminated when that cause is removed. In contrast is the relationship such that when the cause is removed the disease is not eliminated. The classic example is the sword thrust. When the sword is taken away, the disease — the wound — nevertheless remains.

It takes considerable effort for modern readers to view sympathetically the gropings of seventeenth century physicians. They were carrying on the Galenic heritage, an excellent framework in its own context but not adapted for accommodating masses of new data. Disease states were poorly differentiated yet the physicians identified many causal connections, however vague they seem to our eyes. Medical theorists also sought some scope for necessity. Wherein lies the necessity of a causal relation? And how can you relate necessary factors to those that are not necessary? In trying to solve these problems, earlier physicians adopted the Galenic nomenclature and, even though they did not agree completely among themselves, found the multiple categories helpful.

As medicine progressed in the latter half of the seventeenth century and reached a peak in the mid-eighteenth century, the concepts of causation also developed. The Galenic nomenclature persisted but with the dropping out of some categories and, for the remainder, a different emphasis and new insights. Many of the concepts that are latent or barely expressed in Riverius or Sennert became important, even dominant, in the eighteenth century.

Boerhaave

In the first half of the eighteenth century the most influential physician was Hermann Boerhaave, who created a unified system that ranged over all of medicine, from lofty first principles down to specific rules of practice. Boerhaave did not himself make any great discoveries. Instead he rendered orderly the various doctrines and discoveries of the preceding century. In his writings he demonstrated not so much new facts as new relations between facts already known. He wove together concepts that were, in their outlines, quite familiar, synthesizing ideas and data that were current, making them logically coherent and intellectually satisfying. He critically examined the ideas of the times and placed them into an ordered structure. To speak of him as an eclectic is somewhat misleading, for this implies a certain disparagement. Rather we should regard him as a great synthesizer, and thus recognize his creative talents.

As part of his overall system Boerhaave discussed the causes of disease but he also touched on certain broader aspects of causation as a general philosophical problem. It is very difficult to analyze his teachings and offer them as a coherent whole. His own presentation is rather disorderly, for there is considerable jumping back and forth. Then, if we use the standard English translation of the *Academical Lectures,* we must be wary, for this often inserts terms not present in the Latin and sometimes renders the Latin in a wrong sense.[19] Often this is of no great importance, but in dealing with subtle concepts we can be badly misled if we rely only on a translation.

Relevant here is a linguistic point. The Latin provides no distinction between a and the. Earlier in this chapter we have seen the differing implications of a cause and the cause. The standard English translation often applies what I consider to be the wrong particle and thereby distorts the meanings. Often considerable reflection on the Latin text is necessary to know which particle is the more appropriate.

Furthermore, Boerhaave often had the disconcerting trait of qualifying his statements. Thus, in discussing the so-called proximal cause, he said in one place that this is the disease itself — *causa proxima est ipse morbus* — a flat and unequivocal assertion. But elsewhere, again speaking of the proximal cause, he said "It is almost the same as the entire disease itself" (*Est fere idem res ipse integro morbo*).[20] We can translate the Latin *fere* in various ways, such as virtually, or quite, or, more freely, essentially. But there is always the lurking sense of "almost but not quite." Then we are left with the nagging uncertainty, are the two terms, the cause and the disease, the same or not the same? As I shall show later, Boerhaave's entire doctrine of causation indicates that they are the same, but the one word *fere* can really confuse the problem. Part of the confusion may result from the different sources of the two quotations. The one, with the *fere,* comes from Boerhaave's original text; the other, without the *fere,* from one of the notes in Haller's edition. Presumably, Haller, writing thirty years after the first edition, believed that the true sense rested in the omission of *fere.*

In his discussion Boerhaave used the same nomenclature as did Sennert and Riverius, but in rather different senses, much more akin to modern concepts. Boerhaave was indeed a prisoner of conventional terminology, but he was groping to find more comprehensive meanings. In this he was only partially successful, but nevertheless his analysis marks an important step forward in the methodology of science.

In his analysis Boerhaave, like his predecessors, used pairs of contrasting terms: internal and external, remote and proximal, predisposing and exciting (proegumenical and procatarctic). Yet we find that Boerhaave, while retaining the older nomenclature, attended to a smaller number of concepts which acquired a richer meaning than before. The terms had descended from Galen, but their meanings and relative importance changed with the new contexts.

Boerhaave also was deeply concerned with the concept of necessity, of the relations such that, when one thing is given, something else necessarily follows. That this relationship existed, he had no doubt, but he had to express himself with conventional terminology. To the modern viewpoint his ideas seem vague indeed, and any exposition involves considerable interpretation.

The multitude of causes that Sennert had discussed Boerhaave reduced to three main categories, which he enunciated as the remote (or predisposing) cause, the occasional (or procatarctic or inciting) cause, and most difficult of all, the proximal cause. But when we examine the problem more closely, we realize that both the predisposing cause and the inciting cause, while opposed to each other, are both, in a sense, remote, so that there is a basic logical opposition between remote and proximal. To clarify these ideas let us examine Boerhaave's own exposition.[21] Unless otherwise stated, the quotations represent my own translations from the Latin.

As a general definition Boerhaave declared that the cause of the disease is that which produces the present disease (*morbum praesentem facit*). A disease is a physical thing (*ens physicum*), and its cause is also a physical thing (*res physica*), which induces a change in the solids or the fluids of the body. This emphasis on the physical character of disease and of its cause has a special purpose. Boerhaave, in my interpretation, was condemning anything that savored of substantial form or archeus or immaterial substance.

The occurrence of a disease ordinarily involves a predisposing cause that sets the stage; and to this is added some additional factor, the exciting or occasional or procatarctic cause, that actually brings the disease into being. Boerhaave identified predisposing with remote. He said explicitly that the remote cause renders the body capable of receiving the disease (*suscipere morbum*) but some other factor must be added thereto. In this context predisposing cause represents the condition where the remote cause actually inheres in the body, that is, is internal. This might involve such factors as temperaments or a particular state of the humors, like a plethora. A person with a particular composition of humors might be more likely to contract a particular disease than someone of a different humoral composition, when both face the same exciting cause. These vague expressions cover a fully meaningful concept, as we see if we transpose into modern equivalents and speak, say, of excessive cholesterol in the blood, instead of an indefinite cacochymia. The latter may sound comical to modern ears, but nevertheless is a lineal ancestor of the more specific terminology involving identifiable chemical compounds in the blood.

Boerhaave emphasized the point that the remote cause, by itself, is never sufficient to produce a disease. There must supervene some additional factor that forcibly acts on the predisposing cause. (The Latin word is *nocet*. This suggests a disrupting force that brings about a disease from a previously quiescent state.) This accessory factor is the familiar occasional or procatarctic cause. It may be internal or external and ordinarily can be reduced to the nonnaturals, which we will discuss in detail later.

When we examine the concepts so far enunciated, we see that the distinction of internal and external is of little consequence and subordinate to the truly important contrast of predisposing and occasional or exciting. To produce a disease these two must act together; "both together constitute the proximal cause."

Boerhaave gave an excellent example. Imagine, he said, a weight of 200 pounds, to be raised by two men, neither of whom can lift it alone, although together they can do so. If the weight were divided into two, then the first man could raise half, and when the second man came to help, then the entire weight would be raised. Said Boerhaave, physicians would commonly call the first man the remote cause and the second the proximal cause, but this is bad usage, for each is equally near the effect. It is wrong to call one remote and the other proximal and to attribute the effect to the latter. He pointed to a balance with 100 pounds on one side, 99 on the other.[22] The heavier side is down, the lighter side up. If we now add one pound to the up side, then the 100 pound weight will rise, to come to an equilibrium. But you cannot call the addition of one pound the sole cause of the ascent of the balance even though it is the last to be added. It is, however, a cause jointly with the other 99 pounds.

The long and complex note in which this example occurs offers many crucial points for discussion. Boerhaave used the word proximal in two senses: the first, a causal factor that is temporally later than some other factor designated as remote; and second, a meaning where proximal is the equivalent of the disease itself. In reference to the first point Boerhaave made it abundantly clear that this usage is faulty, even though strongly rooted in tradition. Yet despite the impropriety he continued to use this meaning in various other contexts, much to the confusion of later students. He might have advantageously used terms such as causal factors or even partial causes, but such nomenclature was not traditional. Instead of a different nomenclature he kept the same terms but gave them, at times, a different meaning.

The confusion becomes especially acute when we add in some difficulties in translation. He had indicated that the individual factors—the predisposing and the occasional causes—could each be called a remote cause. Each is only a partial cause. Emphasizing the need for both of these to work together to induce the effect, he declared, *Ergo causa remota est causa dimidiata*. The English translation of 1747 renders this, "Therefore the remote cause is but half the cause." A better translation, in my opinion, would be, "Therefore a remote cause is only a partial cause."

We can, perhaps, derive important insight from the word *dimidiata*, which literally means half but might be better rendered as partial. Boerhaave's usage suggests that for any disease there was only one predisposing and one occasional cause. Hence the force of *dimidiata*. Each of the causes produced half the effect and the two together constituted the whole cause. Without doing violence to his thought we can readily transpose this into a more modern sounding format: in the production of disease various factors must combine, factors to which we can give various names—predisposing, occasional, internal, external, remote—any one of which is only partially responsible for the actual appearance of the symptoms.

Boerhaave gave a more precise definition of the proximal cause of a disease: "The entire aggregate [of causes] which directly constitutes the present disease. This, whether simple or complex, is always the entire, sufficient, and present [cause] of the whole disease. Its presence establishes and continues the disease, its absence removes the disease. It is quite the same thing as the entire disease itself."[23]

He reinforced this notion that the proximal cause is the same as the disease, for he said explicitly that the various remote causes, conjoined, are the proximal cause; and that the various conditions that are separately called the causes are, when combined, the disease.[24] We must think of the various causal factors (remote causes) each as *a* cause and reserve the particle *the* for the proximal cause, the conjunction of factors that constitutes the disease.

If we return to Boerhaave's example of the balance we appreciate the ambiguity in the concept of proximal cause. In the one sense we have the notion of a temporal sequence — events take place over a span of time, during which many partial causes occur but do not individually yield the final event — in this instance the equilibrium of the balance. But the addition of the final one pound weight immediately precedes the event (the equilibrium). The additional weight, the last link in a causal chain, was closest to the event, but nevertheless is only one link among many. We see the same mode of thought in the reporting of sports events. We read that Jones won the baseball game with a home run in the last of the ninth, just as if the other eight men on the team had nothing to do with the victory. The home run is the analog of the final one pound weight, while the performance of the other eight men would compare with the 99 pounds already in the balance pan. Boerhaave indicated that the one pound weight in pan A could not bring into equilibrium a weight of 100 pounds in balance pan B. Only when the separate weights in balance pan A aggregate 100 pounds do we have the equilibrium. In Boerhaave's terminology the 100 pounds in pan A represent the proximal cause of achieving equilibrium with the 100 pounds in pan B.

We thus have an equivalence. If the 100 pounds in pan A is the proximal cause, and the equilibrium is the effect, we can see the force of Boerhaave's contention, that the cause — the proximal cause — is the same as the effect. We also see the cause in this sense is the *definition* of the effect. Since 100 pounds is equal to 100 pounds, we have an equilibrium by definition. We have a necessary connection between cause and effect, a necessity that we find only through definition.

Since cause and effect are, for Boerhaave, "really" identical, only our human imperfection makes us think otherwise. Things are different in the mind of God. He declared, "If we could understand the nature of things, like the Creator himself . . . we should not then use the name of cause and effect, but we should see every thing as existing together." But in our limitation we can think only in succession and "for this reason therefore we call the thing first conceived, the cause, and that which comes next, the effect; not because there is any real difference betwixt the cause and effect, since the cause is inseparable from the effect, and the effect from the cause, and differ only with respect to duration in ourselves."[25] Cause and effect are thus really (in the mind of God) simultaneous and only our human imperfection makes us perceive succession.

Boerhaave offered some illustrations. What, he asked, is a "phrenzy" (*phrenitis*)? And he answered, a physical entity that, when it occurs in man, brings about a raging delirium and that is produced by cerebral disturbance with a high fever.[26] Frenzy is associated with inflammation of the brain. But we can go further. Frenzy *is* an acute fever with inflammation of the brain, disturbance of cerebral function, and confusion of ideas. This obviously is the definition, as we might find in a textbook or a dictionary. Boerhaave continued, that if we ask the cause of the frenzy, he would answer, the inflammation; and if anyone objected that the disease is the cause of itself, he would agree. There cannot be an inflammation of the brain without frenzy, he thought, nor can the function of the brain be disturbed without inflammation being present. Therefore, he concluded triumphantly, the whole effect is completely the same as the whole cause.

Boerhaave, apparently, was describing the delirium that may occur in some cases of meningitis or encephalitis. He had noted a set of clinical features and he thought that they were always and necessarily associated with inflammation of the brain. When we have that inflammation, he thought, we have a specific disorder of function, namely, a frenzy—by definition. The inflammation of the brain and the frenzy are completely equivalent. And if we say that the inflammation is the cause of the frenzy, then cause and effect are clearly identical. In Boerhaave's terminology, the inflammation of the brain causes the frenzy; in my terminology it is the defining factor. We today know that a frenzy can occur without cerebral inflammation but Boerhaave did not know that.

An even more illuminating example is apoplexy.[27] This, he said, is a "sudden destruction of the animal functions with retention or even increase of the vital functions," that is, sudden paralysis of the voluntary muscles with persistence of cardio-respiratory function. (For simplicity of discussion I will restrict myself to the paralytic aspects only.) He pointed to what we would call a causal chain of events: if a man is struck on the head with a hammer, and two ounces of blood extravasate, and this blood compresses the brain, then an apoplexy results; if we remove the extravasated blood, we remove the apoplexy, and "therefore the compression of the brain is the cause of the disease." The hammer blow led to the effusion of the blood, and the effusion led to compression of the brain, and this gave an apoplexy immediately, without any further intermediary (whereas the hammer blow did require an intermediary). Just as the inflammation of the brain was the equivalent of a frenzy, so the sudden compression of the brain was for

Boerhaave the immediate equivalent of the apoplexy. We can think of the example of the balance, wherein the sum of 100 pounds, however arrived at, became the immediate equivalent of the 100 pounds in the other pan of the balance — in Boerhaave's terminology, the proximal cause of the equilibrium.

Today we do not consider a sudden compression of the brain substance the equivalent of paralysis, for we can interpolate other factors. One part of the brain is not the same as any other part of the brain, but localization is important. Furthermore, we know a great deal about nerve cells. Cellular function and cerebral localization are factors that Boerhaave did not know about. So, too, we can now speak learnedly about edema and oxygen lack. We can bring in more subtle factors on an ultramicroscopic or biochemical level. All these refinements in knowledge would, in Boerhaave's terminology, represent additional remote causes, and the degree of detail would depend on the degree of our sophistication. But for practical purposes we can say that a sudden extravasation of blood, when it interrupts the function of nerve cells in specific parts of the brain, results in the paralysis we call apoplexy. For those of us sympathetic with eighteenth century thought, this definition is remarkably similar to Boerhaave's proximal cause and entirely comparable to the definitions of apoplexy in any modern dictionary.

But once the definition — the proximal cause — is known, it holds little further interest. If we want to know, say, why a patient died, we find no satisfaction in being told that his heart stopped beating. If we want to know why a patient had a stroke, it is not at all helpful to hear that the function of his motor nerve cells was interrupted. Instead, we want to know the chain of events that led up to the proximal cause and culminated in the extravasation of blood and compression of the brain. To what extent did renal disease play a part? What was the state of the cerebral arteries? What were the emotional stresses? Only the skillful physician will find the answers to these and innumerable similar questions. He will hunt for various predisposing and precipitating factors. Boerhaave realized this as well as does the modern physician, but he sought his answers within the framework of contemporary knowledge — within such internal factors as the temperament, humoral composition, plethora, excessive gluten, configuration of the solids, and the like, and external factors dependent on the environment.

As we have already seen, the environmental factors relevant to health and disease were generally known as the nonnaturals. There is no good simple definition of this term. We can grasp its essence if we think of the question "How can we keep healthy?" Today, the popular newspaper columnists are glad to tell us. They say, in effect, "Eat good food, breathe clean air, get plenty of rest, establish regular bowel habits, avoid worry," and so on. These recommendations, we note, involve degrees: we must avoid too much and too little, and we must choose the degree that is just right. All this constitutes what we call hygiene—the art of preserving health. Boerhaave and his predecessors would have given exactly the same answers as do our columnists today but Boerhaave would have been referring to the nonnaturals. These represent the factors that, properly applied to the body, maintain it in health; but when badly applied will lead to disease.[28]

Disease, then, can result from error or abuse of the nonnaturals, and such errors were regarded as precipitating causes of disease. If we make allowances for the strange terminology, we see that this makes a great deal of sense and that the major differences from today's usage lies with the degree of specificity. Suppose that today we have a gastrointestinal upset. We might say, "It was something I ate." Or we might become progressively more specific: "I had an attack of food poisoning"; or, "I contracted a Salmonella infection"; or, "I was infected by *S. enteritides*." Each statement is more specific than its predecessor. Boerhaave could not have offered these degrees of specificity. He would merely have called the condition "an error of the non-naturals, in the category of the *ingesta*." Between this simple statement, which says only that I ate bad food, and the identification of *S. enteritides*, there is a great difference in precision. Yet if we are seeking the precipitating cause of disease, then "an error in the ingesta" has logical force. Boerhaave differed from the modern physician not in his logic but in the degree of precision he could offer.

Boerhaave described the way he went about studying a patient. First, he had to find out what the disease was. He sought the proximal cause, which comprised the predisposing cause plus the procatarctic or precipitating cause. In regard to the predisposing cause, he queried whether the fault lay in the temperament of the patient. Did it lie, for example, in a plethora? If not, he went on to some other category until he was satisfied about the predisposing and internal cause. Then he went on to consider the external and accessory causes. I quote from the English translation of 1747 which, although not entirely precise, gives a good eighteenth century flavor. "Therefore I ask the patient what he has eat or drank, what medicines he has taken, or whether he has received any infection from people afflicted with contagious disease, or by any other accident; whether he has eaten any bad shellfish, or sallad, upon which toads have spit or spued their froth &c. If there appears no defect in that class, enquiry must be next made, whether there is anything amiss in the excreta or retenta; and in this manner are all the four classes of the accessory causes to be run over, till the true cause is found."[29]

He went on to indicate the great importance of asking the proper questions. "I have seen people who have persuaded themselves for certain, that they have been troubled with the stone in the kidney, because they made bloody urine, which became afterward purulent, and was discharged with great pain: but upon strict enquiry it appeared, that cantharides [an aphrodisiac that may cause intense inflammation of the bladder] had been externally applied to their body. By attending to all these particulars, you will in time become a physician; but without this consideration you will wander altogether in the dark."

Nor did he completely ignore the physical examination. He mentioned the case of an infant "who had a fever without any manifest cause; it cried much, and was convulsed, for which I could find no cause by all my enquiries, till at length I ordered the body of the infant to be undressed or stripped naked, by which means we found a needle thrust through the cloaths into the flesh; by removing it and applying a fomentation, the whole disease was removed. If I had not thus learnt the cause of the disorder, no bleeding or other medicine would have recovered the child to its health." This quite illuminating passage indicates that physical examination of a nude body was rarely performed, and that even in infants attention was paid chiefly to the history.

Boerhaave indicated four categories into which the procatarctic cause of disease would fall: those things that were taken into the body—food, drink, poisons, infections; or performed by the body (including exercise, sleep, emotional states); or retained or excreted, whether normally or abnormally; or applied externally, for example, baths, clothing, wounds, contusions, irritants. This classification did not, however, replace the more traditional six nonnaturals but did loosen the rigidity of the traditional categories.

According to my interpretation, when we allow for the difference in terminology we find a close similarity between Boerhaave's concepts of cause and those that obtain in contemporary textbooks. In this connection we must realize that Boerhaave wrote before David Hume, Thomas Reid, John Stuart Mill, and other philosophers who provided analyses so important for present-day logical theory. In the history of logic Boerhaave certainly deserves a significant place.

Lesser Physicians

Boerhaave, in his *Institutes*, was dealing with the scientific foundations of medicine, but most texts of that era concerned themselves not with basic concepts but rather with details of medical practice. In more or less orderly fashion the authors took up individual diseases and usually made some statements about the causal factors at work. There was a wide variation in the mode of presentation, the degree of detail, and the extent of dogmatism. I will offer two characteristic examples that show how physicians of the second or third rank paid little heed to the subtleties of the causal relationship.

Riverius Reformatus, attributed to one François de la Calmette, was first published in Lyons in 1690, with a second edition in 1696. I have an English translation of 1713.[30] The author aimed to reconcile the practice of Riverius with the "modern philosophy," that is, with the mechanical philosophy. While directed toward practice, the book also contained a fair amount of theory. I will note two diseases.

The understanding of apoplexy, said the author, depends on the principles of anatomy.[31] The "glandules" of the brain separate the "animal spirits" from the blood, and the "small nervous threads coming forth from each glandule, like so many excretory vessels . . . carry off the spirits." If there is some obstruction or compression that hinders the passage of the spirits, then "an abolition of sense and motion must necessarily follow, and consequently an apoplexy."

The author adhered to the conventional terminology. He offered an internal cause: a thick lymph that can impair the filtration of the spirits or hinder the distribution of the spirits within the cavities of the nerves. (The nerves were regarded as hollow tubes.) Inflammation or tumor can squeeze the nervous canals and thus hinder the passage of the spirits. Excessive blood can oppress the substance of the brain. Correlative to the internal are the external causes: whatever thickens the blood or promotes its passage into the head or hinders its reflux therefrom. These factors would all result from an abuse of the nonnaturals. The victim is "deprived of sense and motion; because the influx of the animal spirits, into the noble and sensible parts, is denied" (although respiration is still performed). All this is discussion on a merely verbal plane, dealing with hypothetical entities.

We may compare this account with his exposition of gout.[32] This he defined as a periodically recurrent pain, "proceeding from a sharp saline humor, that falls upon the parts near the joints." There may or may not be a fever. Sometimes there is a hereditary disposition, while another type is "adventitious, and proceeds from errors in diet, or the abuse of the nonnaturals." The "nearest, and joined cause," that is, the proximal and conjoint causes, "can be nothing else, than serous or lymphatic humor, that is very acid, that is impregnated with acid salts, that is very corrosive." This, "falling upon the parts near the joints . . . vellicates, and pricks the same . . . . . whence follow the very intense pains." The "external causes of the gout are victuals, that are gross, of a difficult concoction, acid, salt; drunkenness, immoderate venery, violent exercise, an idle life, much sleep, fear, sadness, care, all which may make an exultation of the acid in the blood and serum." We have here an interesting mixture of concrete observation and hypothetical entities.

Our next example is Johannes Juncker (1679-1759), a disciple of Stahl, who wrote from the Stahlian viewpoint. Each volume he wrote, called a *Conspectus*, presented masses of detail arranged in a rather formal manner. In the *Conspectus Medicinae* he described 138 diseases, each description adhering to a common pattern that gave definition, differentiation, distinguishing signs, subjects (persons likely to contract the disease), causes, prognosis, recommended remedies, and practical observations. We will note his discussions of apoplexy.[33]

In this disease he enumerated the causes in a way that illuminates the usage of terms in the early eighteenth century. The "remote antecedent cause" is the neglect of the customary evacuation, thus resulting in a plethora and thickening of the lymph. The "less remote" antecedent cause is the sudden congestion of the abundant blood, spreading into the cerebrum, the delicate vessels of the choroid plexus, and the immediately adjacent medullary tissues. The "proximal and continuing cause" is the extravasation of the blood and serum around the choroid plexus. The occasional and procatarctic causes are a "bad disposition" of the stomach, advanced age, hereditary disposition, a life given to constant intoxication, and violent injury to the head. This insistence on detailed and proper categorization is closer to the earlier viewpoint, which we have already noted for Sennert and Riverius, in contrast to the more penetrating viewpoint of Boerhaave.

It might be interesting to go over a whole series of diseases, especially various infections and fevers, and study the ways in which various authors of the eighteenth century dealt with the causes of these conditions. Such an exposition, however, might get bogged down in details which, although of great antiquarian interest, would not provide significantly greater insight into the basic thought modes of the eighteenth century.

The cause of disease is a problem that holds major interest for many different groups: philosophers, concerned with logical theory; research scientists, who study the factors that distinguish health from disease; practicing physicians, concerned not with laws and generalizations, but with the care of particular sick patients and with getting them well; various governmental and private agencies, concerned with ecology, planning for the good life, allocation of funds and with the relative values of society; and many others. In this chapter I have attempted only a very limited analysis, dealing with eighteenth century medical usage. It is well, I believe, in view of the great complexity of the subject, to be entirely explicit on the deliberate limitation.

TEN

RATIONALISM AND EMPIRICISM

The earnest student wants to know the how and the why of things. He seeks explanations, causes, and relationships. But having asked the how and the why, and having received his answers, he can make himself quite unpopular if he asks the further question, "But how do you know?" Here we have an implied challenge. The student is not merely curious, he wants not only an answer but a justification of that answer. To his original curiosity he has now added a critical awareness.

To the question, "How do you know?" the reply ordinarily will take one of these three basic forms: "Someone told me"; or, "I saw it myself"; or, "I figured it out." These three separate categories we may call, respectively, authority, observation, and reason.

Reliance on authority forms the basis of education: the child depends on what his parents and teachers tell him; the adult, on the news media and on books; the scientist, on the reports of other scientists; the historian, on his primary documents and the reports of other historians. This reliance on authority involves a faith which may suffer erosion. Thus, personal experience, contrary to authority, may induce doubts whose extent will vary according to the critical bent of the individual. And critical bent is another aspect of reason. In mature persons, beliefs involve all three interdependent features — authority, experience, and reason — which constantly interact. We check authority against experience and reason; experience, against reflection and authority; reflection, against the statements of others as well as our own personal experience.

Of the three factors that condition belief, I want to attend especially to reason and experience and the generalizations known as rationalism and empiricism. It would be extremely difficult to frame satisfactory definitions. Instead of attempting this I will indicate some broad zones of distinction. On the one hand we have a special concern with the abstract and the conceptual, with theories and first principles, with deduction of particular instances from the general rule, with mathematics as the ideal methodology. The contrasting attitude stresses practical activity, sensory experience, direct observation, and the concrete immediacy of particular things. It accepts only limited degrees of abstraction and relies on inferences that remain close to direct observation. Remote and complex inferences have no place in the empiricist camp.

These distinctions, admittedly approximate and quite fluid, were in the seventeenth and eighteenth centuries a little firmer and were often buttressed with metaphysical supports. Nevertheless we cannot make any rigid distinction between the two camps. We deal with questions of more or less, not of absolutes.

To understand rationalism we may, perhaps, point to some modern detective fiction. The great fictional detectives — Sherlock Holmes, Hercule Poirot, Ellery Queen, Nero Wolfe — all rely on reason. Through reflection they invariably penetrate the confused mass of particulars, the intermingling of the important and the irrelevant, and always find the essential feature, that is, the criminal. The detective shows us what logical analysis and ratiocination can do. Reason, acting through the "little grey cells" and functioning with "order and method," will reach the truth.

In all this there is an implied metaphysics: that the universe itself is rational and that reason is a tool adequate to analyze reality and find the interconnection among events. Many professional philosophers have expounded this concept but never more delightfully than did Sherlock Holmes, who compressed a volume of metaphysics into a few sentences. As if to explain his remarkable ability of drawing true inferences from seemingly casual observation, he said, "From a drop of water a logician could infer the possibility of an Atlantic or Niagara without having seen or heard of one or the other. So all life is a great chain, the nature of which is known whenever we are shown a single link." Sherlock Holmes could "figure things out" through reason alone. He could do this because the universe is logical and rational. Events are bound together in a logical chain, and given a single link, the rational person, if his reason is sharp enough, can go forward to predict the future or go backward to identify a cause.[1]

This, of course, is merely a different version of the Renaissance doctrine of macrocosm and microcosm, wherein, because of interrelations and correspondences, a knowledge of the great world (or macrocosm) enables us to tell what will happen to a particular man, the microcosm.[2] This doctrine provided the theoretical basis for the arts of divination, such as astrology, cheiromancy, umbilicomancy, metaposcopy, and kindred practices.[3] Reason, then, can penetrate the secrets of the universe because the universe is rational. Logic will achieve truth in constructing a picture of the universe.

Hoffmann

The rationalist leaned heavily on mathematics and on system formation. We find this view admirably expressed by Friedrich Hoffmann. In his major work, *Medicina Rationalis Systematica*, an important chapter deserves a summarizing exposition.[4]

Just as the mathematical method that geometers use is the best for finding and teaching truth, so also the philosophical physician ought to furnish this type of demonstration to his own discipline. "From principles [that is, axioms] and from simple, clear, and manifest propositions, the geometers draw suitable conclusions and relationships, arrange them in a proper order, and thus they explain what is difficult and discover new truths." So, too, in all the changes that affect the human body, the philosophical physician ought to draw true conclusions and relationships from clear principles.

I would emphasize that the term philosophy in this context refers particularly to physics, as in the phrase natural philosophy. As we have seen in Chapter 5, many physicians wanted to reduce the science of medicine to physics. Physics was a science that could readily be reduced to a few first principles — the axioms of a system — from which the particular details could be derived. Descartes had provided a powerful impetus for this view and his concepts dominated continental philosophy. Cartesian physics, with its three kinds of matter, comprised a systematic formulation adopted by most continental iatromechanists. The physics of Newton, experimentally based, dominated British philosophy and eventually replaced Cartesian physics on the Continent. However, the conflict between Cartesian and Newtonian theories does not affect the point at issue here, that Hoffmann regarded physics as the foundation of medicine. And since physics was a mathematical science, permitting systematic formulation and deductive reasoning, medicine could similarly be a systematic science, with its own first principles and its derivation of particulars through deductive reasoning.

Hoffmann elaborated the rationalist viewpoint. Any scientific discipline, he said, should seek first principles in order that subordinate causes could be connected to them. This should also be done in medical science. In medicine a first principle should be clear, applicable to medical observations and experiments, and the proximal cause of physiological processes, insofar as all these pertain to the cause and cure of diseases. It must be the cause of all actions, movements, and changes that occur in our bodies; it must be easily understood and, furthermore, must really exist in our bodies. The "real existence" of which Hoffmann made mention contrasts with the vitalistic or animistic entities (of Stahl) whose "real" existence was not demonstrated.[5] For Hoffmann the first principle in medicine, the primary and proximal cause of all functions in the human body, is motion.

We must note two distinct features of this exposition: the general framework for medical science that starts with a first principle and permits deductive derivation of subordinate events; and second, the identification of a particular term to serve as this principle. In regard to the latter factor, we may object to Hoffmann's choice but this does not affect the point at issue, namely, that he regarded medicine as a science that could be cast into a system analogous to mathematics. Such a system allowed deduction of particulars, and the deductive process revealed the causes of particular

phenomena. When we read widely in Hoffmann's writings we find inconsistencies and confusion, vast gaps in information, and highly questionable
reasoning. Nevertheless we do have an explicit statement of the rationalist
viewpoint, reflecting Hoffmann's full maturity.

In an earlier work of 1695, now available in English, Hoffmann indicated in a less systematic form some of the ideas that he elaborated later.
"No physician is rational unless he is accomplished in natural philosophy
and has a precise knowledge of natural principles." Otherwise, there will
be only "a refined empiricism, disguised with eloquence and talent, but
making no true knowledge." This, however, is not to be necessarily condemned, for in medicine, apart from science, there are also the problems
of practical judgment and wisdom. Science, he said, is best presented by
the moderns (those who followed the mechanical philosophy) but "judgment and wisdom" are best learned from the ancients. Declared Hoffmann, "I have tried hard to reduce the basic principles of medicine into a
brief system and into a structure arranged by the easiest method, according
to the precepts of sound modern mechanical-chemical philosophy."[6]

As we have seen in earlier chapters, in the late seventeenth century
neo-Galenic doctrines were in full retreat, the iatrophysicists were in
the ascendant, while the chemists had a somewhat equivocal position. The
various proponents disputed abundantly, yet the different doctrines could
equally be called rationalistic. Sennert, for example, made no obeisance to
mathematics nor did he embody the new physics. But he, like Hoffmann,
had a logical system that rested on a few basic or primitive terms, that lent
itself to ready generalization, and that gave great scope to logical inference. If we had to characterize in a single word the rationalism of seventeenth and eighteenth century medicine, I would suggest the word system,
in the sense sketched above. This epithet indicates a logical rigidity. We
might characterize the rationalist as one who leans heavily on logic.

But medicine was more than an intellectual discipline. Physicians had to
treat sick people, an activity commonly called the practice of medicine.
Practice, emphasizing activity, contrasts with theory and its logical elaborations. This contrast was indeed explicit in medical education, wherein
the professorial chair for the Practice of Medicine was quite distinct from
that of the Institutes of Medicine. The difference between theory and practice is crucial. It goes back to antiquity.

Classical Components

Galen provided a basic historical text, "On the Medical Sects: For Be-
ginners," in which he clearly described the empiricist and the rationalist

schools and the differences between them, particularly in regard to experience and reasoning. By the eighteenth century the context of medicine had changed so massively that the details of the ancient Greek sects are only tangential to the later problems. Important, however, is the preliminary distinction: for one school of thought "experience alone is all that our art requires, while to others it seems that also reason or reflection has no small contribution to offer. Those that make experience alone the starting point are, accordingly, called Empiricist, and similarly those who start from reason are called Rationalist."[7]

Attitudes toward the cause of disease also played an important part in the distinction between the sects. The interrelations between theory and practice, reason and experience, and the role of "cause" therein formed an important part in the teachings of Aristotle, whose analysis influenced not only post-Hippocratic Greek medicine but all subsequent medical doctrine. To appreciate the seventeenth and eighteenth century controversies we must note the distinctions that Aristotle made explicit.

The philosophy of Aristotle is probably the most influential body of doctrine in the history of thought, even though the distinctions he made, the shades of meaning on which he insisted, and the terms that he used often seem a little strange at the present time. Especially important for this study are the distinctions between concrete and abstract, particular and universal, experience and knowledge, scientific knowledge (*episteme*) and art (*techne*).

Aristotle had exalted notions of scientific knowledge, which for him dealt with pure contemplation and the study of what is necessary, eternal, and invariable. Examples would be astronomy or mathematics. These, in Aristotle's words "are not capable of being otherwise." We cannot change the course of the stars, nor can we alter the truths of mathematics.[8] Medicine clearly does not belong in this category, for medicine, like architecture and shipbuilding, concerns activity; it involves the contingent rather then the necessary; it requires choice and the possibility of things being otherwise. Where we have such contingency we can still have knowledge, but it has a different character from the pure knowledge that characterizes, say, mathematics. For the conceptual basis of medicine (or of comparable activities) Aristotle used the term *techne*, which has been translated as *ars* in Latin, art in English. But today the terms art and science have such different contexts that the Aristotelian usage can be quite confusing. A still better translation would be science, if restricted to its modern sense. But this would run counter to the Aristotelian usage. I have discussed this problem elsewhere.[9]

To apply these general concepts to medicine let us imagine a patient suffering from a given disease, who receives a remedy and then recovers. Let us suppose that this occurs repeatedly, in different patients. Regarding such a series of events, Aristotle declared, "to have a judgment that when Callias was ill of this disease this did him good, and similarly in the case of Socrates and in many individual cases, is a matter of experience." In Aristotle's sense, through experience we learn what happens. But if we start to generalize from our experience, if we pass from individual instances to an entire class, and if we then can note explicit identifiable properties of that class, we are entering the domain that Aristotle called *techne*. Said Aristotle, continuing the previous quotation, "but to judge that it [the remedy] did good to all persons of a certain constitution, marked off in one class, when they were ill of this disease, e.g., to phlegmatic or bilious people when burning with fever — this is a matter of art" (*techne*). "Art," he said, arises "when from many notions gained by experience one universal judgment about a class of objects is produced." Or, in summarizing fashion, "Experience is knowledge of individuals, art of universals."[10]

First we note that each of several individuals behaves in a certain way; then we generalize that *all* similar cases behave in that way. Although he did not specifically say so, Aristotle here was describing the aphoristic method that formed the basis of Hippocratic medicine and maintained its significance ever since.

Once we deal with universals (or generalizations) instead of particulars, we enter the domain of theory. We can have successive degrees of abstraction, getting more and more remote from the original experience, in a sort of hierarchical manner. With a series of propositions that exhibit logical relationships, we can have syllogistic demonstrations and proof. Moreover, in this connection we can appropriately speak of the why of things, that is, their cause. Said Aristotle, "Men of experience know that a things is so, but do not know why, while the others [those who know the *techne*] know the 'why' and the cause."[11] The knowledge of causes separates the man of *techne* from the man of experience. We might offer the comparison between the scientist and his technician, or between the electrical engineer and the journeyman electrician. *Techne* thus represents the theoretical background of an activity such as medicine. It is the rational component. In contrast, the man of experience, the empiricist, proceeds from case to case; not knowing the theory, he is ignorant of causes.

Generalization proceeds by abstraction. Out of a mass of particulars a class is formed by identifying a few characteristics, welding these into a unity and ignoring all other characteristics. This process of abstraction may involve temporal sequences — for example, the recovery of several individual patients after they have received a particular remedy; or the abstraction may be static, as we find when we classify a miscellaneous collection of animals.

We can have a series of classes ascending in a hierarchy and becoming progressively more abstract as they proceed from species to genera, to family, order, class, phylum, and kingdom. Similarly, we engage in progressive abstraction as we go from clinical observation to first principles. Among the eighteenth century medical rationalists, the passage from the most concrete to the most abstract was relatively brief. Clinical observations were explained by physiological processes, which in turn were explained by laws of mechanics, which in turn could be referred to Cartesian or Newtonian principles.

A rationalist thus organized his classes into a system, and with a system it is easy to assign causes. Hoffmann, as we have seen, found the ultimate cause of biological phenomena in motion, which, accordingly, was his first principle, the apex of his hierarchy. A series of classes allows logical demonstration through syllogistic reasoning.

Aristotle devoted a great deal of attention to the validity of syllogistic reasoning. However, there is a great difference between valid reasoning and truth. Valid syllogisms yield truth only if the premises are true. How do we establish the truth of the initial premise? This we do not by logical demonstration but only by intuition.[12] The initial premise on which our reasoning depends cannot be proven logically but most be inductively established. Through repeated observation of particulars we become aware of the universal implicit in them.[13] But once this intuition is achieved, what is the warrant for accepting it as true?

Aristotle did not have any sound answer to this problem, and the difficulty persisted well into the nineteenth century. Eighteenth century physicians had no clear idea of probability and statistical validity. Hume's analyses had negligible influence on medicine, Kant wrote only in the latter part of the century, and the formulations of J. S. Mill were far in the future. We will see that for the seventeenth and eighteenth centuries analogy was the principal tool whereby a physician could induce acceptance of his intuition.

To understand the conflicts in the seventeenth and eighteenth centuries, we must examine the viewpoint that stressed experience. This we can best approach through the concept of aphorisms, closely connected with so-called natural history of disease. By natural history we mean an objective description of facts, an impartial report stripped of any interpretation. The aphoristic method and the natural history of disease were the mainstay of Hippocratic medicine as well as of the empirically inclined physicians of the seventeenth and eighteenth centuries.

In different writings Hippocrates exhibited both rationalist and empirical aspects.[14] He made careful observations, provided a natural history of many diseases, offered generalizations of varying scope, and propounded explanatory theories. He covered the entire gamut of medicine, with all grades of contrast from the concrete to the abstract, from observation to interpretation, from practice to theory. Yet the empiricist aspects of Hippocratic doctrine have had the most influence. The *Epidemics*, for example, give us careful descriptions of certain diseases, admirable natural history of the type that Sydenham prized so highly more than 2000 years later. Other books such as *Prognosis, Regimen,* and especially *Aphorisms* and *Coan Prognosis* give us correlations, "if . . . then" statements, concrete recommendations based on experience, and generalizations derived from repeated observations. They summarize a vast amount of experience and serve as guide for the physician, who, in his daily practice, must make decisions on his prognosis and treatment. A compendium of past experience tells the physician what he might reasonably expect in the future and thus gives him a base of assurance. These summaries of experience, which we find in Hippocrates, are not merely descriptive. They do more than tell what *has* happened. As generalizations they have a forward reference. They represent an approximate "law of nature" that refers to all cases of a given type — those that have occurred and those that will occur.[15]

Let us note a few examples from Hippocrates: "It is a bad sign if the head, hands, and feet are cold while the belly and sides are warm"; "Sleep that stops delirium is good"; "Unprovoked fatigue means disease"; "The more nourishment you give to a person who has not been purged, the more harm you do"; "Cases of pneumonia which follow pleurisy are safer than those who are pneumonic from the beginning of the illness."[16]

Hippocrates made the inductive leap from some — the cases that he actually observed — to all, that is, a generalization that transcended experience. In the words of Aristotle, Hippocrates had perceived the universal in the numerous particulars, and this universal he framed as an aphorism, expressing generality. In recounting to others his generalized experience of disease, Hippocrates gave us the that and the what, but not the why. He gave us what he considered to be facts but offered no explanation.

Hippocrates was not really aware that his generalizations went beyond experience. He knew that these various events had happened and he assumed that they would happen again in the future. There is an act of faith involved, faith in what we today call the uniformity of nature or, in a more archaic terminology, an insight into the essence of the *physis*.

Recorded experience carries conviction in the degree to which it is confirmed by later experience. But aphorisms could also find justification by theory, that is, by a rationalist schema that tells us the why of things, that shows us how concrete particulars derive logically from more general statements.[17] In some of his writings Hippocrates offered extensive reasons for the phenomena he described. However, the physicians of the seventeenth century who inclined to the empiricist viewpoint could reject the proffered theories and still regard the aphorisms as a satisfactory practical guide. The complex relations between the empirical and the rational components we can study in the writings of Sydenham, Baglivi, and Boerhaave.

Sydenham

Thomas Sydenham (1624-1689), most influential British physician of the late seventeenth century, stands as the model of medical empiricism in its best sense. The epithet English Hippocrates indicates the esteem in which he was held. Dewhurst's indispensable book provides a valuable biography together with important texts and is a necessary supplement to the widely used two volume edition of 1850.[18] Elsewhere I have devoted considerable discussion to Sydenham's doctrines, and here I want to focus only on certain aspects that bear on medical empiricism.[19]

Sydenham, in the empirical tradition of Bacon and Locke, condemned speculation and sought more accurate, more detailed description of nature, more facts. Nature cured disease. The physician's task was to help her, but first he had to observe and know what she was about. This meant the cultivation of natural history. "The whole philosophy of medicine," he said, "consists in working out the histories of disease, and applying the remedies that may dispel them."[20] For this purpose, he continued, "Experience is the sole guide." He was pleading for "commonsense rather than speculation."

Implicit in Sydenham's writings, and sometimes explicit, is the Baconian distrust of theoretical speculation that "flies from the senses and particulars to the most general axioms"; or that "begins at once by establishing certain abstract and useless generalities"; or "the premature hurry of the understanding to leap or fly to universals and principles of things." Thus did Bacon condemn rash generalizations and the detested hypotheses.[21] We must keep in mind that Bacon, as an empirical philosopher, objected not to generalizations as such but to those that went far beyond the evidence. The Hippocratic brand of empiricism propounded generalizations very close to experience, so close that their inferential aspect is easily overlooked. The Hippocratic method is good. Bad, however, is reliance on fragmentary experience, on whose basis a philosopher propounds "the most general principles."

This Baconian attitude Sydenham had thoroughly absorbed, yet he differed in an important point. For Bacon knowledge was power: and knowledge meant sound theory, which, based on sound induction, avoided unwarranted speculation. Bacon had faith that his inductive method would lead to theoretical knowledge, which in turn would give power over nature.

For Sydenham, however, the power over disease depended on experience rather than on eventual theoretical formulation. This separation between power and theory, or differently phrased, between practice and theory, is explicit in Baglivi but certainly implicit in Sydenham.

Of particular interest are two manuscript framents, *De Arte Medica* (1669) and the *Anatomie* (1668), intended as parts of a book that was never published. Even though the handwriting (with the exception of one sentence) is that of John Locke, Dewhurst has convincingly shown that these texts are Sydenham's works. They furnish valuable insight into the relationship of theory and practice, as Sydenham conceived it.[22]

Crucial for Sydenham was the distinction between observation and hypothesis. He took a dim view of medical theory, especially the theory of the ancients, as elaborated in the schools. Theory he equated with the assertions of hidden causes of disease, the attribution of disease to some conceptual entity. He admitted that the human understanding is naturally curious about causes of things (compare Aristotle, "All men by nature desire to know.")[23] and is restless until "it has framed to itself some hypothesis and laid a foundation whereon to establish all its reasonings." He did not blame the ancients "who fashioned to themselves systems and hypotheses" or censure them in any way. But his praise he reserved for their practice, and Sydenham thereby emphasized his reliance on observation. Regarding the ancients, he said somewhat condescendingly, "To them we owe a great number of excellent observations and several ingenious discourses, and there is not any one tool of practice founded upon unbiased observation of which I do not receive."[24] He was willing to accept any observation, of whatever source, that seemed reliable.

However, the ancients were too devoted to speculation—hypothesis—that prevented their inquiries from going any further than "how the phenomena of disease might be explained by these doctrines." All this merely "amused the understanding with fine but useless speculations, and diverted their inquiries from the true and advantageous knowledge of things" (that is, from empirical observation).[25] The conceptual formulation—speculative theorems—do not advance the practice of medicine.

Sydenham was criticizing not only the ancients but the modern schools as well. He condemned equally "the doctrine of the humors" and "the notions of obstruction and putrefaction," and also "the acquaintance . . . with sulfur and mercury." In contrast he referred to "true knowledge," which depended on "experience and rational operations," by which he presumably meant sound inference. Had physicians only continued to use this method and "add their own trials to the observation of others," then physick would be "in a far better condition that now it is." Then he continued, "but proud man, not content with that knowledge he was capable of and was useful to him, would needs penetrate into the hidden causes of things, lay down principles and establish maxims to himself about the operations of nature, and then vainly expect that nature, or in truth God himself, should proceed according to those laws his maxims had prescribed."[26]

Human vanity and empty speculations hindered the growth of practical knowledge. Sydenham praised the mechanics—in Aristotle's terms, the men of experience—who found out how to do things but did not know the causes and the why. Whoever wants a fine garden does better "to consult the experience of the dull plowman and unread gardener than the profound philosopher."[27] Sydenham, like Aristotle, was regarding medicine as a practical art, whose goal was the cure of disease. But people differed on the way that this end could best be achieved.

In the empiricist camp we can note two divergent trends. One involved faith in the ultimate value of sound theory but recognized that system formation and rationalist speculation must be replaced by rigorous induction. This was the Baconian viewpoint. We might place Robert Boyle in this camp, for Boyle, although adopting the corpuscularian philosophy for his overall principles, nevertheless had the most profound respect for experience. He constantly insisted on the primacy of observation, the need for experiment, the importance of observations made by rude and unlettered mechanics. Boyle usually insisted on critical examination of data. Yet with this empirical bent he had faith in the ultimate validity of scientific principles and of eventual deductive formulations from established principles. Boyle combined the best of the seventeenth century rationalists and empiricists.

On the other hand there were those who had doubts regarding the validity of any rationalistic formulation. Physicians should aim at practical results, and the way to achieve these was to observe clearly the empirical sequences that led to cures. Sydenham inclined toward this view although he was by no means free of rationlistic trends.

Dewhurst has made available the text *Anatomie* in which Sydenham refused to accord value to scientific investigations that had no direct relevance to patient care. He could see no merit in anatomical research and indulged in sarcasm to make his point. Assume that the anatomist had a sharpness of knife and keenness of vision that could let him demonstrate the shape of the pores in liver and kidney, the size and configuration of the particles of urine or bile. How, he asked, could this "direct him in the cure either of the jaundice or stoppage of urine?" "A diligent observation of these diseases, of their beginning, progress, and ways of cure, would be better." Sydenham lacked faith that anatomy—pure research—could ever lead to practical results. "If therefore anatomy shew us neither the causes nor cures of most diseases I think it is not very likely to bring any great advantages for removing the pains and maladies of mankind."[28]

He pointed to particular examples of research, such as the attempts to discover the uses of the spleen. We know nothing of its function, he said, despite the experimental removals in animals. He spoke of the "inflated opinion of our own knowledge" and he did not believe that anatomy will ever "instruct" us how disordered functions of whatever organs could be corrected. Painstaking anatomical research, like tracing the fine vessels of liver or kidney, does not bring us "one jot nearer the cause nor manner of their operation." "After all our porings and mangling the parts of animals we know nothing but the gross parts, see not the tools and contrivances by which nature works, and are as far off from the discovery we aim at as ever."[29]

Sydenham continued with great eloquence, ringing the changes on this theme, that multiplying dissections and poring over the parts do not give us any knowledge of function nor help us cure disease. Furthermore, there is little hope for the future. The failure of "so many learned, ingenious, industrious and able men" arises "not for want of any skill or sagacity in them, but because the matters they handle did not bear it, the tools wherewith nature works and the changes she produces in these particles being too small and too subtle for the observation of our senses."[30] Sydenham lacked faith in the ultimate power of science to untangle the inmost workings of nature. Anatomical investigation has not helped in the cure of patients. He believed it never would. Therefore, the physician should devote his energies to clinical observations and correlations. This, perhaps, is the essence of Sydenham's empiricism and his reliance on the aphoristic method. Scientific investigation would not help cure diseases; close clinical observation would.

Baglivi

The writings of Giorgio Baglivi (1668-1706) show the difficulties in making any sharp distinction between rationalism and empiricism.[31] Baglivi praised both reason and experience and insisted on the need for both in medicine. Reason correlates with theory, experience with practice. The rationalists we might identify as those who had special concern with theory, while the empirical physicians had special concern for practice. With this rough criterion we would certainly consider Baglivi as an empiricist.

His fame rests principally on the book *Practice of Physick*, published originally in 1696. The title is quite illuminating: *The Practice of Physick, reduced to the ancient way of observations, containing a just parallel between the wisdom and experience of the ancients, and the hypotheses of the modern physicians. Intermixed with many practical remarks upon most distempers.* This title, although ponderous, foreshadows his key points: distinction between the ancients and the moderns, respect for the wisdom and experience of the ancients, and praise for the theory of the moderns.

The so-called battle between the ancients and the moderns is interwoven into the intellectual currents of the seventeenth century and part of the eighteenth. Jones' magnificent work is a standard exposition. In a previous book I have discussed some of the medical aspects and some of the antagonists important in medical history.[32]

What had started as a literary quarrel—do the modern writers compare in merit with the giants of the ancient world?—spread into a more general comparison of the moderns and the ancients. The new science of the sixteenth and seventeenth centuries, had toppled the authority of Aristotle in physics, of Ptolemy in astronomy, of Galen in physiology. Did all the traditions and values of the ancient world also tumble before the new science and its mechanical explanations? When phrased in this wider fashion the quarrel between ancients and moderns merges into the perpetual struggle between old and new, between conservatives and proponents of change. Baglivi, in the first part of his *Practice of Physick,* takes up some aspects of this conflict in a broader sense, but he addressed himself to quite specific medical problems.

The influx of the new scientific ideas, he said, had seriously impaired the simplicity and harmony of medical practice. Whereas other sciences—presumably he was referring to physics, astronomy, and mathematics—were becoming more and more splendid, the practice of medicine was becoming "meaner and more despicable." This loss of status, claimed Baglivi, stems from the unbridled speculations of the theorists—in Baglivi's words, from the physicians "addicting themselves entirely to systems and hypotheses, their being so solicitous, not so much to discern and cure diseases, as to assign them handsome and specious reasons."[33] This quotation reveals the burden of the book: criticism of the hypotheses of the moderns, and of their impact on medicine.

Like Sydenham, Baglivi conceived of medicine not as a science in its own right, but as an activity concerned primarily with getting sick people well. Baglivi defined medicine—physick—as the "apprehending and perceiving the several kinds of disease, and explaining them by such things as it has observed and taken notice of for a long tract of time." Against these diseases medicine provides remedies, not those indicated by probable hypothesis but by proven effectiveness over a long time. Baglivi was condemning not the activity of reason as such, but only the speculation or conjectures of "unbridled" reason. He repeatedly compared the proven merits of the ancient practice, drawn from observation and embodied in aphorisms, and the speculations that modern hypotheses had impressed on the art of medicine.[34]

In an important passage he rejected any opposition between reason as such and experience. Each has its place. We should not attribute too much to reason. We cannot give it credit for those aspects of medicine acquired "by trial and use continued through long progress of time." But neither is it proper to exclude reason. And then he provided a significant definition. By reason he did not mean "that faculty of the mind which, investigating the obscure features of nature, is called invention or a devising, and which belongs rather to physics; but rather Reason, queen and mistress of all, through which the physician perceives consequences, makes conjectural interpretation of principles and causes of diseases, and from the present state of affairs foresees and comprehends progress and outcome, and looks forward to the future."[35]

In medicine reason has as its function the ordering of observations, whereby probable outcome can be foretold. Penetration into the obscurities of nature is the task of physics. In medicine reason can conjecture the first principles and causes, but this seems a secondary activity. Reason has a practical function, to bring greater order into observations and make them more useful in treating disease and predicting its outcome. This contrasts with the function so dear to the rationalists, namely, to unlock the secrets of the universe. "The two chief pilars of physick are reason and observation," but observation is the dominant partner. Neither can be relied upon exclusively. Each has definite limitations. Said Baglivi firmly, "We are, and for ever will be, ignorant of the minute subtle texture of the solid as well as the fluid parts of a living body, which is altogether out of reach not only of our senses, but even of reason."[36] Experience, unless guided by reason, can be deceived. Reason and experience can each lead to error unless they illuminate each other.

Baglivi emphasized that medicine rested on "certain rules, confirmed by repeated experience." This was the Hippocratic method. Observation shows that diseases have some constant characteristics, while other characteristics are variable and nonspecific. The characteristics of disease are sometimes obvious, sometimes obscure. But in any event they should be noted and described, thus providing a reliable natural history. The obscurities are manifold. Since we cannot penetrate to the nature of these obscurities through reason, it is the part of wisdom to note the practical outcome and then accordingly frame precepts that would be suitable for practice.[37]

In concluding this chapter, Baglivi emphasized again that reason must be joined to observation. Disease is so complex, there are such innumerable causes, there are so many variations and circumstances "and an infinity of other things that concur towards the production or removal of diseases . . . that it is a hard matter to trace the truth, unless the complexion of them all be weighed and illustrated by a discrete use of reason."[38] Reason thus has practical use but must be subservient to experience.

Since Baglivi distinguished rather sharply between theory and practice, he could neatly straddle the issue whether the moderns surpassed the ancients or the ancients surpassed the moderns. His answer was that the moderns were better in their theory, the ancients better in their practice.

Modern theory, he said, "is grounded upon experiments made with diligence and repetition, and drawn from the storehouse of natural philosophy: it lays down, and demonstrates the causes and symptoms of diseases, not by uncertain conjectures, but by mathematical truths, that shine clear as the sun." Far otherwise was the theory of the Galenists, which "not only seduce[s] weak minds from the true road of practice, by an idle train of questions; but by a nauseous repetition of things already said, a barrenness of invention, and an ostentation of logical quibbles in refuting and retorting arguments, covers its practice with the greatest obscurity."[39]

On the other hand, the practice of the Galenists "is infinitely preferable to that of the moderns," owing chiefly "to that immortal patience in making observations . . . in a grave, discrete, and mature order." And these observations have been confirmed over a long period of time. He was referring to the method of Hippocrates, who, "in his enquiries after nature, consulted rather nature her self than his own thoughts."[40]

The moderns, however, did things differently. Through experiments they had achieved sound theory, but then they thought that theoretic certainty would yield conclusions for the cure of disease. The moderns had devoted themselves too much to theory and "decided on their practice according to the dictates of theory." And this has been the root evil "of all the pernicious errors that physick groans under at this day."[41] To offer a modern paraphrase: the moderns did not realize that we cannot formulate rules of practice by deduction but must rely on empirically based induction.

Baglivi further described the function of reason: to account for the phenomena appearing in disease, to compare the past with the present, investigate the hidden causes of disease and their origins, and provide explanations so that the physicians can be more clear in determining what remedies are needed. Reason, and the theories to which it leads, guard the physician from being an empiric, who acts blindly, without knowing the reasons for what he does. Baglivi could not in any sense be accounted an empiric. For him theory was important but only to illuminate and clarify practice. Furthermore, theory at all times remained closely tied to experience. If theory went beyond experience, it was denigrated as hypothesis—a thorough condemnation.

Practice had the function of providing remedies in accordance with the "indications." But practice must act "pursuant to the laws of experience. He who pursues a contrary course, and promiscuously forms his notions of practice from the rules of theory, will never be a happy practitioner."[42] Theory thus justified practice and served to explain what the physician had learned through experience but was nevertheless subordinate to practice at all points.

Let us examine some of the theory to which Baglivi subscribed. He was, in essence, an iatromechanist. The human body, he said, "is truly nothing else but a complex of chymico-mechanical motions, depending on such principles as are purely mathematical." Whoever regards the human body attentively will really (*profecto*) find shears in the jawbones and teeth, a phiol (*phialam*—a shallow vessel or receptacle) in the stomach, hydraulic tubes in the blood vessels, a piston (*embolum*, which the 1723 text wrongly translates as wedge) in the heart, seives in the viscera, bellows in the lungs, levers in the muscles, and the like. He rejected the explanations of the chemists but attributed bodily actions "to the force of a wedge, balance, lever, spring, and such like mechanical principles."[43] And what was true for physiological processes he also would apply to what was pathological.

But then he made an explicit qualification of extreme importance, which negated much of his iatromechanism. If, he said, disease really did arise from disorders of the solids, the explanations of disease would unquestionably accord with the mechanical principles he had just mentioned. However, the greater part of disease "owes its origin to various alterations in the fluids." Hence we must not be surprised that we will never be able to find the true cause of disease. Even those persons who are the most skilled must admit "that they will never be able to find or determine, by any art of speculation, the ultimate components of the humors of the human body, whether in health or disease." And whatever the physicians tried to say on the subject is nothing else than a will-o'-wisp (*ignes fatui*), which does not even touch the surface of things.[44]

Nevertheless, even if we can never know the ultimate configuration and texture of the humors, experience will suffice for achieving cures. Through experience we can know the progress, outcome, and variations (*declinationes*) in nature, all of which reveal to us the true indications for exhibiting this or that remedy, that is, show us what circumstances call for which remedies. And again he repeated that practice was more important than theory in the cure of disease.

We must not consider concepts true until they have stood the test of experience, and what has proven true through repeated experience, we can accept. Men think of many things that they consider consonant with rea-son but that, when actually tested, prove to be absurd or impossible. And contrariwise, many things when first proposed are judged contrary to reason and useless, because they do not harmonize with our theories; yet if they are put on trial, we find them useful and certain.[45] Baglivi thus in-sisted that all theories should be tested by experience. This test, however, concerned the practical benefits in the cure of disease, rather than verification as a phase of scientific method in the modern sense.

What we learn from experience we should embody in aphorisms that have practical value in curing disease. It is difficult, however, to frame aphorisms that are both reliable and sound. To provide guidance Baglivi indicated four steps, which remind us of Francis Bacon: collect observa-tions; arrange them in due order; digest them; and finally, from the obser-vations thus prepared, draw precepts and general axioms. Observations should be collected without discrimination or analysis. "Let him [the ob-server] set down the minutest, meanest, and most useless circumstances: let him add nothing of his own . . . but like a faithful scribe, he must diligently collect the laws enacted by nature, and describe them in the same very manner in which nature spoke them."[46] The collection resulting from this "unpolished way of observation" is like a storehouse of information, to be dipped into when we want to construct axioms or cure diseases.

We must know "the minutest circumstances of time and place, the sea-son of the year, the antecedent and concommitant causes, the method of cure, and the remedies made use of: in a word, all things that are either antecedents, concommitants, or consequents of the disease."[47] A tall order, indeed! We must not omit "the very least circumstance," while anything doubtful or uncertain should be plainly described under the heading of caution or remarks.

The multitude of observations must then be classified. "After the histo-rian has made a thousand or two thousand observations of the colic," for example, he then divides the observations under various heads: causes, in-fluences, seasons, weather, symptoms, constant concommitants, outcome, success of particular remedies, and so on.[48] This lays the ground for an or-derly induction.

There is no need to belabor the obvious drawbacks of these recommen-dations. However defective, they are at least clear. Unfortunately, for the next step, the digestion, Baglivi was not so clear. He did not indicate how the process should be carried out, and although he noted a few particular instances, he failed to give general rules. We must be cautious regarding doubtful things, which have an analogy with another disease. We must reject what is false or inconsistent—but all is left very vague. Nor did he give much help for achieving generalizations. In flowery language he indicated that the observer must rely on his judgment which, like a divine fire, can light up the vast wilderness of confusion, entanglement, and ambiguities. By use of such judgment we may gradually ascend to the highest aspects of nature, and then we may descend again by easy stages to practice.[49]

In essence he was pleading, in Baconian fashion, for close attention to experience and massive collection of data. Like Bacon he recommended formation of an academy for research into medical phenomena. But, after masses of data had been collected, only the use of judgment — illumination — could yield any advance. He did not commit the Baconian error of thinking that his method would place all wits on a level. He realized the need for judgment and insight, but to facilitate this insight he could give no better advice than a few vapid recommendations: proceed cautiously and gradually, make constant reference to the mass of particulars that had been collected, rely on experience rather than on logic. In any history of the inductive method Baglivi stands intermediate between Francis Bacon and John Stuart Mill, but much closer to Bacon.

When we study Baglivi we realize the futility of any sharp distinction between rationalism and empiricism. However we define the terms, Baglivi had characteristics of both. He stressed both reason and observation, but observation enjoyed primacy. Because he depended so much on experience he was relatively critical. He demanded evidence, wanted to evaluate that evidence, and refused credence to conceptual elaborations that did not accord with experience. At least, this was his program. Actually, when we examine his doctrines, we find far too much credulity and lack of critical sense. He did not practice what he preached. Yet he did emphasize the importance of judgment and, even if only by indirection, concerned himself with those all-important questions "How good is the evidence?" and "How do you know?" Baglivi's writings make us realize that in the history of medical thought the presence of critical acumen is important, the distinction between rationalism and empiricism is not.

Boerhaave

Boerhaave criticized Galenic doctrine because it relied too much on imagination. "Galen's entire theory rests on foundations constructed from imagination and metaphysical subtlety which led his followers into abstractions. Meanwhile, nature escaped from the hands of those who were grasping the clouds." Medicine requires not imagination but experience and reason, whose interrelationships are complex. Among the ancients, said Boerhaave, medicine was constituted first of all by accurate observations. Afterwards physicians thought about the causes of experience, which they investigated through rational disputation. The former—the experiential aspect—is always the same and not subject to error. The latter, the theory, is doubtful and inconstant and differed from one sect to another.[50]

In great detail the notes explained Boerhaave's meanings. By sect he meant "a probable opinion which has been received by many people, but yet is not so evident as to compel every reasonable person, skilled in his profession, to allow it for true; but it is of utmost consequence to distinguish what relates to the sect or opinion from observation or matter of fact."[51] Observation and opinion are highly charged words, whose many relationships we must untangle if we want to understand Boerhaave's thoughts. From scattered passages we can build up a sketch of his philosophy of science.

Observation reflects experience and implies facts. Boerhaave was fond of the word *experimentum*, which usually is best translated as experience, the equivalent of *experientia*. However, to make things confusing, there is also the translation experiment in the modern sense. In any given passage the translation requires subjective interpretation. But fortunately, Boerhaave offered some definitions. He used *experimentum* in the sense of "any bodily phenomenon whatsoever, observable by the aid of the senses. Our mind adds nothing to the phenomenon beyond its bare perception."[52] *Experimentum*, which I here translate experience, is the presentation to the mind of something "out there," something to which the mind is passive. Any such presentation is indubitable, and not subject to error. It serves as raw material for further elaboration. We do not know to what extent Boerhaave was familiar with Locke's philosophy and the concept of simple and complex ideas, and ideas of relation. But Boerhaave's concept of *experimentum* bears some kinship to the simple ideas.

Yet by referring to phenomena he immediately introduced a complexity that involves multiple factors and also a time span, quite different from simple ideas. Unlike Locke, Boerhaave did not distinguish adequately between simple sensation and complex events. He had naive concepts of what the mind might contribute to perception. Experience is that which is presented, whether it be simple or complex. He stated explicitly, as we have already seen, that the mind adds nothing to a phenomenon other than the bare perception. He had no inkling that the mind determined the perception of a phenomenon just as much as did the reality.

Boerhaave contrasted experience and opinion: the former compelled acceptance, the latter was something fallible. Opinion, if I interpret him correctly, is an inadequate functioning of reason. Through reason "the data of experience are tested, examined in all their characteristics, then scrupulously compared with each other, to reveal the agreements and differences; and then, most cautiously, everything is noted that is clearly implicit therein and can be inferred therefrom." He gave a further clarification. We speak of reason "when we compare among themselves all those ideas arising in experience, so that we perceive distinctly all those notions of which the ideas are composed, and then can judge what these ideas have in common and wherein they differ." And then he continued, "Nor is anything else required for science than this comparison patiently carried out."[53]

It is interesting to compare his definition of reason with that of Baglivi. Reason has essentially an analytic function. It identifies similarities and differences and makes comparisons. It examines and manipulates the data of experience. We must also allow it some sort of synthesizing function, for through the analytical process reason produces positive judgments.

Of utmost importance is the relationship between experience and reason. A proper relationship would lead to truth, and an improper one to error. Boerhaave pointed to the early medical sects. He declared that the ancient art of medicine was established solely by the careful collection of observations, that is, through experience. Then, however, the ancient physicians engaged in a process of reasoning that investigated the causes of the experience (*experimentorum*) through disputation. Experience, he emphasized, is always the same and does not err. The latter — the process of reasoning — is doubtful and uncertain, and each sect offered different explanations. Nevertheless, by a suitable use of reason the results can be as assured as the original empirical data.[54]

If the reasoning is sound it can penetrate to the causes of disease, and the conclusions thus derived can be just as reliable as experience. Thus, the good physician observes carefully. He "considers accurately every separate thing affecting the patient that may be learned by observation; compares them all with each other and collates them with the phenomena that occur in health; and then by rigorous and disciplined reasoning [he] achieves knowledge of the proximal cause [of disease] and remedies suitable for removing it."[55] Thus, the physician must observe accurately, reflect carefully, and reason soundly.

In a different passage Boerhaave again claimed complete validity for sound reasoning. In a commentary on the need for both observation and inference in medicine, he declared, "Nor will this latter [that is, inferences] be less reliable or dependable than the former [empirical data]." Or, again, he declared that the art of medicine should rest on experience, and then he continued a little less dogmatically than before, "but indeed we should not refuse belief to those propositions that follow by a clear chain [of reasoning] from the sensory phenomena." The powers of reason are great, but the reasoning must be sound. If not, then error results.[56]

Before we proceed to Boerhaave's analysis of error, we can profitably note two instances taken from other authors. These examples reveal forcefully the strong points and the weak points of the reasoning process.

Galileo gave a splendid instance of cogent reasoning.[57] He faced the problem, what would happen when a stone was dropped from the mast of a moving ship? In one of the *Dialogues* the character Salviata, relying on the laws of physics, the principles of motion, and the process of reasoning, provided an answer to this question without having any direct experiment. Yet he was absolutely confident of the validity of his answer. "I am assured that the effect will ensue as I tell you, for it is necessary that it should, and . . . it cannot fall out otherwise." There is a logical necessity in applying the laws of motion, a necessity which the power of reason perceives. Reason, which has penetrated into the reality of things, renders actual observation unnecessary. When skeptics did perform the experiment, it turned out exactly as Salviata had predicted. This was a triumph of rationalism.

On the other hand, other exercises in rational inference might not turn out so well. In the early eighteenth century there was widespread belief that the planets might be inhabited. Fontanelle, especially, popularized this view.[58] The philosopher Christian Wolf, disciple of Leibniz and a pillar of continental rationalism, wrote on this subject. He thought he could determine, by reason, the actual size of the inhabitants of Jupiter. With admirable logic he reasoned as follows: the pupil of the eye dilates or contracts according to the intensity of the light. But the light on Jupiter is much more dim than on earth, because Jupiter is much further from the sun. Hence the inhabitants of Jupiter must have pupils much larger than men on earth have. Experience indicates that the diameter of the pupil is proportional to the size of the eye. And the size of the eye, in turn, bears a proportion to the size of the body—the larger the pupil, the larger the eye and the larger the body. Since in distance from the sun the earth and Jupiter stand to each other in the ratio of 5:26, Wolf made appropriate calculations. He concluded that the inhabitants of Jupiter were somewhat more than 13 feet in height. This reasoning process is described by Condillac.[59]

Here we have two striking examples of reasoning, one sound, the other fallacious. Boerhaave, although he did not refer to either of these instances, tried to give some sort of criteria by which he could tell sound reasoning from unsound. Without being in any way systematic, he pointed to a few sources of error whereby reason might go astray. For example, experience may be interpreted according to preconceptions, or conclusions may be rationally drawn from too few data. Or, once we have valid conclusions derived from one set of data, we may fall into error if we apply these conclusions to another set of data. Thus, any changes that chemistry describes as occurring under the influence of fire are true. But if we extrapolate these conclusions from the laboratory and assert that the same changes take place in the human economy, we may err. Without using the particular phrases, Boerhaave cautioned us against applying *in vivo* the conclusions derived *in vitro*. Similarly, we can err if we apply the laws established in one area of knowledge to other areas that have not been sufficiently studied. Thus, although the laws of mechanics are eternally true, they do not explain the behavior of a magnet.

What is true under one set of circumstances may not be true if the circumstances change. The remedies may be effective in a given disease, but if you apply a given remedy to a case which manifests some other disease, or even to the same disease under different circumstances, error can arise. In all these examples Boerhaave indicated that we may not safely apply established laws to new instances unless we know that the new cases are similar to those from which the law was originally derived. A law, he said, may apply to a thousand instances and yet there may be an exception in the very next one. But he did not indicate how we can be confident of similarity, nor how we can safely make inductive generalizations with reasonable assurance.[60]

Even worse than assuming similarity when none in fact exists, is excessive haste in drawing conclusions. Errors arise not so much from weakness of reason as from impatience. We must not assert relationships before we have sufficiently examined the data. We should suspend judgment until the necessary data are available. For example, the ancients had claimed the heart as the source of body heat. They drew wrong conclusions from the evidence and eventually Harvey demonstrated their mistake. The ancients had generalized too hastily and should have delayed the drawing of conclusions. This, Boerhaave admitted, would have been difficult. "Who indeed would suspend his judgment throughout the twenty two hundred years which have elapsed from the time of Hippocrates? This would be confessing ignorance concerning something of outstanding importance. But [he continued with complete disregard of realities] it should have been done anyway for only by such patience can medicine be purged of its errors."

When we face uncertainties we must, he continued wait for concrete observational data, rather than filling in the gaps by hypotheses. To be sure, the inferences attained by solid reasoning may have the force of experience and command assent. Yet Boerhaave emphasized, "Where there are doubts which cannot be resolved by hypothesis, we must proceed very slowly, and realize that future generations will resolve the uncertainty when experiments, which we have not yet made, will have kindled the light for them."[61] To show how he himself was willing to exert caution and not hurry into premature inference, he indicated areas where no conclusions should be drawn: the function of the spleen, the medicinal virtues of many plants, the cause of plague and smallpox. Concerning these we should remain without any opinion until time shall have brought forth the truth.

Boerhaave did not have any consistent theory of error, but we must realize that the eighteenth century had little insight into the problems of induction. Despite the work of Bacon, with which Boerhaave seems to have been at least partially familiar, physicians of the eighteenth century had no systematic analysis of induction. Instead, a facade of logical respectability came from system formation, with deduction from the first principles. But these first principles of a medical system had no rigorous support, and there was no empirical demonstration. Logical consistency took the place of empirical evidence.

I suggest some factors to account for this. First, physicians concerned themselves with ultimate concepts as first principles of a system. This was a heritage of the seventeenth century, and of the neo-Galenic, the corpuscularian, and the chemical philosophies that dominated the period. Then, experimental methods were crude indeed and did not allow a precision sufficient to decide between disputed points or to furnish hard data to support the allegations of the system. Thus, however much the physicians might praise the need for concrete demonstration or stress a caution in drawing inferences, there was no way to provide evidence that might be decisive. Differences of opinion were disputed by logic and analogy, rather than by direct evidence. Only when the concern for first principles receded, and interest centered on limited and concrete aspects of reality (as with Morgagni, for example) could inductive reasoning make progress. Such a change in goal then could find ready integration with the limited technical abilities.

The physicians had kept their sights too high, a height to which technical abilities could not reach. When the attitude changed and interests centered on limited objectives rather than overall systems, inductive reasoning could make significant progress. This transition began to acquire momentum in the 1740s, but specific analysis of the whole movement would constitute a major study beyond the realm of the present book.

The Process of Analogy

In the seventeenth and early eighteenth centuries the principal tool of reason was analogy, and to this process we must now turn. In a recent publication I noted three different senses of analogy.[62] The first I called *declarative:* this includes figures of speech, such as a simile that points to a factual similarity but draws no conclusions. "Your cheeks are like the rose" makes a statement of fact. The cheeks and the rose are both red, but there is no further inference. The similarity does not impel us to infer that therefore the nose is like a thorn. A similarity in one respect does not imply similarity in any other respect.

A second subdivision is the *illustrative* analogy, to clarify an obscure point. We may offer an illustrative example that brings some familiarity into a situation that is unfamiliar. We thereby relate the unknown to the known, but without drawing any conclusions. There is merely a rough and ready illustration that has some explanatory and clarifying value.

The third type of analogy I call *inductive*. It attends to two or more events, situations, or objects, compares them, identifies certain similarities that we can directly observe, and then implies certain other similarities that we do not directly observe. Similarities that we note with the corporeal eye lead us to infer certain other similarities that we perceive only with the eye of reason.

In any analogy whatever there are similarities, but there are also differences as well. The force of analogy depends on an assumption: the similarities are significant, while the differences we can dismiss as unimportant. If this proves to be truly the case, then the analogy is sound. If, on the other hand, the observed similarities turn out to be trivial and the differences profound, then the analogy fails or is unsound. On the basis of the observed similarities, how reliably can we go from the known to the unknown? This question summarizes the whole problem of inference.

Analogy can lead to many absurdities. In one famous example, a sixteenth century monk, Francisco Giorgi, tried to bring together in one schema the planets and angels, spirits and souls, and relate them to the music of the spheres and the mathematical relationships of music. He found a series of mathematical analogies on which his whole case rested. The signs of the zodiac, for example, and the Apostles must be in some way connected because there are 12 of each.[63] There are indeed twelve signs of the zodiac and twelve apostles. The similarity, that the number 12 occurs in each case, led Giorgi to infer an interconnection between astrological concepts and religious concepts. All the differences he ignored. He tried to pass from the known to the unknown on the basis of similarities that were utterly trivial.

Sound analogy penetrates, somehow, to the essence of things and takes as its point of departure certain properties that share in the essence. An observer tries to identify particular features that relate to the essence; these he follows with the eye of reason until he reaches the more central core, deeper and more essential. To distinguish the essential properties from the accidental or trivial requires judgment on the one hand, empirical study on the other. Whoever fails in either of these respects will fail in his analogies.

Modern medical science also depends on analogy. Are the findings in animals transferrable to man? For example, do dietary experiments on experimental arteriosclerosis in rabbits apply to man? The answer depends on the further question, are the similarities between man and rabbit more significant than the differences? Comparable considerations apply to the *in vitro* observations. Can we apply these to the living body? The physiologists of the seventeenth and eighteenth centuries who in the laboratory investigated the properties of blood were fully aware of the pitfalls that attended any extension of data from the "furnace" to the animal body.[64] So, too, with the modern scientific passion for models as the means for extending our knowledge.[65] However, we must not try to use twentieth century methodology in a discussion of eighteenth century medicine.

How can we tell the difference between good and bad analogies? Eighteenth century workers were fully aware of this problem. Baglivi devoted a chapter to what he called "false simile's, or a false sort of analogies." He knew that scientists had to hunt for "similitudes." To argue from the anatomy of insects to that of animals and thence to man was, he thought, sound reasoning, for "the attributes of the one are exactly answerable to those of the other . . . are exactly of a piece with them."[66] Furthermore, he felt that physicians reasoned soundly when they argued from the laws of mechanics to the structure of the living body. However, as we have seen, analogies that rested on chemistry he considered fallacious.

In their innumerable disputes, physicians of the eighteenth century would criticize the analogies of their opponents. Each physician was willing to accept some analogies, while rejecting others. There were always similarities, always differences. To argue against your opponent you needed only to emphasize the differences. To bolster your own case you emphasized the similarities. Baglivi, for example, praised the use of analogical arguments in general, but he wanted "to see them managed with more judgment." Analogy he recognized as an aspect of induction, and sound induction required a "long and manifest series of experiments" from which general axioms could be collected.[67]

In retrospect we can see the major pitfalls in analogical reasoning of the eighteenth century, and the crucial difference between eighteenth and twentieth century science. The older authors did not feel any urgency to pass from a verbal to a factual level, or to confirm the inferences in experience. We must realize, however, that for most inferences there was no method of proof. We find an interesting example in the writings of Strother, a vigorous iatromechanist.[68]

In discussing jaundice he pointed out truly that in this "disease" the liver was often hard and shrunken. Brandy drinkers often got jaundice and their livers often became "hardened irreparably." He tried to explain this by analogy. He pointed to the fact that if we mix brandy with serum, the latter becomes hard, like a jelly. Today we would say that the serum was denatured by the alcohol. Strother pointed out further that the same thing happened with fire. Today, again, we would say that the serum was denatured by heat as well as by alcohol. Strother explained the properties of brandy by reference to heat. He declared, "We may conclude by analogy, that the active particles it [the brandy] consists of raise a motion in the serum, and evaporates so many of its watery parts, as to leave it a jelly." He was asserting that alcohol denatures protein in the same way as does heat, and that in both cases this occurred through evaporation of water.

When Strother wrote there was no way to either confirm or refute his claim. Even if he had wanted to test his statements empirically, he could not have possibly achieved any answer. We can only say that his assertion was plausible, considering the theories of the day. It did not contradict any established scientific principles. But this absence of contradiction established only the possibility, not the actuality. Had Strother declared, "This *may* be the mechanism or the cause," there would have been no dispute. But there is a vast gulf between "It may be" and "It is." The failure to make this distinction impaired most of the analogical reasoning of the eighteenth century.

There were two alternative approaches. One was skepticism, the deliberate withholding of assent, the willingness to remain in a state of indecision until some definitive answer might be forthcoming. This Boerhaave had recommended but the method found few or no enthusiasts. He himself did not in any way follow his own suggestion. The other alternative was a retreat from grandiose overall formulations, with closer attention to small details, to limited investigations, to orderly progression from the better known to the less well known, as Bacon had recommended. This did, indeed, take place, but only over a long time span.

Yet the entire problem of rationalism and empiricism can be fitted into a different formulation, apparently simple but actually infinitely complex, involving the questions: what do you consider significant? or conversely, what do you consider trivial? These might be rephrased: to what will you pay attention and what will you ignore? And this is simply another way of asking the question with which Aristotle wrestled so vigorously: what is *essential* and what is *accidental?* Correlative to this is a cognate problem: what do you take for granted, and what will you question, examine, and try to verify? If we could answer these questions — which are all interrelated — we would have a splendid insight into the entire history of ideas. Meanwhile, we must realize that the squabbles between rationalists and empiricists are far less important than the problem: how did a critical sense, a critical judgment, develop in medical science and medical practice?

NOTES

1. THE OLD ORDER CHANGETH

1. *Le médecin malgré lui,* Act II, scene 6. The translations are mine.

2. *Monsieur de Pourceaugnac,* Act I, scene 8.

3. *Le malade imaginaire,* Intermezzo following Act III.

4. Joh. Conrad Peyer, *Merycologia* (Basel, 1685), pp. 251-255. The translations are mine.

5. Georges Gusdorf, *Dieu, la nature, l'homme au siècle des lumières* (Paris: Payot, 1972), p. 427; Voltaire, "Médecins," in *Dictionnaire philosophique. Oeuvres complètes,* 35 vols. (Paris, 1859-1861), XIV, 185, 161, articles "Médecins," "Maladie."

6. Mary B. Hesse, *Forces and Fields: The Concept of Action at a Distance in the History of Physics* (Totowa, N.J.: Littlefield, Adams & Co., 1965), p. 74.

7. Thomas S. Kuhn, *The Structure of Scientific Revolutions* (Chicago, University of Chicago Press, 1962), 2nd ed. enlarged (Chicago, 1970).

8. Lester S. King, *The Road to Medical Enlightenment, 1650-1695* (New York: American Elsevier, 1970), pp. 5-7.

9. Imre Lakatos and Alan Musgrave, eds., *Criticism and the Growth of Knowledge* (Cambridge: Cambridge University Press, 1970).

10. Margaret Masterman, "The Nature of a Paradigm," in Lakatos and Musgrave, *Criticism and Growth,* pp. 59-89.

11. Kuhn, *Structure of Scientific Revolutions* (1970), pp. 231-278.

12. Kuhn, *Structure of Scientific Revolutions* (1970), pp. 174-210.

13. Walter Pagel, "The Historical Dimension of Philosophy: Review of *Historisches Wörterbuch der Philosophie,* by Rudolph Eisler," *History of Science 11:* 231-235 (1973).

2. THE CONCEPT OF NATURE

1. Max Neuburger, *Die Lehre von der Heilkraft der Natur im Wandel der Zeiten* (Stuttgart: Ferdinand Enke, 1926); *The Doctrine of the Healing Power of Nature throughout the Course of Time,* tr. Linn J. Boyd (New York, n.p., n.d.).

2. Robert Boyle, "A Free Inquiry into the Vulgarly Received Notion of Nature," in *The Works of the Honorable Robert Boyle,* 6 vols., ed. Thomas Birch (London, 1772; reprinted Hildesheim: Georg Olms, 1966), V, 158, 160. See also Basil Willey, *The Eighteenth Century Background* (London: Chatto and Windus, 1950).

3. Aristotle, *Metaphysics,* 1014b16-1015a15; *Physics,* 192b8-193b22.

4. Boyle, "A Free Inquiry," p. 169; see also pp. 167-168, 219.

5. Peter Gassendi, "Syntagmatis Philosophici Pars Secunda," in *Petri Gassendi Opera Omnia in Sex Tomos Divisa* (Lyons, 1668), I, 125.

6. Hippocrates, "The Sacred Disease," in *The Medical Works of Hippocrates*, tr. John Chadwick and W. N. Mann (Oxford: Blackwell, 1950), p. 179.

7. Edward Fitzgerald, tr., *Rubáiyat of Omar Khayyám* (fifth ed. of translation), stanza 72.

8. Emma J. Edelstein and Ludwig Edelstein, *Asclepius: A Collection and Interpretation of the Testimonies*, 2 vols. (Baltimore: The Johns Hopkins Press, 1945). See also Lester S. King, *The Growth of Medical Thought* (Chicago: University of Chicago Press, 1963), pp. 11-17.

9. R. Hooykaas, *Religion and the Rise of Modern Science* (Edinburgh: Scottish Academic Press, 1972), p. 2.

10. Some of the important secondary sources are: John Tulloch, *Rational Theology and Christian Philosophy in England in the Seventeenth Century*, 2 vols. (London, 1872), vol. II, *The Cambridge Platonists;* Frederick J. Powicke, *The Cambridge Platonists* (Cambridge, Mass.: Harvard University Press, 1926); G. P. H. Pawson, *The Cambridge Platonists and Their Place in Religious Thought* (London: Society for promoting Christian Knowledge, 1930); John M. Muirhead, *The Platonic Tradition in Anglo-Saxon Philosophy* (New York: Macmillan Co., 1931); Rosalie L. Colie, *Light and Enlightenment: A Study of the Cambridge Platonists and the Dutch Arminians* (Cambridge: Cambridge University Press, 1957); Gerald R. Cragg, ed., *The Cambridge Platonists* (Oxford: Oxford University Press, 1968); C. A. Patrides, ed., *The Cambridge Platonists* (London: Edward Arnold, 1969).

11. Ralph Cudworth, *The Intellectual System of the Universe* (London, 1678).

12. Cudworth, p. 195.

13. Ibid., p. 136.

14. Ibid., p. 145.

15. Ibid., pp. 98, 131.

16. Ibid., p. 147.

17. Hooykaas, p. 8; see also p. 29.

18. Cudworth, p. 147.

19. Ibid., pp. 151, 150.

20. Ibid., pp. 156, 156 bis, 158, 160, 163.

21. Ibid., p. 167.

22. *Plotinus: The Enneads,* tr. Stephen MacKenna, 2nd ed., rev. B. S. Page (London: Faber and Faber, 1956). The references are given by Ennead, tractate, paragraph, and page reference. For a general overview, the reader can profitably consult William Ralph Inge, *The Philosophy of Plotinus*, 2 vols., 2nd ed. (London: Longmans, Green, and Co., 1923).

23. Plotinus 5. 3-15, 397; 4. 8-6, 362.

24. Ibid., 4. 3-9, 268.

25. Ibid., 4. 4-13, 298; Arthur O. Lovejoy has expressed this hierarchical concept in his *The Great Chain of Being: A Study of the History of an Idea* (Cambridge, Mass.: Harvard University Press, 1957).

26. François Bernier, *Abrégé de la philosophie de Gassendi*, 8 vols. (Lyons, 1678).

27. There are good overall expositions in P.-Félix Thomas, *La Philosophie de Gassendi* (Paris, 1889; reprint ed., New York: Burt Franklin, 1967); and Kurd Lasswitz, *Geschichte der Atomistik vom Mittelalter bis Newton*, 2 vols. (Leipzig, 1890; reprint ed., Hildesheim: Olms, 1963), II, 126-187. The work of G. S. Brett, *The Philosophy of Gassendi* (London: Macmillan & Co., 1908), has been justly criticized by Robert Hugh Kargon, *Atomism in England from Hariot to Newton* (Oxford: Clarendon Press, 1966) and can be safely ignored. Gassendi's controversy with Descartes (Elizabeth S. Haldane and G. R. T. Ross, *The Philosophical Works of Descartes Rendered into English*, 2 vols. [New York: Dover Publications, 1955], II, 135-233) stands outside this study. Richard H. Popkin, *The History of Scepticism from Erasmus to Descartes* (Assen, Netherlands: Van Gorcum and Co., 1960), stressed Gassendi's role in the skeptical movement of the time; and Kargon, *Atomism*, the seminal influence on seventeenth century scientific thought, especially in regard to Boyle and British atomism. Jacques Roger, *Les sciences de la vie dans la pensée française du XVIIIe siècle* (Paris: Armand Colin, 1963), has discussed the biological views. Oliver René Bloch, *La philosophie de Gassendi: Nominalisme, matérialisme et métaphysique* (La Haye: Martinus Nijhoff, 1971), has studied much manuscript material and collated this with various published works. These studies provide splendid bibliographies. A recent work by Craig B. Brush, ed. and trans., *The Selected Works of Pierre Gassendi* (New York: Johnson Reprint Corp., 1966), offers a limited selection of Gassendi's writings in English. A recent reprint of Walter Charleton, *Physiologia Epicuro-Gassendo-Charltoniana* (original ed., London, 1654), with intro. by Robert Hugh Kargon (New York: Johnson Reprint Corp., 1966), provides a useful text. Perhaps in the not too distant future Gassendi may assume a stature comparable to what Descartes now enjoys.

28. "De materiali principio, sive materia prima rerum," in Gassendi, I, 229-282. Book IV deals with causation.

29. Ibid., p. 231.

30. Ibid., p. 232.

31. Ibid., pp. 259, 268.

32. Ibid., pp. 269-270, 272.

33. Ibid., pp. 273, 280.

34. Ibid., pp. 280, 282.

35. Kargon, *Atomism*.

36. Boyle, "A Free Inquiry."

37. Boyle, V, 177, 178.

38. Ibid., p. 166. See also p. 215.

39. Ibid., p. 175.

40. Ibid., p. 211.

41. Ibid., pp. 189, 214, 215.

42. Ibid., p. 216.

43. Ibid.

44. Ibid., pp. 208, 238-239.

45. Ibid., p. 230.

46. Ibid., p. 232.

47. Ibid., pp. 236-238.

Notes to Pages 35-42

48. Different printings show varying dates from 1718 to 1741. I have used a uniformly bound set, Friedrich Hoffmann, *Medicina Rationalis Systematica,* 4 vols. (vols. I and II, 2nd ed., Halle, 1729-1734).

49. Friedrich Hoffmann, *Fundamenta Medicinae* (Halle, 1695); ibid., tr. Lester S. King (New York: American Elsevier, 1971); see also King, *The Road to Medical Enlightenment,* which includes a survey of the text and a perspective on the background.

50. Hoffmann, *Fundamenta Medicinae.* (The references indicate Book, chapter, and paragraphs.) I, 2, 1; I, 2, 4; I, 2, 9; I, 2, 8-20.

51. Ibid., I, 3, 4.

52. Ibid., I, 3, 6; I, 3, 21-24.

53. Ibid., I, 5, 45-47.

54. Ibid., I, 6, 2-3.

55. Ibid., I, 6, 42.

56. H. R. Trevor-Roper, *The Crisis of the Seventeenth Century: Religion, the Reformation and Social Change* (New York: Harper and Row; 1968), pp. 90-192; Keith Thomas, *Religion and the Decline of Magic* (London: Weidenfeld and Nicolson, 1971); Wayne Shumaker, *The Occult Sciences in the Renaissance: A Study in Intellectual Patterns* (Berkeley: University of California Press, 1972); Paul Boyer and Stephen Nissenbaum, *Salem Possessed: The Social Origins of Witchcraft* (Cambridge, Mass.: Harvard University Press, 1974); H. C. E. Midelfort, *Witch Hunting in Southwestern Germany, 1562-1684: The Social and Intellectual Foundations* (Stanford: Stanford University Press, 1972); Alan C. Kors and Edward Peters, eds., *Witchcraft in Europe, 1100-1700: A Documentary History* (London: J. M. Dent and Sons, 1973).

57. *The Malleus Maleficarum of Heinrich Kramer and James Sprenger,* tr. Montague Summers (New York: Dover, 1971).

58. (6 vols., with two supplements, 11 vols. Geneva, 1741-1750), V, 94-103. The title is here altered to *De Diaboli Potentia in Corpore.* Büching's name has been eliminated and the text, when compared to the 1703 original, shows some stylistic improvements together with correction of misprints.

59. *De diaboli,* Sec. 1. References indicate the numbered section of *Opera Omnia* version. The 1703 original has errors in numbering.

60. Ibid., Sec. 5.

61. Ibid., Sec. 6.

62. Ibid., Sec. 7.

63. Ibid., Sec. 4.

64. Ibid., Sec. 10.

65. Ibid., Sec. 14.

3. SUBSTANTIAL FORMS

1. Julien Offray de la Mettrie, *Man A Machine* (French-English edition. La Salle, Ill.: Open Court Publishing Co., 1943), pp. 69, 140; Aram Vartanian, *La Mettrie's L'Homme Machine: A Study in the Origins of an Idea* (Princeton: Princeton University Press, 1960), p. 189.

2. Lazar Riverius, *The Universal Body of Physick,* tr. William Carr (London, 1657), p. 3. For critical analysis the Latin is essential. I use the edition *Opera Medica Universa* (Geneva, 1728). Subsequent references will be distinguished by indicating the date.

3. "Tanquam materia quaedam in dissimilarium compage & coagmentatione," John Fernel, *Physiologia,* Book II, "De Elementis," Ch. 1, in *Universa Medicina,* 2 vols. (Leyden, 1645), I, 106.

4. Daniel Sennert, *Epitomes Scientiae Naturalis,* Book I, Ch. 3, in *Opera,* 3 vols. (Lyons, 1650), I, 10 Aa. The capital letter refers to the column, the lower case letter to the position in the column.

5. Peter Gassendi, "De Materiali Principio, sive Materia Prima Rerum," Book III, Ch. 4, of the *Physica,* in *Opera Omnia,* 6 vols. (Lyons, 1658), I, 248.

6. Sennert, *Hypomnemata Physica,* Book I, Ch. 3, *Opera* I, 143 Bb.

7. Fernel, *De Abditis Rerum Causis,* Book I, Ch. 3, *Universa Medicina,* II, p. 24. Fernel used the term *nominis species* rather than *forma.*

8. Riverius (1657), p. 9.

9. Sennert, *Hypomnemata,* p. 143 B.

10. Ibid., p. 143 B-144 Aa.

11. Sennert, *Epitomes,* Book I, Ch. 3, I, 10 Ac, Ad.

12. Ibid., p. 10 Bb.

13. Aristotle, *Metaphysics,* esp. Book VII (Zeta); W. D. Ross, *Aristotle* (London: Methuen, 1923); John Herman Randall, Jr., *Aristotle* (New York: Columbia University Press, 1960); A. E. Taylor, *Aristotle* (New York: Dodge Publishing Co., n.d.); Albert L. Hammond, *Ideas about Substance* (Baltimore: Johns Hopkins Press, 1969). On this topic of substance and accident, the older works on logic are far more informative than the modern ones. Preeminent among the older texts is H. W. B. Joseph, *An Introduction to Logic* (2nd ed. Oxford: Clarendon Press, 1950).

14. Aristotle, *Physics,* Book I, Ch. 5, 188a 25-28.

15. Sennert, *Epitomes,* p. 7 Ad; Gassendi, *Physica,* Book III, Ch. 4. Gassendi has a particularly clear discussion of principles in which he follows Aristotle quite closely.

16. Aristotle, *Physics,* 188b 20-25.

17. Ibid., p. 188b 2-5.

18. Sennert, *Epitomes,* p. 7 Bc.

19. See Randall, p. 180; Ross, pp. 64-65.

20. Sennert, *Epitomes,* p. 8 Ad.

21. Ibid., p. 8 Ba.

22. Ibid., p. 8 Ac.

23. Ibid., p. 15 Ac.

24. Ibid., p. 15 Ac-Bc.

25. Ibid., p. 18 Aa.

26. Ibid., p. 18 Ab.

27. Sennert, *De Morbis Occultis,* Pt. I, Ch. I, *Opera,* III, 521 Aa.

28. *Hypomnemata,* I, 148 Ac.

29. Ibid., p. 148 Ba.

30. *Epitomes,* I, 18 Ac.

31. See "De qualitatum occultarum Origine," in *De Morbis Occultis,* Pt. I, Ch. IV, III, 524-531.

32. *Hypomnemata,* I, 147 Bc.

33. Lynn Thorndyke, "Three Texts on Degrees of Medicine (*De Gradibus*)," *Bull. Hist. Med., 38,* 533-537 (1964). See also Fernel, *Therapeutices Universalis,* Book IV, Ch. 2 (Leyden, 1644), p. 122.

34. Riverius, *Universal Body of Physick* (1657), p. 7; (1728), p. 3.

35. Sennert, I, 150 (misnumbered 250).

36. Riverius, *Universal Body of Physick* (1657), p. 7; (1728) p. 3.

37. Sennert, I, 148 Bc., 149 Ab.

38. Sennert, I, 153 Ba-155 Ac; III, 527 Ba-528 Bc.

39. Ibid., III, 521 Bd-522 Aa.

40. Ibid., I, 154 Aa.

41. Ibid., III, 528 Ac.

42. Ibid., I, 154 Ac-Ba; III, 528 Ad-Ba.

43. Ibid., I, 154 Bd-155 Ab.

44. Ibid., I, 155 Ac; III, 528 Bb.

45. Ibid., I, 151 Bb; III, 525 Aa.

46. Ibid., III, 524 Ac.

47. Ibid., I, 151B-152 A; see also III, 525 Ac-526 Bd.

48. Ibid., III, 525 Bc-526 Aa.

49. Ibid., III, 526 Ab, c.

4. IATROCHEMISTRY

1. Lester S. King, *The Growth of Medical Thought* (Chicago: University of Chicago Press, 1963), pp. 86-138.

2. Ibid., p. 134.

3. Walter Pagel, *Paracelsus: An Introduction to Philosophical Medicine in the Era of the Renaissance* (Basel: S. Karger, 1958), p. 103.

4. King, *Growth of Medical Thought,* p. 136.

5. Aristotle, *Physics,* 188 a 26-28.

6. Sennert, *Epitomes,* Book I, Ch. 3, *Opera* (1650), I, 7 Ab.

7. Gassendi, *Physica,* Book III, Ch. 1, *Opera Omnia* (1658), I, 229 Bc. For a slightly different expression, see p. 248 Ab.

8. Sennert, *Epitomes,* I, 50 Bd.

9. Ibid., I, 40 Ac.

10. Allen G. Debus, "Fire Analysis and the Elements in the Sixteenth and the Seventeenth Centuries," *Annals of Science 23:* 127-147 (1967).

11. Sennert, *De Chymicorum cum Aristotelicis & Galenicis Consensu ac Dissensu.* On a different page the title reads, *Tractatus de Consensu et Dissensu Galenicorum et Peripateticorum cum Chymicis, Opera,* III, 697-862.

12. Rembert Ramsauer, *Die Atomistik des Daniel Sennert* (Braunschweig: Vieweg & Sohn, 1935); Robert Hugh Kargon, *Atomism in England from Hariot to Newton* (Oxford: Clarendon Press, 1966); Allen G. Debus, *The Chemical Philosophy: Paracelsian Science and Medicine in the Sixteenth and Seventeenth Centuries* (in press); Kurd Lasswitz, *Geschichte der Atomistik vom Mittelalter bis Newton,* 2

vols. (originally published, 1890; Hildesheim: Georg Olms, 1963), I, 436-454.

13. Daniel Sennertus, Nich. Culpeper, and Abdiah Cole, *Chymistrie Made Easie and Useful. Or, The Agreement and Disagreement of the Chymists and Galenists* (London, 1662).

14. Sennert, *Opera,* III, 755 Aa.

15. Ibid., p. 755 Ac.

16. Ibid., p. 754 Bd.

17. Ibid., p. 752 Ad-Ba; p. 757 Ac.

18. Ibid., pp. 757 Bb-758 Aa.

19. Riverius (1657), pp. 7-8.

20. Frederic L. Holmes, "Analysis by Fire and Solvent Extractions: The Metamorphosis of a Tradition," *Isis 63:*129-148 (1971); Allen G. Debus, "Fire Analysis"; R. Hooykaas, "Die Elementenlehre der Iatrochemiker," *Janus 41:*1-28 (1937). Also important in this connection are Hélène Metzger, *Newton, Stahl, Boerhaave et la doctrine chimique* (Paris: Alcan, 1930); Metzger, *Les doctrines chimiques en France du début de XVIIᵉ à fin du XVIIIᵉ siècle,* reprint (Paris: Blanchard, 1969); J. R. Partington, *A History of Chemistry,* vols. II, III (London: Macmillan & Co., 1961, 1962); Allen G. Debus, *The Chemical Philosophy.*

21. Marin Mersenne, *La verité des sciences contre les septiques ou Pyrrhoniens* (facsimile of 1625 edition, Stuttgart: Fromann, 1969), pp. 79-84; Lynn Thorndyke, *A History of Magic and Experimental Science,* vol. VII, *The Seventeenth Century* (New York: Columbia University Press, 1964), 185-187; Robert P. Multauf, *The Origins of Chemistry* (New York: Watts, 1966), pp. 276-277; Debus, *The Chemical Philosophy.*

22. Van Helmont's works are collected in his *Ortus Medicinae,* edited by his son, F. M. van Helmont. There are many editions, of which I have used the fourth (Leiden, 1667). More commonly in use, among scholars, is the English translation by J. C[handler], *Oriatrike or, Physick Refined* (London, 1662). To simplify the references, I identify all quotations by the title of the treatise and the numbered paragraphs rather than by page. For convenience I give the titles as Chandler translates them. The translations of text material, however, unless otherwise indicated, are mine, from the Latin of 1667.

23. King, *Road to Medical Enlightenment,* pp. 37-62.

24. "The Causes and Beginnings of Natural Things," Sec. 23.

25. "The Fiction of Elementary Complexions and Mixtures," Sec. 30.

26. King, *Road to Medical Enlightenment,* pp. 47-55; "Heat doth not digest efficiently, but excitingly onely," Sec. 28.

27. "The Fiction of Elementary Complexions . . . ," Sec. 12.

28. "The Image of the Ferment . . . ," Sec. 23.

29. "The Causes and Beginnings of Natural Things," Sec. 6; Sec. 8, (Chandler's translation); "*Archeus Faber* or the Master Workman," Sec. 3.

30. King, *Road to Medical Enlightenment,* pp. 93-112.

31. Molière, *L'amour médecin,* Act III, Scene 5.

32. [Boerhaave], *A New Method of Chemistry, Translated from the Original Latin of Dr. Boerhaave's Elementa Chemiae, by Peter Shaw,* 2nd ed., 2 vols. (London, 1741), I, 36.

33. Erwin H. Ackerknecht, *Therapeutics from the Primitives to the 20th Century* (New York: Hafner, 1973); Chauncey D. Leake, *An Historical Account of*

Pharmacology to the 20th Century (Springfield, Ill.: Charles C. Thomas, 1975).

34. Sir Henry Thomas, "The Society of Chymical Physitians," in E. Ashworth Underwood, ed., *Science, Medicine and History,* 2 vols. (Oxford: Oxford University Press, 1953), II, 58.

35. See, for example, Sir George Clarke, A. M. Cooke, *A History of the Royal College of Physicians,* 3 vols. (vols. 1 and 2 by Clarke, vol. 3 by Cooke; Oxford: Clarendon Press, 1964, 1966, 1972); Lester S. King, *The Medical World of the Eighteenth Century* (Chicago: University of Chicago Press, 1958), esp. pp. 1-58, King, *Road to Medical Enlightenment,* pp. 145-154; Allen G. Debus, *The English Paracelsians* (London: Oldbourne, 1965).

36. See note 20, above.

37. Partington, *History of Chemistry,* III, 17; see also pp. 17-24.

38. Nicasius le Febure, *A Compleat Body of Chymistry,* tr. P. D. C. (London, 1664), p. 1.

39. Ibid., pp. 6-8.

40. Ibid., p. 9.

41. Ibid., p. 10.

42. Thomas Willis, *Of Fermentation,* in *The Remaining Medical Works of that Famous and Renowned Physician Dr. Thomas Willis,* tr. S[amuel] P[ordage] (London, 1681). This in turn is included in the larger volume, *Dr. Willis's Practice of Physick, Being the Whole Works of that Renowned and Famous Physician* (London, 1684). For the original Latin I used the text *De Fermentatione,* in *Thomas Willis Opera Omnia,* 2 vols. in one (Venice, 1720), I, 1-27.

43. Willis, *Of Fermentation* (1681), p. 2.

44. *De Fermentatione,* p. 2. The translation is mine. The rendition of Pordage (1681, p. 3), is barbarous.

45. Willis, *Of Fermentation,* p. 2.

46. Hansruedi Isler, *Thomas Willis, 1621-1675, Doctor and Scientist* (New York: Hafner, 1968), p. 60.

47. Willis (1681), p. 1.

48. This is my own translation of the Latin, "Fermentatio est motus intestinus particularum, seu principiorum cujusvis corporis, cum tendentia ad perfectionem ejusdem corporis, vel propter mutationem in aliud" (1720, p. 5). The translations of Pordage (1681, p. 9) I feel are unsatisfactory.

49. Ibid., (1681), p. 10.

50. Ibid., p. 12.

51. Ibid., p. 13.

52. Ibid., p. 19.

53. Ibid., p. 26; (1720), p. 14. Recourse to the original Latin clarifies the meaning of Pordage's often obscure translation.

54. Ibid., (1681), p. 27.

55. Ibid., p. 29.

56. Ibid., p. 18.

57. Robert Boyle, "Some Specimens of an Attempt to make Chymical Experiments useful to illustrate the notions of the Corpuscular Philosophy. The Preface," in *Works* (1772, facsimile reprint, Hildesheim: Georg Olms, 1965), I, 354.

58. Boyle, "Of the Usefulness of Natural Philosophy," *Works,* II, 169.

59. "Some Specimens . . . The Preface," I, 354.

60. Ibid., p. 358.

61. Thomas Shadwell, *The Virtuoso,* ed. Marjorie Hope Nicolson and David Stuart Rodes (London: Edward Arnold, 1966), Act II, scene 2, p. 47.

62. "Reflections upon the Hypothesis of Alcali and Acidum," *Works,* IV, 288.

63. Boyle, "Some Specimens," I, 359.

64. John F. Fulton, *A Bibliography of the Honourable Robert Boyle,* 2nd ed. (Oxford: Clarendon Press, 1961), p. 37.

65. "Usefulness . . . ," *Works,* II, 75, 76, 79.

66. Ibid., p. 80.

67. Ibid., pp. 83, 84.

68. Ibid., pp. 103-122.

69. *Works,* IV, 273-292.

70. *The Sceptical Chymist, Works,* I, 544.

71. "Of the Imperfections of the Chemist's Doctrine of Qualities," *Works,* IV, 275.

72. Ibid., p. 276, 277.

73. "About the Excellency . . . ," IV, 73.

74. Bayle and Thillaye, *Biographie Medicale par ordre chronologique,* 2 vols. (Paris, 1855), II, 267-268.

75. Antonio Deidier, *Institutiones Médicinae Theoricae Physiologiam et Pathologiam complectentes,* Montpellier, 1711; August Hirsch, ed., *Biographisches Lexicon der Hervorragenden Artze,* 6 vols. (Munich: Urban and Schwarzenberg, 1962), II, 204.

76. Partington, III, 28-41.

77. *A Course of Chymistry,* tr. Walter Harris (London, 1677); and the 4th ed., translator not recorded (London, 1720). In regard to this latter, Partington (p. 30) states that the 11th French edition was "the last revised by the author" but gave the date as 1730. The 10th edition, with exactly the same pagination, was published in 1713. Presumably the 11th edition was merely a reprinting of the 10th. The 4th English edition must have been translated from the French edition of 1713, that is, the 10th, and not the 11th as stated on the title page.

78. 1720, p. 3.

79. Ibid., p. 4.

80. Deidier, *Institutiones,* Proemium, unpaginated, Sig a2 v-a3 v.

81. Ibid., p. 1.

82. Ibid., pp. 3-8.

83. Ibid., pp. 9-14.

84. Ibid., p. 9.

85. Boyle, "Some Specimens of an Attempt to make Chymical Experiments useful to illustrate the notions of the Corpuscular Philosophy: The Preface," *Works,* I, 355-356.

5. IATROMECHANISM

1. Albrecht von Haller, *Bibliotheca Medicinae Practicae,* ed. J. D. Brandis, 4 vols. (Berne, 1776-1788), III, 24; IV, 38; IV, 261; III, 268; IV, 57; III, 483; IV, 257; III, 536.

2. Kurt Sprengel *Versuch einer pragmatischen Geschichte der Arzniekunde,* 5 vols., 1st and 2nd eds. mixed (Halle, 1799-1803), IV, 321-469.

3. Ibid., p. 470.

4. Ibid., p. 519.

5. Ibid., pp. 504, 544-545.

6. Charles Daremberg, *Histoire des sciences médicales,* 2 vols. (Paris, 1870).

7. Ibid., II, 849.

8. Ibid., pp. 735-736, 889.

9. Maurice Crosland, "The Development of Chemistry in the Eighteenth Century," in *Studies on Voltaire and the Eighteenth Century,* ed. Theodore Besterman (Geneva: Institut Voltaire, 1963), XXIV, 371-372.

10. I. B. Cohen, *Franklin and Newton* (Cambridge, Mass.: Harvard University Press, 1973); Cohen, "Newton in the Light of Recent Scholarship," *Isis 51:*489-514 (1960); Robert Hugh Kargon, *Atomism in England from Hariot to Newton* (Oxford: Clarendon Press, 1966); Robert E. Schofield, *Mechanism and Materialism: British Natural Philosophy in an Age of Reason* (Princeton: Princeton University Press, 1970); Arnold Thackray, *Atoms and Powers: An Essay on Newtonian Matter: Theory and the Development of Chemistry* (Cambridge, Mass.: Harvard University Press, 1970).

11. John Freind, *Praelectiones Chymicae,* in *Opera Omnia Medica,* 2nd ed. (Paris, 1735), pp. 1-58.

12. Crosland, *Development of Chemistry,* p. 394.

13. I have used the Neapolitan edition of 1734. The references will indicate the chapter and proposition, as well as the page.

14. Sig b1 v.

15. Howard B. Adelmann, *Marcello Malpighi and the Evolution of Embryology,* 5 vols. (Ithaca, N.Y.: Cornell University Press, 1966), I.

16. Borelli, Part II, Ch. 3, Prop. 23, p. 214; Prop. 24, p. 215; Prop. 26, p. 217.

17. Ibid., Prop. 27, pp. 217-218.

18. Ibid., Prop. 28, pp. 218-222.

19. Ibid., Ch. 9, Prop. 134, p. 318.

20. Ibid.

21. Ibid., Prop. 135, p. 319.

22. Ibid., pp. 319-320.

23. Ibid., p. 320.

24. Ibid., Prop. 136, p. 321.

25. Ibid., Prop. 138 (137 *bis*), pp. 322-323.

26. Ibid., Prop. 139, p. 324.

27. Ibid., Prop. 140, p. 325.

28. Theodore M. Brown, "The Mechanical Philosophy and the 'Animal Oeconomy': A Study in the Development of English Physiology in the Seventeenth and Early Eighteenth Century" (Ph.D. dissertation, Princeton University, 1968; Ann Arbor: University Microfilms, 1969).

29. *Dictionary of National Biography* (Oxford: Oxford University Press, 1959-1960), XV, 1221-1223.

30. I have used the Latin text in the *Opuscula Medica,* 3rd ed. (Rotterdam, 1714), bound with the *Elementa Medicinae* (The Hague, 1718). The translations are in *The Whole Works of Dr. Archibald Pitcairn,* tr. George Sewell and I. T. Desaguliers, 2nd ed. (London, 1727).

31. Archibald Pitcairn, *The Philosophical and Mathematical Elements of Physick* (London, 1718). The translator is not identified in the first edition, but in the second edition of 1745 John Quincy is named as translator. The exposition in the next several paragraphs relies on pp. iv-xiv of the translator's preface of the 1718 edition.

32. This address is reference 30 above. I translate from the Latin version of 1718. The references give the numbered paragraphs.

33. Par. 3.

34. Ibid., par. 4.

35. Ibid., par. 5.

36. Ibid., par. 7.

37. Ibid., par. 8.

38. Ibid., par. 9.

39. Ibid., par. 12.

40. Pitcairn, *The Whole Works,* p. 57.

41. *The Elements of Physick,* p. 338.

42. *The Whole Works,* pp. 110-112.

43. Ibid., pp. 117-118.

44. *Elements of Physick,* p. 36.

45. *The Whole Works,* p. 120.

46. *Elements of Physick,* p. 36.

47. Ibid., pp. 28, 29.

48. *The Whole Works,* p. 222.

49. Ibid., p. 57.

50. Ibid., p. 199.

51. Haller, *Bibliotheca Medicinae,* IV, 38.

52. Friedrich Hoffmann, *Fundamenta Medicinae,* tr. and intro. by Lester S. King (London and New York, 1971), p. 5, par. 1; p. 6, par. 2; p. 7, par. 20.

53. Ibid., p. 9, par. 55; p. 17, par. 37; p. 18, par. 53.

54. Ibid., p. 20, pars. 12-23; p. 28, pars. 4-6; p. 29, par. 11.

55. Ibid., pp. 31-32, par. 39; pp. 32-33, pars. 50-52.

56. Ibid., p. 30, pars. 20-21.

57. Ibid., pp. 48-49, par. 12.

58. Everett Mendelsohn, in his *Heat and Life: The Development of the Theory of Animal Heat* (Cambridge, Mass.: Harvard University Press, 1964), notes the views of Pitcairn but does not mention Hoffmann.

59. G. A. Lindeboom, *Herman Boerhaave: The Man and His Work* (London: Methuen, 1968), pp. 61-67.

60. Herman Boerhaave, *De Usu Ratiocinii Mechanici in Medicina* (Leyden, 1703). This is the first edition, which I have not seen. It has been frequently reprinted. See G. A. Lindeboom, *Bibliographia Boerhaaviana* (Lieden: Brill, 1959), pp. 19-21. I have used the text in Boerhaave's *Opera Omnia* (Venice, 1751; Linde-

boom, *Bibliographia,* #521) as well as that in the *Opuscula Omnia* (Lindeboom, #526). Quite useful is the reprint with French translation, printed in *Opuscula selecta Neerlandicorum de arte Medica* (Amsterdam: F. van Rossen, 1907), pp. 143-199. The page references are from this edition, identified as *Opuscula Selecta.*

61. *Opuscula Selecta,* p. 142. My translation differs markedly from that of Lindeboom (1968, p. 66).

62. Ibid., p. 144.

63. Ibid., p. 146.

64. Ibid., p. 158.

65. Ibid., p. 162.

66. Ibid., pp. 166, 170.

67. Ibid., p. 172.

68. Ibid., p. 190.

6. SOUL, MIND, AND BODY

1. See Chapter 4, note 22. All translations are mine, from the Latin, unless otherwise stated.

2. See Lester S. King, *Road to Medical Enlightenment,* pp. 37-62.

3. Walter Pagel, "The Religious and Philosophical Aspects of van Helmont's Science and Medicine," *Supplements to the Bulletin of the History of Medicine,* no. 2 (Baltimore: The Johns Hopkins Press, 1944).

4. "Knitting of the Sensitive Soul and Mind," par. 6. The references will indicate the tractate in its English title (as Chandler renders it) and the numbered paragraph. However, all translations are mine, unless otherwise indicated.

5. "A Mad or Foolish Idea," par. 4.

6. "The Seat of the Soul," pars. 23, 24. See also "A Treatise of the Soul," "The Distinction of the Mind from the Sensitive Soul," and "Of the Immortality of the Soul."

7. "The Birth or Originall of Forms," par. 67.

8. "The Image of the Mind," pars. 11, 12.

9. "The Birth or Originall of Forms," pars. 70-72.

10. King, *Road to Medical Enlightenment,* pp. 42-49.

11. "Birth or Originall of Forms," pars. 71, 72.

12. Ibid., par. 74.

13. Ibid., par. 61. The Latin is *fracidum fermentum arripere.* The word *fracescere* has several distinct meanings: to soften, to ripen, and to rot or decay, and all these meanings occur in van Helmont's writings. Chandler, unfortunately, disregards context and uses throughout the single (and utterly baffling) translation "putrefy by continuance."

14. Ibid., par. 62.

15. Ibid., pars. 63, 64.

16. "Image of the Mind," par. 17; "Birth or Originall of Forms," par. 81; "Knitting of the Sensitive Soul and Mind," esp. pars. 8-10.

17. "A Mad or Foolish Idea," par. 12.

18. Ibid., par. 13.

19. King, *Medical World of the Eighteenth Century,* pp. 163-165.

20. "The Seat of the Soul," par. 13.

21. Ibid., par 32 (see also "From the Seat of the Soul unto Diseases," pars. 10, 11, 12); "The Authority or Priviledge of the Duumvirate," par. 8.

22. "The Seat of the Soul," par. 32; "The Authority or Priviledge of the Duumvirate," pars. 35, 36. Here it is especially important to consult the Latin text and not rely on Chandler's translation.

23. "Birth or Originall of Forms," par. 76.

24. Ibid., par. 79; "The Knitting or Conjoyning of the Sensitive Soul and Mind," par. 13.

25. *Pathologiae Cerebri et Nervosi Generis Specimen* (London, 1667) and *Affectionum quae Dicuntur Hystericae et Hypochondriacae Pathologia Spasmodica Vindicata* (London, 1670).

26. The translation, with its own pagination, is included in the *Dr. Willis's Practice of Physick* (London, 1684); for the Latin I have used the *Opera Omnia* (Venice, 1720).

27. Hansruedi Isler, *Thomas Willis, 1621-1675* (New York: Hafner, 1968).

28. (1684), p. 4; (1720), p. 7 Ac. In reference to Willis I give the page number of the English edition (1684). However, the text has been closely collated with the Latin and where I do not agree with Pordage's rendition I provide my own and note this in the reference. Where I feel it is important to indicate the Latin reference, I give the page, column, and position in the column of the 1720 edition.

29. (1684), p. 22; (1720), p. 20 Ab; (1684), p. 7.

30. (1684), p. 6; (1720), p. 8 Ad.

31. (1684), ibid.; (1720), p. 8 Ba.

32. (1720), p. 8 Bd-p. 9 Aa.

33. (1684), p. 22.

34. (1720), p. 21 Ab; (1684), p. 23.

35. (1720), p. 21 Ac.

36. (1684), pp. 24-25; (1720), p. 21 Bd.

37. (1684), p. 25.

38. My translations (1720), p. 26 Ab—the English of Pordage (1684), p. 29, J consider inadequate; (1720), p. 28 Aa; (1684), p. 32.

39. (1684), p. 33; (1720), p. 28 Bc.

40. (1684), p. 34; (1720), pp. 28 Bd-29 Aa.

41. (1684), p. 37; (1720), p. 31 Ac; (1684), p. 38.

42. (1684), p. 39; (1720), p. 31 Bd.

43. (1684), pp. 39, 40.

44. (1684), pp. 40, 41.

45. (1720), p. 33 Ad; (1684), p. 41.

46. (1684), p. 41; (1720), p. 33 Ba. The translation of Pordage is reasonably accurate and conveys the seventeenth century flavor without textual distortion.

47. (1684), pp. 41-42; (1720), p. 33 Ba-Bb.

48. (1684), p. 42; (1720), pp. 33 Bd-34 Aa.

49. (1684), p. 42; (1720), p. 34 Aa.

50. (1684), p. 42.

51. Bernward Josef Gottlieb, "Bedeutung und Answirkung des hallischen Professors . . . Georg Ernst Stahl," *Nova Acta Leopoldina,* new series *12:*423-502 (1943).

52. Ibid., p. 428.

53. Article, "Stahlianisme," in *Dictionnaire des sciences médicales, par une société de médicins et de churgiens,* 60 vols. (Paris, 1812-1822), LII, 405.

54. Lester S. King, "Stahl and Hoffmann: A Study in Eighteenth Century Animism," *J. Hist. Med. 19:*118-130 (1964); "Basic Concepts of Eighteenth Century Animism," *Amer. J. Psychiat. 124:*797-807 (1967); article, "Stahl," in *Dictionary of Scientific Biography,* ed. C. C. Gillispie, 14 vols. (New York: Scribner's, 1970-1976), XII, 599-606 (1975). In this last essay I indicate the major secondary sources.

55. Albert Lemoine, *Le vitalisme et l'animisme de Stahl* (Paris, 1864), pp. 31, 33-74.

56. For Stahl's significance in modern psychiatry, see Karl A. Menninger's discussion of King, "Basic Concepts of Animism" (1967), p. 802.

57. *Disquisitio de mechanisme et organismi diversitate* (Halle, 1706); *Paraenesis ad aliena a medica doctrina arcendum* (Halle, 1706); *De vera diversitate corporis mixte et vivi . . . demonstratio* (Halle, 1707). I have used principally the second edition of the work, *Theoria medica vera, physiologiam et pathologiam . . . sistens* (Halle, 1737), but have also consulted the first editions of the treatises mentioned. In the *Theoria Vera* the titles of the treatises show some transposition of words and there are some very minor textual differences between the earlier and the later editions. The 1737 edition, however, provides numbers for the separate paragraphs, and for simplicity I will make reference to the treatise and the paragraph number, rather than the page.

58. *Negotium Otiosum seu SKIAMACHIA* (Halle, 1720). Gottfried Wilhelm Leibnitz, *Opera Omnia,* 6 vols., ed. L. Dutens (Geneva, 1768), vol. II, pt. 2, pp. 131-161.

59. *De vera diversitate . . . demonstratio* (hereafter referred to as *De diversitate*), par. 93.

60. *Disquisitio de mechanismi et organismi diversitate* (hereafter *Disquisitio*), par. 68; *De diversitate,* pars. 10, 29, 30, *et seq.; Paraenesis,* par. 20.

61. *Disquisitio,* pars. 69-71; par. 48. See also *Physiologia,* Sec. I, Membrum I, par. 3, and *De diversitate,* par. 51.

62. *Disquisitio,* pars. 31, 33.

63. Ibid., pars. 36, 39, 41.

64. Ibid., pars. 45, 47; see also pars. 64, 65 and *Negotium Otiosum,* p. 90.

65. L. J. Rather, "G. E. Stahl's Psychological Physiology," *Bull. Hist. Med. 45:*37-49 (1961).

66. *De diversitate,* par. 90.

67. Ibid., par. 63; see *Paraenesis,* par. 32 *bis.*

68. *De diversitate,* pars. 63, 64. The translation is mine.

69. *Physiologia,* Sec. I, par. 5, p. 200.

70. Ibid., Sec. I, Membrum I, par. 3, p. 202; par. 5, p. 203; par. 7, p. 203; see also *De diversitate,* par. 123.

71. *Physiologia,* par. 7, p. 204.

72. L. J. Rather and J. B. Frerichs, "The Leibniz-Stahl Controversy: I, Leibniz's opening objections to the *Theoria Medica Vera,*" *Clio Medica 3:*21-40 (1968); Rather and Frerichs, "The Leibniz-Stahl Controversy: II, Stahl's Survey of the Principal Points of Doubt," *Clio Medica, 5:*53-67 (1970).

73. *Negotium,* p. 95.

74. Ibid., p. 96.

75. Ibid., pp. 97-100.

76. King, *Growth of Medical Thought,* pp. 104-105; E. R. Dodds, *Proclus: The Elements of Theology* (Oxford: Clarendon Press, 1933), app. 2, esp. pp. 313 and 318.

77. *Physiologia,* Sec. I, Membrum I, par. 16, p. 207.

78. Walter Pagel, "Helmont, Liebniz, Stahl," *Arch, Gesch. Med. 24:*19-59 (1931).

79. *Physiologia,* pars. 19-24, pp. 208-209; see also *Disquisitio,* par. 90.

80. *Disquisitio,* par. 84; *De diversitate,* par. 123.

81. *De diversitate,* par. 83; *Disquisitio,* par. 97.

82. Max Neuburger, *Die Lehre von der Heilkraft der Natur im Wandel der Zieten* (Stuttgart: Ferdinand Enke, 1926), pp. 65-75.

83. *De diversitate,* pars. 63, 70; *Disquisitio,* par. 91.

84. *Paraenesis,* pars. 27-34.

7. THE POWER OF THE IMAGINATION

1. Friedrich Hoffmann, *Fundamenta Medicinae,* tr. Lester S. King (New York: American Elsevier, 1971), ch. 6, pars. 46, 47, p. 28.

2. Some recent studies on the history of embryology and cognate topics are: Peter J. Bowler, "Bonnet and Buffon: Theories of Generation and the Problem of Species," *J. Hist. Biol. 6:*259-281 (1973); F. J. Cole, *Early Theories of Sexual Generation* (New York, Oxford University Press 1930); Frederick B. Churchill, "The History of Embryology as Intellectual History," *J. Hist. Biol.* 3:155-181 (1970); J. Needham, *History of Embryology,* 2nd ed. (Chicago: University of Chicago Press, 1959); Elizabeth B. Gasking, *Investigations Into Generation, 1651-1828* (Baltimore: The Johns Hopkins Press, n.d.); Jacques Roger, *Les sciences de la vie dans la pensée francaise du XVIIIᵉ siècle* (Paris: Armand Colin 1963); Charles W. Bodemer, "Embryological Thought in Seventeenth Century England," in *Medical Investigations in Seventeenth Century England* (Los Angeles: William Andrews Clark Memorial Library, 1968); Howard B. Adelman, *Marcello Malpighi and the Evolution of Embryology,* 5 vols. (Ithaca: Cornell University Press, 1966); Jane M. Oppenheimer, *Essays in the History of Embryology and Biology* (Cambridge, Mass.: M. I. T. Press, 1967).

3. G. S. Rousseau, "Science and the Discovery of the Imagination in Enlightened England," in *Eighteenth Century Studies 3:*108-135 (1969); "Pineapples, Pregnancy, Pica, and Peregrene Pickle," in *Tobias Smollett: Bicentennial Essays Presented to Lewis M. Knapp,* ed. G. S. Rousseau and P. G. Boucé (New York: Oxford University Press, 1971), pp. 79-109.

4. Sennert's analysis is found in his Chapter 14, "De viribus imaginationis,"

of his *De Consensu et Dissensu Galenicorum et Peripateticorum cum Chymicis.* I have used the text in Sennert's *Opera,* 3 vols. (Lyons, 1650), III, 786-791. In the references I give page, column, and position in the column.

5. 787 Ab-c.

6. 787 Ad.

7. 787 Ba.

8. 787 Bb.

9. L. J. Rather, "Thomas Fienus' (1567-1631) Dialectical Investigation of the Imagination as Cause and Cure of Bodily Disease," *Bull. Hist. Med. 41:*349-367 (1967).

10. Sennert, 787 Bc-788 Ac.

11. 788 Bb-c-d.

12. Lester S. King, "The Road to Scientific Therapy: 'Signatures,' 'Sympathy,' and Controlled Experiment," *JAMA 197:*250-256 (1966).

13. Sennert, 788 Bc.

14. 789 Ab.

15. 787 Ac.

16. 789 Bc-d.

17. 790 Aa-b.

18. 790 Ad.

19. The most convenient edition is René Descartes, *Treatise of Man,* French text with translation and commentary by Thomas Steele Hall (Cambridge, Mass.: Harvard University Press, 1972).

20. Descartes, *Treatise of Man,* p. 87, note 136.

21. Descartes, *Oeuvres Philosophiques,* vol. I, 1618-1637 (Paris: Garnier, 1963), p. 699.

22. Elizabeth S. Haldane and G. R. T. Ross, *The Philosophical Works of Descartes,* 2 vols. (New York: Dover, 1931), I, 391, article 136.

23. Malebranche, *De la recherche de la verité,* ed. G. Rodis-Lewis, 3 vols. (Paris: J. Vrin, 1962). All translations are mine.

24. Ibid., I, 119.

25. Ibid.

26. Ibid., p. 121.

27. Ibid., pp. 122-123.

28. Ibid., p. 124.

29. Ibid., "Introduction," pp. ix, x.

30. For the various editions and translations, see G. A. Lindeboom, *Bibliographia Boerhaaviana* (Leiden: E. J. Brill, 1959), pp. 28-40.

31. I have used the Latin edition, 5 vols. (Turin, 1742-1745), Lindeboom, p. 38, no. 116; and the English edition, *Dr. Boerhaave's Academical Lectures on the Theory of Physic,* 6 vols., 1st and 2nd eds. mixed (London, 1741-1751), Lindeboom, p. 38, #121, #122 mixed.

32. For the various editions, see Lindeboom, *Bibliographia Boerhaaviana,* pp. 41-54. I have used the original Latin text, without commentaries, H. Boerhaave, *Aphorismi de cognoscendis et curandis morbis,* 6th ed. (Louvain, 1752), Lindeboom, p. 45, no. 178; and the English translation of text and commentaries,

in Baron van Swieten, *Commentaries upon Boerhaave's Aphorisms Concerning the Knowledge and Cure of Diseases,* 18 vols. (Edinburgh, 1776), Lindeboom, p. 51, #245.

33. *Praelectiones,* par. 694, IV, 261-262.

34. Ibid., IV, 262; *Academical Lectures,* V, 241.

35. *Praelectiones,* IV, 264.

36. Ibid., IV, 267; *Academical Lectures,* V, 243.

37. *Aphorismi,* par. 1075; van Swieten, X, 314.

38. For the concept of acrimony, see King, *Medical World of the Eighteenth Century,* pp. 79-82.

39. Van Swieten, X, 317.

40. Ibid., p. 319.

41. Daniel Turner, *De Morbis Cutaneis: A Treatise of Diseases Incident to the Skin.* This was originally published in 1726. I have had access only to the second edition (London, 1733), pp. 155-190.

42. (London, 1729). This exchange between Turner and Blondel has been well discussed by G. S. Rousseau (1971) although his approach is quite different from that pursued here.

43. Blondel, 1729, Preface, p. vi.

44. Ibid., p. 2.

45. Ibid., p. 3.

46. Ibid., p. 6.

47. Ibid., p. 11.

48. Ibid., p. 13.

49. Ibid., pp. 20-22.

50. Ibid., p. 55.

51. Ibid., pp. 93-94.

52. Ibid., pp. 109-111.

53. Ibid., p. 130.

54. Ibid., Preface, p. x.

55. Robert E. Schofield, *Mechanism and Materialism: British Natural Philosophy in an Age of Reason* (Princeton: Princeton University Press, 1970).

56. Bentley Glass, "Maupertuis, Pioneer of Genetics and Evolution," in *Forerunners of Darwin, 1745-1859,* ed. Bentley Glass, Owsei Temkin, and William L. Straus, Jr. (Baltimore: The Johns Hopkins Press, 1959), pp. 51-83.

57. See note 2 above.

58. I have used the text in *Oeuvres de Mr de Maupertuis,* 4 vols. (Lyons, 1756), II, 3-133.

59. Pp. 75-79.

60. Buffon, *Histoire générale des animaux,* in *Oeuvres philosophiques de Buffon,* ed. Jean Piveteau (Paris: Presses Universitaires de France, 1954).

61. Ibid., pp. 250-252.

62. This discussion occurs in Chapter 11 of the *Histoire,* entitled "Du développement et de l'accroissement du foetus," which is not reprinted in the Presses Universitaires edition. I have used the text given in the *Oeuvres complètes de Buffon,* ed. M. Flourens, 12 vols. (Paris, 1853-1855), I, 627-654, esp. pp. 642-647.

63. *Elementa Physiologiae Corporis Humani,* 8 vols. (Lausanne, 1757-1766), vol. VIII.

64. Ibid., p. 132.

65. Ibid., p. 133.

66. Ibid., p. 136.

67. Ibid., pp. 139, 142.

68. Ibid., p. 148.

69. Ibid., pp. 149-150.

70. (Paris, 1788). I have so far been unable to uncover biographical material on Bablot.

71. Ibid., p. 42.

72. Ibid., pp. 97-104.

73. Ibid., pp. 104-110.

74. Ibid., p. 111.

75. Ibid., pp. 126-131.

76. Ibid., pp. 143-147.

77. Ibid., p. 195.

78. Ibid., p. 196.

79. *Encyclopedia Britannica, or, a Dictionary of Arts and Sciences,* by a Society of Gentlemen in Scotland, 3 vols. (Edinburgh, 1771; facsimile reprint, 1971), II, 671.

8. THE PROCESS OF EXPLANATION

1. I prefer these terms to the *explanandum* and *explanans* of Hempel. See Carl G. Hempel, *Aspects of Scientific Explanation and Other Essays in the Philosophy of Science* (New York: The Free Press, 1965), pp. 247-251.

2. Carl L. Becker, *The Heavenly City of the Eighteenth Century Philosophers* (New Haven: Yale University Press, 1955), p. 29.

3. Basil Willey, *The Seventeenth Century Background* (London: Chatto and Windus, 1957), p. 2.

4. Francis Bacon, *Aphorisms Concerning the Interpretations of Nature,* Aphorisms 58, 60, 44.

5. David Hume, *A Treatise of Human Nature,* ed. L. A. Selby-Bigge (Oxford: Clarendon Press, 1951), p. 224.

6. The details of this theory are described in all textbooks of medical history. I have a partiality for my own discussion in *Growth of Medical Thought,* pp. 27-34.

7. Lester S. King and Marjorie C. Meehan, "A History of the Autopsy," *American Journal of Pathology 73:*514-544 (1973).

8. Martin Lister, *Dissertatio de Humoribus* (Amsterdam, 1711), pp. 343-344.

9. Herman Boerhaave, *Praelectiones Academicae,* 5 vols. (Turin, 1743), II, 12, par. 246.

10. King, *Medical World of the Eighteenth Century,* pp. 77-81, 91-92.

11. Ibid., pp. 65-70.

12. Francis Bacon, Aphorisms 20, 14.

13. John Baptist Morgagni, *The Seats and Causes of Disease,* tr. Benjamin Alexander, 3 vols. (London, 1769).

14. Theophilus Bonetus, *Sepulchretum sive Anatomica Practica ex Cadaveribus Morbo Denatis,* 2nd ed., 3 vols. (Geneva, 1700). The first edition was published in 1679.

15. Morgagni, I, 90, 100. I give only a small part of the total clinical description.

16. Erwin H. Ackerknecht, *Medicine at the Paris Hospital, 1794-1848.* (Baltimore: The Johns Hopkins Press, 1967).

17. King, *Growth of Medical Thought,* pp. 181-182; King, *Medical World of the Eighteenth Century,* Chapter 3; Herman Boerhaave, *Academical Lectures on the Theory of Physic,* 6 vols. (London, 1741-1747), II, 97, 99, par. 200, notes 9, 12, 13.

18. King, *Growth of Medical Thought,* pp. 182-183.

19. For a more general discussion of glands, see Herman Boerhaave, "De Fabrica Glandularum in Corpore Humano: Epistola Anatomica ad Fredericum Ruysch," in *Opera Omnia* (Venice, 1751), pp. 415-436; Luigi Belloni, "Boerhaave et la doctrine de la glande," in *Boerhaave and His Time,* ed. G. A. Lindeboom (Leiden: E. J. Brill, 1970), pp. 69-82.

20. The discussion of these two theories is drawn from the *Academical Lectures,* II, 239-244, pars. 255-256. The quotations are from the published translations.

21. Ibid., par. 253 and notes, pp. 234-238.

22. Ibid., par. 254, p. 239.

23. Godofredus Bueching, *De potentia diaboli in corpore* (Halle, 1703); see Chapter 2 above. In the present chapter I use the text as printed in Hoffmann's *Opera Omnia,* (notes 67, 68 in Chapter 2), where the wording of the title is slightly different. The notes indicate the numbered sections in the *Opera Omnia* version.

24. *De diaboli potentia,* Sec. 6.

25. Ibid., Secs. 4, 10.

26. Ibid., Secs. 14, 15.

27. Ibid., Sec. 17.

28. Hoffmann, *Fundamenta Medicinae,* p. 70, par. 38; ibid., p. 71, par. 41; *De diaboli,* Sec. 18.

29. *De diaboli,* Sec. 19.

30. *Fundamenta,* p. 74, par. 80.

31. *De diaboli,* Secs. 22, 23.

32. Ibid., Sec. 24.

9. THE CAUSE OF DISEASE

1. Paul B. Beeson and Walsh McDermott, eds., *Textbook of Medicine* (Philadelphia: W. B. Saunders Co., 1975), pp. 360, 472.

2. William Osler, *The Principles and Practice of Medicine,* 3rd ed. (New York, 1899), p. 203.

3. Ibid., p. 207.

4. H. A. Lechevalier and Morris Solotorovsky, *Three Centuries of Microbiology* (New York: McGraw-Hill, 1965), pp. 414-427.

5. Thomas Watson, *Lectures on the Principles and Practice of Physic,* 2 vols., 4th ed. (London, 1847).

6. I, 745, 746.

7. I, 766.

8. Beeson and McDermott, pp. 1647-1660; A. McGehee Harvey et al., eds., *The Principles and Practice of Medicine* (New York: Appleton-Century-Crofts, 1976), pp. 1422-1428; James B. Wyngaarden and William N. Kelley, *Gout and Hyperuricemia* (New York: Grune and Stratton, 1976).

9. Thomas Clifford Albutt, ed., *A System of Medicine,* 8 vols. (New York: Macmillian and Co., 1900), III, 166.

10. Ibid., pp. 181-184.

11. John Mason Good, *The Study of Medicine,* 5 vols., 4th American ed. (Boston, 1826), II, 621-625.

12. Lazar Riverius, "De causae morbificae natura," in *Opera Medica Universa* (Geneva, 1728), p. 39. An English version in *The Universal Body of Physick,* tr. William Carr (London, 1657), p. 102, provides a translation which I consider entirely unsatisfactory.

13. John Herman Randall, Jr., *Aristotle* (New York: Columbia University Press, 1960), pp. 123-124.

14. Daniel Sennert, "De Caussis Morborum," in *Opera Omnia,* 3 vols. (Lyons, 1650), I, 340 Bd-341b.

15. This analysis of Riverius is found in "De càusarum differentiis," pp. 39 Bd-40 Bc.

16. L. J. Rather, "The 'Six Things Non-Natural'," *Clio Medica 3:*333-347 (1968); Saul Jarcho, "Galen's Six Non-Naturals," *Bull. Hist. Med. 44:*372-377 (1970); Jerome J. Bylebyl, "Galen on the Non-Natural Causes of Variation in the Pulse," *Bull. Hist. Med. 45:*482-485 (1971); P. H. Niebyl, "The Non-Naturals," *Bull. Hist. Med. 45:*486-492 (1971); William Coleman, "Health and Hygiene in the *Encyclopédie,*" *Hist. Med. 29:*399-421 (1974).

17. H. W. B. Joseph, *An Introduction to Logic,* 2nd ed. (Oxford: Clarendon Press, 1950), p. 478.

18. Sennert provides a general discussion of causation in his chapter, "De caussis morborum in genere," *Opera Omnia,* I, 340-344, esp. 341 Bb to 342 Bd.

19. See notes 30, 31 in Chapter 7.

20. *Institutiones,* par. 737, note *realis;* par. 740.

21. The discussion is drawn from the *Institutiones,* pars. 737-743.

22. Ibid., par. 740, note. The English text (*Academical Lectures*) uses the word steelyard, which is a bad translation of the Latin *lanx.* This term would really signify the pan of an apparatus for weighing; a steelyard is such an apparatus but is asymmetrical, so that the weights on the two sides are not equal. Boerhaave's example depends for its force on a symmetrical balance, with the fulcrum at the midpoint of the beam.

23. Ibid., par. 740. Because of the extreme importance of this concept, I append the entire Latin text: "Causa proxima morbi appellatur tota illa simul,

quae totum jam presentem directe constituit; haec semper est integra, sufficiens, praesens, totius morbi, sive simplex fuerit, sive composita. Hujus praesentia ponit, continuat, morbum. Hujus absentia eum tollit. Est fere eadem res ipsi integro morbo." The Turin edition that I used for the Latin text has a semicolon after *praesens,* but this is apparently a misprint, evident if we consult other Latin editions. The English translation in the *Academical Lectures* is not satisfactory.

24. Ibid., par. 740, note, and 741, note.

25. Ibid., par. 737. I have here quoted the published English translation of 1747.

26. Ibid., par. 737, note *causa.*

27. Ibid., par. 737, note *realis.*

28. Ibid., par. 744, note *non naturales.*

29. Ibid., par. 744, note *corporis.*

30. *Riverius Reformatus: Or the Modern Riverius; Containing the Modern Practice of Physick* (London, 1713).

31. Ibid., pp. 185-186.

32. Ibid., pp. 373-375.

33. Johan. Juncker, *Conspectus Medicinae,* 3rd ed. (Halle, 1734), pp. 901-902.

10. RATIONALISM AND EMPIRICISM

1. A Conan Doyle, "A Study in Scarlet," in *The Complete Sherlock Holmes* (Garden City, N.Y.: Doubleday and Co., n.d.), pp. 23, 83-84.

2. Allen G. Debus, *The English Paracelsians* (London: Oldbourne, 1965); "The Chemical Debates of the Seventeenth Century: The Reaction to Robert Fludd and Jean Baptiste van Helmont," in *Reason, Experiment, and Mysticism in the Scientific Revolution,* ed. M. L. Righini and Wm. R. Shea (New York: Science History Publications 1975), pp. 18-47, 291-298; *The Chemical Philosophy: Paracelsian Science and Medicine in the Sixteenth and Seventeenth Century* (in press).

3. Lester S. King, "Metaposcopy and Kindred Arts," *JAMA* 224:42-46 (1973).

4. Friedrich Hoffmann, "Philosophiae Corporis Humanis Vivi et Sani Liber Primus," in *Medicinae Rationalis Systematicae . . . ,* 4 vols., 1st and 2nd eds., mixed (Halle, 1732-1739), Chap. 8 of the "Prolegomena," I, 42-47.

5. For the conflicts between Hoffmann and Stahl see Lester S. King, "Stahl and Hoffmann: A Study in Eighteenth Century Animism," *J. Hist. Med. 19*:118-130 (1964); "Basic Concepts of Eighteenth Century Animism," *Am. J. Psychiat. 124*:797-807 (1967).

6. Hoffmann, *Fundamenta Medicinae,* pp. 2-3.

7. In *Greek Medicine,* tr. Authur J. Brock (London: J. M. Dent and Sons, 1929), pp. 130-151.

8. *Ethica Nicomachea,* 1139b13-b34.

9. King, *Growth of Medical Thought,* pp. 38-40.

10. *Metaphysics,* 981a5-a17.

11. Ibid., 981a28-a30.

12. In this connection see *Ethica Nicomachea,* 1139b29-b30, *Posterior Analytics,* 100b3-b17.

13. John Herman Randall, Jr., *Aristotle* (New York: Columbia University Press, 1960), pp. 42-43.

14. King, *Growth of Medical Thought,* pp. 17-42.

15. In my exposition I use the word law in the naive sense prevalent before Hume.

16. *The Medical Works of Hippocrates,* tr. John Chadwick and W. N. Mann (Oxford: Blackwell, 1950), p. 116 (*Prognosis*), p. 151 (*Aphorisms*), p. 252 (*Coan Prognosis*).

17. Particularly relevent here is Hempel's concept of the "Covering Law." See Carl G. Hempel, *Aspects of Scientific Explanation* (New York: The Free Press, 1965), pp. 229-496.

18. Kenneth Dewhurst, *Dr. Thomas Sydenham (1624-1689): His Life and Original Writings* (Berkeley: University of California Press, 1966); *The Works of Thomas Sydenham,* tr. R. G. Latham, 2 vols. (London, 1848-1850).

19. King, *Road to Medical Enlightenment,* pp. 113-133; "Empiricism and Rationalism in the Works of Thomas Sydenham," *Bull. Hist. Med. 44*:1-11 (1970).

20. *Works,* II, 182.

21. Francis Bacon, "Aphorisms Concerning the Interpretation of Nature," Aphorisms 19, 22, 24, 69.

22. Dewhurst, *Dr. Thomas Sydenham,* pp. 79-84; 85-93, 73.

23. *Metaphysics,* 980a20.

24. Dewhurst, *Dr. Thomas Sydenham,* p. 80. In all the quotations from Sydenham, I have modernized the seventeenth century spelling which Dewhurst gives.

25. Ibid., p. 81.

26. Ibid., pp. 81-82.

27. Ibid., p. 82.

28. Ibid., p. 86.

29. Ibid., p. 87.

30. Ibid., p. 89.

31. I have used his *Opera Omnia Medico-Practica,* 8th ed. (Lyons, 1714); of the little that has been translated, the most important is *The Practice of Physick.* I have the second edition (London, 1723). In the subsequent references I will identify the source by the date, 1714 for the Latin, 1723 for the English. I always compare the published translations with the original Latin.

32. Richard Foster Jones, *Ancients and Moderns: A Study of the Rise of the Scientific Movement in Seventeenth Century England,* 2nd ed. (St. Louis: Washington University Press, 1961); King, *Road to Medical Enlightenment,* pp. 139-180.

33. Baglivi, 1723, Preface, Sig. B 5v. In quotations from this translation I eliminate the capricious use of capitals and dispense with contractions like 'em for them.

34. 1723, p. 4. In this connection, see 1714, p. 3, Sec. VIII.

35. 1714, p. 4, Sec. XII. The translation is mine.

36. 1723, pp. 9, 10.

37. 1723, p. 11; 1714, pp. 6, 7.

38. 1723, pp. 14, 15.

39. Ibid., pp. 114-115.

40. Ibid., p. 116.

41. 1714, p. 124, my translation; 1723, p. 116.

42. 1723, p. 117.

43. 1723, p. 120; 1714, p. 126.

44. 1714, pp. 126-127.

45. 1723, p. 122; 1714, p. 127.

46. 1723, p. 202.

47. Ibid., p. 204.

48. Ibid., p. 205.

49. Ibid., p. 208; 1714, p. 174.

50. Boerhaave, *Praelectiones Academicae,* par. 15, note *damni;* par. 19.

51. *Academical Lectures,* vol. I, p. 43, par. 19, note 2. The words "or opinion" and "or matter of fact" do not occur in the Latin.

52. *Praelectiones,* par. 24, note *sensibus.*

53. Ibid., par. 24; par. 24, note *ratiocinatione.*

54. Ibid., par. 19. The translation in *Academical Lectures* is excessively free and adds phrases not present in the Latin.

55. H. Boerhaave, *Aphorismi de Cognoscendis et Curandis Morbis,* 6th ed. (Louvain, 1752), p. 3, Aphorism 13.

56. *Institutiones,* par. 24; par. 239, note *mirum.*

57. Giorgio de Santillana, *Galileo Galilei: Dialogues on the Great World Systems* (Chicago: University of Chicago Press, 1953), p. 159; see also Allen G. Debus, "Pierre Gassendi and the 'Scientific Expedition' of 1640," *Arch. Internat. d'Histoire des Sciences 16:*129-142 (1963).

58. Fontanelle, *Entretiens sur la pluralite des mondes,* ed. Robert Shackleton (Oxford: Clarendon Press, 1955), pp. 121-122.

59. *Oeuvres philosophiques de Condillac,* ed. Georges Le Roy (Corpus General des Philosophes Francais, Auteurs Modernes, XXXIII), 3 vols. (Paris: Presses Universitaires de France, 1947-1951), I, 133, note.

60. All these examples are drawn from *Institutiones,* par. 19, note *secta.* The translations are mine.

61. Ibid., par. 19, note *posteriorem.* The translations are mine.

62. Lester S. King, "Evidence and Its Evaluation in Eighteenth-Century Medicine," *Bull. Hist. Med. 50:*174-190 (1976).

63. D. P. Walker, *Spiritual and Domestic Magic from Ficino to Campanella* (London: The Warburg Institute, 1958), p. 116.

64. See, for example, J. A. Borelli, *De Motu Animalium* (Naples, 1734), p. 314; Baglivi, *Practice of Physick* (London, 1723), p. 34; Herman Boerhaave, "Sermo Academicus, de Chemia Suos Errores Expurgante," in *Opera Omnia* (Venice, 1751), pp. 487-496.

65. Mary B. Hesse, *Models and Analogies in Science* (Notre Dame: University of Indiana Press, 1966).

66. Baglivi, 1723, pp. 33-34.

67. Ibid., pp. 37-38.

68. Edward Strother, *An Essay on Sickness and Health* (London, 1725), p. 76.

INDEX

THIS VOLUME MAY CIRCULATE FOR 2 WEEKS
Renewals May Be Made In Person Or By Phone:
x 5300; from outside 472-5300

DATE DUE	DATE RETURNED
AUG 1 1978	JUL 2 0 1978
DEC 3 1979	DEC 4 1979
JAN 2 0 1981	FEB 3 1981
JAN 1 0 1983	JAN 3 1 1983